Contemporary Topics in Radiation Medicine, Part II: Disease Sites

Editors

RAVI A. CHANDRA
LISA A. KACHNIC
CHARLES R. THOMAS Jr

HEMATOLOGY/ONCOLOGY CLINICS OF NORTH AMERICA

www.hemonc.theclinics.com

Consulting Editors
GEORGE P. CANELLOS
EDWARD J. BENZ Jr

February 2020 • Volume 34 • Number 1

JEREMY M. BROWNSTEIN, MD
Radiation Oncology Fellow, Francis H. Burr Proton Beam Therapy Center, Massachusetts General Hospital, Boston, Massachusetts, USA; Department of Radiation Oncology, Comprehensive Cancer Center, The Ohio State University, Columbus, Ohio, USA

TIFFANY W. CHEN, MD
Resident, Department of Radiation Oncology, The University of Texas Health Science Center at San Antonio, San Antonio, Texas, USA

STEVEN J. CHMURA, MD, PhD
Assistant Professor, Department of Radiation and Cellular Oncology, The University of Chicago, Chicago, Illinois, USA

ANTHONY V. D'AMICO, MD, PhD
Department of Radiation Oncology, Brigham and Women's Hospital/Dana-Farber Cancer Institute, Harvard Medical School, Boston, Massachusetts, USA

SHRADDHA MAHESH DALWADI, MD, MBA
Resident, Department of Radiation Oncology, Baylor College of Medicine, Houston, Texas, USA

PRAJNAN DAS, MD, MS, MPH
Professor and Chief of Gastrointestinal Radiation Oncology Section, Department of Radiation Oncology, The University of Texas MD Anderson Cancer Center, Houston, Texas, USA

JOHN DE GROOT, MD
Professor, Neuro-Oncology Department, The University of Texas MD Anderson Cancer Center, Houston, Texas, USA

ROY H. DECKER, MD, PhD
Department of Therapeutic Radiology, Smilow Cancer Center, Yale University, New Haven, Connecticut, USA

THOMAS F. DeLANEY, MD
Radiation Oncologist, Department of Radiation Oncology, Andres Soriano Professor of Radiation Oncology, Harvard Medical School, Associate Medical Director, Francis H. Burr Proton Therapy Center, Massachusetts General Hospital, Boston, Massachusetts, USA

BAHER ELGOHARI, MD, MSc
Department of Radiation Oncology, The University of Texas MD Anderson Cancer Center, Houston, Texas, USA

HESHAM ELHALAWANI, MD, MSc
Department of Radiation Oncology, The University of Texas MD Anderson Cancer Center, Houston, Texas, USA

JACLYN EMMETT, MSN, CNRP
Nurse Practitioner, Inpatient Oncology, Department of Hematology/Oncology, Massachusetts General Hospital, Boston, Massachusetts, USA

TONY Y. ENG, MD
Professor, Radiation Oncology Department, Winship Cancer Institute of Emory University, Atlanta, Georgia, USA

AHSAN FAROOQI, MD, PhD
Resident Physician, Radiation Oncology Department, The University of Texas MD Anderson Cancer Center, Houston, Texas, USA

CLIFTON DAVID FULLER, MD, PhD
Department of Radiation Oncology, The University of Texas MD Anderson Cancer Center, Houston, Texas, USA

SARAH J. GAO, MD
Department of Therapeutic Radiology, Smilow Cancer Center, Yale University, New Haven, Connecticut, USA

ALIREZA FOTOUHI GHIAM, MD, MSc
Physician, Department of Radiation Oncology, British Columbia Cancer Agency (BCCA), University of British Columbia, Victoria, British Columbia, Canada

STANLEY I. GUTIONTOV, MD
Resident Physician, Department of Radiation and Cellular Oncology, The University of Chicago, Chicago, Illinois, USA

D. NEIL HAYES, MD, MS, MPH
Van Vleet Endowed Professor and Assistant Dean for Cancer Research, Division Chief, Hematology/Oncology, Departments of Medicine, Genetics/Genomics/Informatics, Preventive Medicine, and Pathology, The University of Tennessee Health Science Center College of Medicine, Adjunct Professor, Department of Computational Biology, St. Jude Children's Research Hospital, Memphis, Tennessee, USA

JOSEPH M. HERMAN, MD, MSc, MSHCM
Professor and Division Head, Department of Radiation Oncology, The University of Texas MD Anderson Cancer Center, Houston, Texas, USA

EMMA B. HOLLIDAY, MD
Assistant Professor, Department of Radiation Oncology, The University of Texas MD Anderson Cancer Center, Houston, Texas, USA

YONG JIANG, MD, PhD
Clinical Oncology Center, The University of Hong Kong-Shenzhen Hospital, Shenzhen, China

JOSHUA A. JONES, MD, MA, FAAHPM
Chief, Palliative Radiotherapy Service, Director of Quality Assurance/Quality Improvement, Department of Radiation Oncology, University of Pennsylvania Health System, Philadelphia, Pennsylvania, USA

SOPHIA C. KAMRAN, MD
Department of Radiation Oncology, Massachusetts General Hospital, Harvard Medical School, Boston, Massachusetts, USA

KENDALL KISER, MS
Department of Radiation Oncology, The University of Texas MD Anderson Cancer Center, Houston, Texas, USA

FENG-MING (SPRING) KONG, MD, PhD
Department of Clinical Oncology, La Ka Shing Faculty of Medicine, The University of Hong Kong, Queen Mary Hospital, Hong Kong, China

YOUNG KWOK, MD
Professor, Department of Radiation Oncology, University of Maryland School of Medicine, Baltimore, Maryland, USA

VICTOR HO-FUN LEE, MD
Department of Clinical Oncology, La Ka Shing Faculty of Medicine, The University of Hong Kong, Queen Mary Hospital, Hong Kong, China

JING LI, MD, PhD
Associate Professor, Radiation Oncology Department, The University of Texas MD Anderson Cancer Center, Houston, Texas, USA

NADIA ROXANNE LIVINGSTONE, BA
Department of Radiation Oncology, The University of Texas MD Anderson Cancer Center, Houston, Texas, USA

NICHOLAS MADDEN, MD
Resident, Radiation Oncology Department, Winship Cancer Institute of Emory University, Atlanta, Georgia, USA

BRIGID McDONALD, BS
Department of Radiation Oncology, The University of Texas MD Anderson Cancer Center, Houston, Texas, USA

MARK MISHRA, MD
Associate Professor, Department of Radiation Oncology, University of Maryland School of Medicine, Baltimore, Maryland, USA

ABDALLAH SHERIF RADWAN MOHAMED, MD, MSc
Department of Radiation Oncology, The University of Texas MD Anderson Cancer Center, Houston, Texas, USA

PRANSHU MOHINDRA, MD
Associate Professor, Department of Radiation Oncology, University of Maryland School of Medicine, Baltimore, Maryland, USA

TIFFANY MORGAN, MD
Resident, Radiation Oncology Department, Winship Cancer Institute of Emory University, Atlanta, Georgia, USA

MANNAT NARANG
Department of Radiation Oncology, University of Maryland School of Medicine, Baltimore, Maryland, USA

ANDREA K. NG, MD, MPH
Professor, Department of Radiation Oncology, Dana-Farber/Brigham and Women's Cancer Center, Harvard Medical School, Boston, Massachusetts, USA

BENJAMIN E. ONDERDONK, MD
Resident Physician, Department of Radiation and Cellular Oncology, The University of Chicago, Chicago, Illinois, USA

WILLIAM REGINE, MD
Professor, Department of Radiation Oncology, University of Maryland School of Medicine, Baltimore, Maryland, USA

DAVID L. SCHWARTZ, MD, FACR
Professor and Chair, Departments of Radiation Oncology and Preventive Medicine, The University of Tennessee Health Science Center College of Medicine, Memphis, Tennessee, USA

SONJA STIEB, MD
Department of Radiation Oncology, The University of Texas MD Anderson Cancer Center, Houston, Texas, USA

GITA SUNEJA, MD, MSHP
Associate Professor, Department of Radiation Oncology and Population Health Science, University of Utah, Salt Lake City, Utah, USA

DANIEL TANENBAUM, MD
Resident, Radiation Oncology Department, Winship Cancer Institute of Emory University, Atlanta, Georgia, USA

YOLANDA D. TSENG, MPhil, MD
Assistant Professor of Radiation, Department of Radiation Oncology, Seattle Cancer Care Alliance Proton Therapy Center, University of Washington School of Medicine, Seattle, Washington, USA

LISANNE VAN DIJK, PhD
Department of Radiation Oncology, The University of Texas MD Anderson Cancer Center, Houston, Texas, USA

JUAN VENTURA, BS
Department of Radiation Oncology, The University of Texas MD Anderson Cancer Center, Houston, Texas, USA

AKILA VISWANATHAN, MD, MPH, MSc
Department of Radiation Oncology and Molecular Radiation Sciences, Professor and Interim Director, Johns Hopkins Medicine, The Sidney Kimmel Comprehensive Cancer Center, Baltimore, Maryland, USA

NARINE WANDREY, MD
Resident, Department of Radiation Oncology, The University of Texas Health Science Center at San Antonio, San Antonio, Texas, USA

SARAH WESTERGAARD, MD
Resident, Radiation Oncology Department, Winship Cancer Institute of Emory University, Atlanta, Georgia, USA

KAREN XU, MD
Resident, Radiation Oncology Department, Winship Cancer Institute of Emory University, Atlanta, Georgia, USA

LI YANG, MD
Clinical Oncology Center, The University of Hong Kong-Shenzhen Hospital, Shenzhen, China

DEBRA NANA YEBOA, MD
Assistant Professor, Radiation Oncology Department and Health Services Research Department, The University of Texas MD Anderson Cancer Center, Houston, Texas, USA

TORUNN I. YOCK, MD, MCH
Department of Radiation Oncology, Massachusetts General Hospital/Harvard Medical School, Francis H. Burr Proton Therapy Center, Boston, Massachusetts, USA

Contents

A series of landmark studies have increasingly emphasized the role of adjuvant radiotherapy for the definitive management of breast cancer. Although regional nodal irradiation, including the internal mammary nodes, was typically reserved for high-risk patients, there is now evidence of benefit to this approach even for those with a limited nodal disease burden. Similarly, low-risk disease has historically been treated with whole-breast tangents, although contemporary studies now support accelerated partial breast irradiation or the omission of radiotherapy in select cases. This article presents recent data informing these contemporary developments in the radiotherapeutic management of breast cancer.

The 2016 World Health Organization classification of central nervous system (CNS) tumors underwent significant restructuring and for the first time gliomas are classified according to both molecular and histologic parameters which guides glioma management. Radiation for intermediate-risk meningiomas improves the progression-free survival from historical controls, and studies are ongoing for atypical meningiomas. For brain metastases, use of stereotactic radiosurgery for a higher number of lesions has become clinical practice. Additionally, hippocampal-sparing whole brain radiation shows promise in preserving neuro-cognitive function. This article summarizes the evolving role of radiation therapy in the management of malignant CNS neoplasms.

Over the past 2 decades, major technical advances in radiation therapy planning and delivery have made it possible to deliver higher doses to select high-risk volumes. This has helped to expand the role of radiation therapy in the treatment of gastrointestinal malignancies. Whereas dose escalation was previously limited by the radiosensitivity of normal tissues within and adjacent to the gastrointestinal tract, advances in target delineation, patient immobilization, treatment planning, and image-guided treatment delivery have greatly improved the therapeutic ratio. More conformal radiation modalities can offer further dose optimization to target volumes while sparing normal tissue from toxicity.

Randomized controlled trials provide evidence-driven clinical decision making in the management of newly diagnosed nonmetastatic and oligometastatic prostate cancer. Advances in technology (eg, multiparametric MRI, MR/transrectal ultrasound fusion biopsy, image-guided radiation therapy, stereotactic body radiation therapy) have transformed diagnosis and treatment of prostate cancer while improving cancer control and quality-of-life outcomes. Exciting breakthroughs are revealing possible new indications for radiotherapy, particularly with respect to oligometastatic prostate cancer. Ongoing studies using next-generation androgen receptor–targeted agents hold promise to continue to improve important clinical outcomes, including metastasis-free prostate cancer–specific and overall survival in addition to health-related quality of life.

Gynecologic malignancies are among the most prevalent cancers affecting women worldwide, but they are heterogeneous diseases with varying risk factors, management paradigms, and outcomes. Gynecologic cancers mediated by human papillomavirus (HPV) are preventable and curable with early detection and treatment. Dramatic reductions in cervical cancer incidence and mortality have been achieved through cancer screening and HPV vaccination. Radiotherapy plays a central role in the management of gynecologic malignancies. For some cancers, radiotherapy alone can be curative. More often, radiotherapy is used in conjunction with surgery and systemic therapy to improve locoregional control and extend overall survival. This chapter reviews recent advances in radiotherapeutic management of gynecologic malignancies.

The length and quality of head and neck cancer survivorship continues to meaningfully improve. Radiotherapy has been central to this process through advances in treatment delivery, fractionation schemas, radiosensitizing systemic therapy, and thoughtful interplay with technical surgical improvements. The future looks brighter still, with ongoing progress in targeted biologic therapy, immuno-oncology, and molecular-genetic tumor characterization for personalized treatment. Head and neck cancer, a disease once fraught with nihilism and failure, is evolving into a major success story of modern multidisciplinary cancer care.

Radiotherapy is the most commonly used nonsurgical modality in treatment of lung cancers, non–small cell lung cancer (NSCLC) in particular. Radiation therapy has been increasingly used as definitive radical treatment, either alone or in combination with concurrent chemoradiation for locally advanced disease. More recently with the advent of novel radiation techniques and modalities such as stereotactic radiotherapy and proton therapy, radiotherapy can now be used as sole radical treatment of small solitary tumors. This article reviews the current indications and future directions of radiotherapy in lung cancer management.

Radiation therapy plays a critical role in the management of a wide range of hematologic malignancies. The optimal radiation dose and target volume, and safe and effective ways of integrating radiation with systemic agents, vary depending on the histologic subtypes, stage at presentation, patient performance status, response to systemic therapy if given, treatment intent, and patient preferences. Limiting doses to surrounding organs without sacrificing disease control is of paramount importance. Reducing radiation doses and treatment volume in selected cases, and the use of advanced radiotherapy technology, can improve the therapeutic ratio of patients receiving radiation therapy for hematologic malignancies.

In pediatric brain tumors, the intensification of chemotherapy has allowed for a reduction in radiotherapy (RT) volume to an involved field approach, particularly in patients with medulloblastoma. For patients with low-grade gliomas, the trend has remained to delay RT with chemotherapy; however, when RT is used, typically smaller clinical target volume margins are used. For patients with extracranial tumors, intensive chemotherapy to address systemic disease with local control is considered standard. Proton beam therapy shows significant promise in addressing both short-term and long-term toxicities in both central nervous system (CNS) and non-CNS pediatric tumors.

Soft-tissue sarcomas are cancerous growths of mesenchymal tissues, most commonly arising from fat, muscles, and other connective tissues. Sarcomas are rare, representing only a small fraction of solid malignant tumors. Because of their scarcity and a relative paucity of data, the management of sarcomas can be challenging, especially for those who infrequently encounter these tumors. Herein, the authors review the current literature regarding the diagnosis, workup, and treatment of adult soft-tissue sarcomas.

Bone sarcomas are rare tumors arising in bone, representing only a small fraction of solid malignant tumors. Desmoids are benign, infiltrative soft tissue neoplasms. Because of their scarcity and a paucity of data, the management of these tumors can be challenging, especially for clinicians who

symptom relief and minimize impact on patients. Patients referred for palliative radiotherapy have many concerns beyond radiotherapy; often, these concerns are not fully addressed in traditional radiotherapy clinics. Discussions of prognosis, patient goals, and concerns are areas for improved collaboration. Innovative, dedicated palliative radiotherapy programs have developed over the past 20 years to provide holistic care to patients referred for palliative radiotherapy and have improved patient-focused outcomes. Advanced radiotherapy techniques may provide opportunities to further improve palliative radiotherapy outcomes.

HEMATOLOGY/ONCOLOGY
CLINICS OF NORTH AMERICA

FORTHCOMING ISSUES

April 2020
Myelodysplastic Syndromes
David P. Steensma, *Editor*

June 2020
**Blastic Plasmacytoid Dendritic Cell
Neoplasm**
Andrew A. Lane, *Editor*

August 2020
Follicular Lymphoma
Jonathan W. Friedberg, *Editor*

RECENT ISSUES

December 2019
**Contemporary Topics in Radiation Medicine,
Part I: Current Issues and Techniques**
Ravi A. Chandra, Lisa A. Kachnic, and
Charles R. Thomas, Jr., *Editors*

October 2019
Transfusion Medicine
Eric A. Gehrie and Edward L. Snyder,
Editors

August 2019
Non-Hodgkin's Lymphoma
Caron A. Jacobson, *Editor*

SERIES OF RELATED INTEREST

Surgical Oncology Clinics of North America
https://www.surgonc.theclinics.com/

Preface

Disease Sites

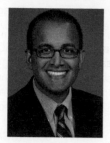 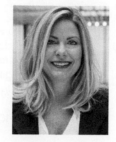 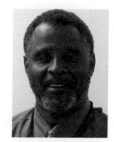

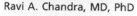

Ravi A. Chandra, MD, PhD   Lisa A. Kachnic, MD, FASTRO   Charles R. Thomas Jr, MD

Editors

Radiotherapy remains one of the most common, although misunderstood, tools in the oncology management arsenal as up to two-thirds of all patients receive this modality at some point during their cancer continuum. Radiation Oncology is a rapidly evolving specialty, with substantial innovation in the technical and clinical aspects of radiation treatment over recent years. This 2-part series aims to update practicing oncologists and associated care team members on many of the exciting changes that are taking place in this field.

This issue of *Hematology/Oncology Clinics of North America* discusses the role of radiation medicine as part of curative and palliative management for both solid and hematologic malignancies. It updates readers on current clinical trials that include radiotherapy as an integral component of management. The contributors comprise the brightest minds within our specialty. Moreover, they have written each article with the expressed intent of educating nonradiation medicine clinicians on the topic at hand with an eye toward the future.

We would like to thank all of our authors for their efforts in making this a successful endeavor. We would also like to acknowledge Kristen Helm, Stacy Eastman, and the team at Elsevier for their generous contributions of time, talent, expertise, and discipline to ensure an outstanding pair of issues of the *Hematology/Oncology Clinics of North America*.

Ravi A. Chandra, MD, PhD
Department of Radiation Medicine
Oregon Health & Science University
3181 SW Sam Jackson Park Road
Portland, OR 97239, USA

Lisa A. Kachnic, MD, FASTRO
Department of Radiation Oncology
Vagelos College of Physicians and Surgeons
Columbia University Irving Medical Center
622 West 168th Street
CHONY North, B Level, Room 11
New York, NY 10032, USA

Charles R. Thomas Jr, MD
Department of Radiation Medicine
Oregon Health & Science University
3181 SW Sam Jackson Park Road
Portland, OR 97239, USA

E-mail addresses:
chandrra@ohsu.edu (R.A. Chandra)
lak2187@cumc.columbia.edu (L.A. Kachnic)
thomasch@ohsu.edu (C.R. Thomas)

Contemporary Issues in Breast Cancer Radiotherapy

Lior Z. Braunstein, MD[a], Jennifer R. Bellon, MD[b],*

KEYWORDS

- Breast cancer • Radiotherapy • Breast conservation • Lumpectomy
- Adjuvant therapy • Postmastectomy radiation • Regional nodal irradiation

KEY POINTS

- Regional nodal irradiation has the potential to improve disease-free survival among patients with limited axillary disease.
- Accelerated partial breast irradiation is a convenient and effective adjuvant radiotherapy (RT) approach for appropriately selected patients.
- RT omission: certain subgroups of patients are of sufficiently low risk to forego adjuvant radiotherapy. Studies in this domain are ongoing.

Breast radiotherapy (RT) has played a pivotal role in definitively managing breast cancer since the demise of the radical mastectomy.[1] The role of RT in breast conserving therapy (BCT) and in the postmastectomy setting with substantial lymph node burden has been well described. In the last decade, studies have further tailored the use of RT across the entire risk spectrum of this disease. For example, regional nodal irradiation has seen expanded use in light of a measurable disease-free survival benefit, even among patients with limited axillary involvement following axillary lymph node dissection.[2,3] In contrast, for very early lower-risk disease, select patients may be eligible to have the RT omitted,[4] or to receive accelerated partial breast irradiation,[5] further mitigating the risk and inconvenience of adjuvant therapy. These recent developments are supported by a growing body of literature, as reviewed here.

Disclosure: L.Z. Braunstein has received support from the American Society of Clinical Oncology, the Lois Green TNBC Fund, and the MSKCC Imaging and Radiation Sciences Program. J.R. Bellon receives honorarium from UpToDate; Wolters Kluwer; The International Journal of Radiation Oncology, Biology, and Physics; Leidos Pharmaceuticals; Accuray; and research funding from Prosigna.
[a] Department of Radiation Oncology, Memorial Sloan Kettering Cancer Center, 1275 York Avenue Box 22, New York, NY 10065, USA; [b] Department of Radiation Oncology, Dana-Farber Cancer Institute, 450 Brookline Avenue, Boston, MA 02115, USA
* Corresponding author.
E-mail address: Jennifer_Bellon@dfci.harvard.edu

Hematol Oncol Clin N Am 34 (2020) 1–12
https://doi.org/10.1016/j.hoc.2019.08.014
0889-8588/20/© 2019 Elsevier Inc. All rights reserved.

REGIONAL NODAL IRRADIATION

Management of the regional lymph nodes in women with early-stage, clinically node-negative breast cancer has dramatically evolved in the last 20 years. Axillary dissection had been standard for all women with invasive disease; however, although an effective procedure for both cancer staging and local control of the axilla, it carries a risk of both lymphedema and shoulder dysfunction.[6] This technique was largely eliminated as an initial axillary treatment with the advent of sentinel node biopsy, which showed modest false-negative rates and no compromise in survival.[7] Until recently, women with a positive sentinel node were still recommended to undergo completion dissection. However, several modern studies in women with limited nodal involvement have shown no loss of local control or survival when an axillary dissection is omitted.[8–11] Although not completing the dissection has become accepted as standard practice, the optimal radiation targets in this setting remain unclear.

The landmark ACOSOG Z0011[8] was a practice-changing study despite multiple limitations. Patients with clinically node-negative stage I or II disease, with 1 or 2 positive sentinel nodes and without gross extranodal extension, were randomized to completion axillary dissection or no further surgery. Tangential RT to the breast was designated in the protocol, but no details were provided regarding dose or specifics of the radiation targets. Ten-year follow-up was reported in 2017.[9] Overall survival was 86.3% in women randomized to sentinel node alone compared with 83.6% in those undergoing axillary dissection (hazard ratio [HR], 0.85; 95% confidence interval [CI], 0–1.16; noninferiority $P = .02$). There was also no statistically significant difference in local-regional control. Critics have noted that this was a highly select group of patients, and therefore the results should not be applied to all eligible patients. Only 27% of patients in the dissection arm had additional nodal disease and 46% of positive sentinel nodes contained only micrometastatic (<2 mm) foci. In an attempt to validate these findings in an unselected population, Morrow and colleagues[12] prospectively studied 793 consecutive patients at the Memorial Sloan Kettering Cancer Center who met Z0011 eligibility. Among these, 84% did not undergo dissection and experienced no isolated axillary recurrences.

Three additional studies also investigated omitting axillary dissection in select women, and uniformly showed no compromise in axillary recurrence rates or overall survival. The IBCSG 23-01[10] trial similarly randomized 934 women with T1 or T2 primary tumors and positive sentinel nodes to completion dissection or no additional axillary surgery. Unlike Z0011, all nodal metastases were smaller than 2 mm without extranodal extension. With 9.7 years' median follow-up, disease-free survival in the no-dissection arm was noninferior to completion dissection. As expected, lymphedema rates were lower with sentinel node alone compared with axillary dissection (4% with sentinel node alone compared with 13% with dissection). Similarly, the EORTC (European Organisation for Research and Treatment of Cancer) AMAROS (After Mapping of the Axilla: Radiotherapy or Surgery) trial[11] randomized women with a clinically negative axilla and a positive sentinel node to axillary dissection or no further surgery. Ninety-five percent of women had 1 or 2 involved nodes, although, in contrast with the IBCSG trial, macrometastases were permitted. Of 1425 patients with a positive sentinel node, axillary recurrence rates at 10 years were 0.93% with axillary dissection and 1.82% without dissection ($P = .37$); similarly, there was no statistically significant difference in overall survival. As in the IBCSG trial, 5-year rates of lymphedema were increased with dissection (23% vs 11%; $P<.0001$). In addition, the Hungarian OTOASOR (Optimal Treatment of the Axilla: Surgery or Radiation[13]) trial also randomized 526 women with positive sentinel nodes to completion axillary dissection or regional nodal irradiation. With a median follow-up of 8 years, axillary recurrence was 1.0% in the completion axillary dissection arm and 1.7% among those randomized to radiation ($P = 1.0$). Overall survival was 77.9% in the dissection arm and 84.8% in the no-dissection arm ($P = .06$).

Although these trials generally indicate that most women with clinically negative axillae and 1 or 2 positive sentinel nodes do not benefit from additional axillary surgery, it is possible that there remain select women at high risk for local and regional recurrence (LRR) with sentinel node alone despite having met entry criteria for the trials previously discussed. Krishnan and colleagues[14] argue that there may even be a small high-risk subset with a survival benefit to dissection. The tumor and/or patient characteristics that identify these higher-risk patients remain to be determined.

Although the previously described trials suggest that most patients can avoid the morbidity of completion dissection, the optimal radiation fields remain unclear. Irradiating the regional lymph nodes is a consequential decision, because radiation to the nodes typically increases the risk of lymphedema, as well as the volume of exposed heart and lung compared with breast irradiation alone. In a prospective cohort study, Warren and colleagues[15] noted an HR of 1.7 ($P = .025$) for lymphedema when comparing patients who received regional nodal irradiation compared with whole breast alone. ACOSOG Z0011 specified tangential radiation to the breast alone, but did not detail the precise dose or require central quality assurance.[8] In a retrospective review of available radiation records by Jagsi and colleagues,[16] there was considerable variability. Fifty percent of patients received high tangential fields (defined as extended to within 1.0 cm of the humeral head), which likely included a large portion of axillary level 1. Nineteen percent of patients had a separate nodal field including the supraclavicular nodes. In contrast, AMAROS[11] required supraclavicular and axillary radiation in patients randomized to omit completion dissection (and also in those with 4 or more involved nodes even if randomized to axillary dissection). Although these patients were on average slightly higher risk than those enrolled in Z0011 (33% of women randomized to dissection had additional nodal disease compared with 27% in Z0011), there was substantial overlap in eligibility.

Two additional trials specifically tested the potential benefit of nodal irradiation. MA.20[2] randomized node-positive or high-risk node-negative patients (>5.0 cm, or >2.0 cm with high-grade or lymphovascular space invasion, or estrogen receptor [ER] negative) to breast-only radiation or breast and supraclavicular and internal mammary (IM) nodal irradiation. In contrast with AMAROS, all node-positive patients had a full axillary dissection. Patients randomized to nodal irradiation had improved local-regional recurrence rates (6.8% vs 4.3%; $P = .009$) and disease-free survival (77.0% vs 82.0%; $P = .01$) compared with those randomized to breast-only radiation. There was no statistically significant difference in overall survival. Although all subsets benefitted from nodal irradiation, there was a suggestion of greater benefit in women with ER-negative tumors, but the interaction between receptor and nodal irradiation did not reach significance for overall survival. These data were strengthened by a similar study from the EORTC (22922), which also randomized women to receive comprehensive nodal irradiation.[17] In contrast with only 10% of patients enrolled on MA.20, 44% of patients on the EORTC trial had negative axillary nodes (eligible by medial or central tumor location), and 24% had a mastectomy. Fifteen-year results showed an improvement in breast cancer–specific mortality with nodal irradiation (16.0% vs 19.8%; $P = .0055$) but no difference in overall survival. These studies were unable to test the relative benefit of supraclavicular and IM node irradiation. This finding is particularly relevant given the large subset of women who were axillary node negative (notably in the EORTC trial given their large number), but nonetheless were treated with supraclavicular and IM irradiation.

The Hennequin trial from France[18] solely assessed IM irradiation. Women with positive axillary nodes or medial/central tumors with negative axillary nodes were randomized following mastectomy to chest wall and supraclavicular irradiation with or without IM treatment. The trial did not show a survival benefit to IM irradiation, but was underpowered to show a difference. In contrast, the Danish nonrandomized prospective study[19] did show a survival improvement with IM irradiation (75.9% vs 72.2%; $P = .005$). In this cohort study, women with left-sided primary tumors did not receive IM irradiation because of concerns for cardiac toxicity, but women with right-sided cancers did receive treatment to the IM nodes. Although not randomized, it is difficult to imagine there were substantial differences in either the tumor or treatment based solely on tumor laterality.

Despite the success of MA.20 and the EORTC trial, several unanswered questions regarding the optimal nodal radiation fields remain. Both trials required supraclavicular and IM nodal irradiation in the experimental arm. Although there did not seem to be a subset who did not benefit from nodal treatment, this requires further study. This point is particularly relevant when patient comorbidities or unusual anatomy increases the cost of additional treatment. Moreover, the benefit of nodal irradiation is likely to change as systemic therapy improves. It is conceivable that improved systemic therapy, which has been shown to decrease the rate of LRR,[20,21] could diminish the need for RT. This possibility may be particularly relevant in women with HER2 (human epidermal growth factor receptor 2)-positive disease, for whom there have been multiple recent advances in systemic therapy that are not reflected in these randomized trials.[22,23] In addition, the biological subgroup most likely to benefit remains unclear. Although there was a suggestion of a greater benefit to nodal RT in MA.20 among women with ER-negative tumors,[2] this was not seen in women with triple-negative tumors in the Danish randomized postmastectomy radiation trials.[24] Genomic assays designed to predict benefit from systemic therapy but also shown to be prognostic for local recurrence (LR) may prove helpful in tailoring treatment to women most likely to benefit.[25,26] This possibility is currently being tested in a prospective randomized trial (MA.39/TAILOR-RT; NCT 03488693) in which node-positive women with oncotype scores of less than 18 are randomized to breast and nodal irradiation or breast alone following breast conservation, and postmastectomy irradiation (including the chest wall and comprehensive regional nodes) following mastectomy.

ACCELERATED PARTIAL BREAST IRRADIATION

Although initial studies of BCT used approximately 5 to 7 weeks of adjuvant whole-breast RT, this regimen represents a significant burden to patients such that fewer than half of those who are candidates ultimately receive breast conservation.[27] Hypofractionation is a feasible alternative for early-stage patients, but still requires 3 to 4 weeks to complete.[28,29] The observation that most recurrences arise proximate to the tumor bed[30–32] ultimately prompted interest in accelerated partial breast irradiation (APBI), which is typically administered in less than 2 weeks. Early brachytherapy trials establishing this paradigm showed promising outcomes.[33–35]

Despite encouraging results, the optimal technical aspects of APBI remained unclear. Moreover, although APBI has been studied for many years, most reports focused on brachytherapy and some showed mixed toxicity and efficacy results.[5,36] More recently, advances in treatment planning and image guidance have allowed the development of external beam APBI techniques that may be well tolerated and more convenient than brachytherapy.[37]

Recent reports of several landmark trials serve to elucidate the appropriate role of external beam APBI in the breast cancer landscape. NSABP B-39/RTOG 0413 conducted by NRG Oncology randomized 4216 patients to APBI or whole-breast irradiation. External beam APBI on this study was administered as 38.5 Gy in 10 twice-daily fractions based on extant radiobiological models suggesting an equivalence to doses of 50 Gy in 25 once-daily fractions. Although the absolute difference in 10-year in-breast tumor recurrence (IBTR) was only 0.7% (4.6% with APBI vs 3.9% with whole-breast RT), APBI did not meet the prespecified statistical criteria for equivalence to whole-breast RT.[38] Interestingly, unplanned subset analysis showed that APBI recurrence rates were higher among patients receiving brachytherapy than among those receiving external beam APBI. As a result, these findings have been interpreted by proponents of external beam APBI as sufficient evidence to offer APBI among appropriately selected patients.

The concurrent report of the RAPID trial yielded consistent results.[39] Patients on this study (n = 2135) were similarly randomized to APBI (38.5 Gy in 10 twice-daily fractions) or whole-breast RT. Eight-year IBTR rates were similarly low as in B-39 (3.0% for APBI vs 2.8% for whole-breast RT); however, adverse cosmesis at 3 years was higher with APBI (29% vs 17%; P<.001), overall suggesting that APBI was noninferior from a disease control standpoint.

In an effort to improve on cosmetic outcomes and the added convenience of daily fractionation (as opposed to twice-daily treatment on B-39 and RAPID), 2 recent studies contributed additional feasible external beam APBI regimens. The British IMPORT LOW trial administered 40 Gy in 15 daily fractions showing that this regimen, when targeting the partial breast, was not inferior to targeting the whole breast (local relapse at 5 years: 1.1% whole breast vs 0.5% partial breast).[40] Moreover, comprehensive cosmesis assessments also showed that treating the partial breast yielded significantly fewer adverse effects with regard to breast appearance and firmness. Building on this experience, an institutional trial at the Memorial Sloan Kettering Cancer Center studied 40-Gy APBI administered in 10 daily fractions.[41] Among 106 patients, only 2 instances of grade 3 toxicity were reported, and 3 recurrences were noted, consistent with the low rate of disease events reported on the large randomized trials earlier.

Taken together, recent studies of external beam APBI offer several feasible regimens that include both once-daily and twice-daily fractionation, affording appropriately selected patients both a low risk of recurrence and excellent cosmetic outcome. ASTRO consensus guidelines outline the emergent literature for APBI candidacy.[42]

OMISSION OF ADJUVANT RADIOTHERAPY FOLLOWING BREAST CONSERVING SURGERY

Adjuvant RT following lumpectomy (whether whole breast or APBI) reduces recurrences for patients with invasive breast cancer.[43–45] This finding has now been seen in numerous studies, establishing adjuvant RT as a standard component of BCT. Although it is well tolerated and effective, RT may be inconvenient, confers financial toxicity, and carries long-term risks. Moreover, large analyses[45] and smaller reports suggest that not all patients benefit equally from RT.[3] Several attempts have sought to identify low-risk patients who may forego RT.

In an early such effort, several Harvard centers accrued 87 early-stage node-negative patients with T1N0 invasive breast cancer who underwent lumpectomy alone without RT.[46,47] Although they were selected for favorable features (ie, unicentric, margins $\geq$1 cm, no lymphovascular invasion), the LR rate was an unacceptable 23% at a median follow-up of 86 months. This rate was worse than permissible for a low-risk group, further supporting the continued use of postoperative RT among these patients. Of note, this trial did include several patients less than 50 years of age, and their ER status was unknown in 50% of cases because of the era of treatment.

In a parallel effort, the National Surgical Adjuvant Breast and Bowel Project (NSABP) B-21 trial evaluated whether the use of tamoxifen could obviate adjuvant RT in patients with small, node-negative tumors.[43] In B-21, 1009 lumpectomy patients were randomized to adjuvant tamoxifen, radiation, or both. The cumulative incidence of LR at 8 years was 16.5% for those treated with tamoxifen alone, 9.3% for radiation alone, and 2.8% for those who received both (P = .01). Therefore, despite careful selection and the use of tamoxifen, this population showed sufficient risk to continue receiving adjuvant RT. Note that, despite the use of tamoxifen, ER status was not known in nearly one-third of enrolled patients.

Advanced age at breast cancer diagnosis has long been associated with more favorable breast cancer outcomes, prompting a Canadian trial that included only women 50 years of age or older.[44] From 1992 to 2000, 769 women with early, localized, node-negative breast cancers were randomized to tamoxifen alone or in combination with RT. At 5 years, the rate of LR was 7.7% for those who received tamoxifen alone versus 0.6% for those receiving the combination ($P<$.001), again highlighting the local benefit of RT. Subgroup analyses of only the most favorable patients with T1 ER+ tumors showed that the LR rate at 8 years remained unacceptable at 15.2%.

Numerous smaller studies have also attempted to forego RT for select subgroups of patients. A Finnish trial of 264 lumpectomy patients with unifocal lesions randomized patients to receive RT or not.[48] After a median of 12 years, LR was noted in 12% of those who received RT versus 27% without RT. A similar trial used a 2 × 2 factorial design to study the independent influences of RT and tamoxifen on LR.[49] Although the study was not powered to detect an interaction between tamoxifen and radiation, the 10-year rate of LR was 34% for those who underwent lumpectomy alone versus 10% for those who also received adjuvant RT. Notably, adding tamoxifen decreased these rates to 7% without RT and 5% with RT. Another Italian study of nearly 600 lumpectomy patients with tumors less than 2.5 cm randomized subjects to adjuvant RT.[50] The cumulative incidence of LR at 10 years was 5.8% for those treated with RT versus 23.5% for those without ($P<$.001). The noted difference was particularly large among those less than or equal to 45 years of age, whereas no difference was noted among those more than 65 years old (P = .326). An important overarching consideration is that these studies could not rigorously evaluate tumor ER status and none used any contemporary expression profiling. The use of recently validated biomarkers has significantly improved the ability to risk stratify patients, and molecular testing is now a routine component of systemic therapy decision making.

More recently, the Cancer and Leukemia Group B (CALGB) conducted a practice-changing study showing the feasibility of omitting RT after lumpectomy.[4,51] CALGB 9343 enrolled more than 600 women in the early 1990s, all of whom were more than 70 years of age, with small ER+ tumors. After lumpectomy, all patients were to receive tamoxifen, and were further randomized to RT or not. At 10 years, the rate of LRR was significantly different between the two groups (2% for tamoxifen plus RT vs 10% for tamoxifen alone). No significant differences were seen for distant metastasis or overall survival between treatment arms. Although the increased risk of LRR without RT was significant, the small absolute benefit to RT, in conjunction with the absence of a survival difference, showed that foregoing RT might be feasible among these appropriately selected patients. To date, there are limited data to guide this approach for younger women.

Many of the aforementioned studies were conducted in an era of now-outdated therapies. Advances in imaging, chemotherapy, endocrine therapy, and surgery have changed the BCT landscape, reducing LRR rates for early breast cancer to less than 5% to 10% in many reports.[52–54] The studies summarized earlier that were designed to identify low-risk subgroups were largely conducted with approaches that are no longer standard, yielding increased rates of LRR even among highly favorable patients. Therapies and risk-stratification approaches have since been refined considerably, with ongoing efforts to de-escalate treatment of the lowest-risk patients.[55]

Enabling these efforts, molecular profiling findings have shown that breast cancer is not a single disease entity but a class of distinct biological subtypes. These subtypes carry prognostic and predictive significance, with a discrete natural history characterizing each.[56–59] Given the complexity associated with comprehensive transcriptional profiling, surrogate methods using widespread immunohistochemical (IHC) and histologic techniques have been correlated with the relevant transcriptional profiles; these have been largely based on staining for the ER, progesterone receptor (PR), Her2neu overexpression (HER2), and the Ki-67 proliferation marker, along with an assessment of histologic grade. Among the intrinsic biological subtypes distinguished by these markers, the most favorable is luminal A, typically defined by immunohistochemistry showing ER+, PR+, and Her2−, along with a low histologic grade and/or low Ki-67 proliferation rate.[52,60,61] Accordingly, luminal A tumors have the lowest risk of LRR among all breast cancers and the most indolent biology.

With the widespread adoption of IHC-based subtype approximation, some information is lost that can only be inferred from larger panels of expression profiles. As a result, researchers have sought to develop more comprehensive and standardized assays to reliably and reproducibly characterize biological subtype.

PAM-50 (Prediction Analysis of Microarray–50) is a molecular diagnostic test, performed on RNA extracted from formalin-fixed paraffin-embedded (FFPE) breast tumor tissue samples. FFPE samples are typically produced in the course of standard clinical care, requiring no additional tissue collection. The assay technology chemically labels each messenger RNA transcript in the sample with a molecular "barcode," facilitating analysis of the expression profile of 50 predictive genes. A classifier algorithm then assigns the resultant expression profile a score and 1 of 4 breast cancer biological subtypes (luminal A, luminal B, HER2, or basal) in accordance with prior validation cohorts.

To date, studies using PAM-50 in breast cancer have shown the potential to accurately identify those patients who stand to benefit from antiestrogen therapy or chemotherapy,[62–64] while similarly informing which patients might feasibly forego these treatments. The PRECISON (Profiling Early Breast Cancer for Radiotherapy Omission; NCT02653755) trial is currently studying this assay for risk stratification and RT decision making. Provided that other favorable clinicopathologic features are present, patients whose tumors show a low risk-of-recurrence score are eligible to enroll and forego RT. The EXPERT (Examining Personalised Radiation Therapy for Low-risk Early Breast Trial; ClinicalTrials.gov NCT02889874) trial, being conducted in Australia and New Zealand, is a phase III study also examining the utility of PAM-50 in identifying appropriate patients for RT omission using a larger and randomized study design.

The IDEA (Individualized Decisions for Endocrine Therapy Alone) study is a multi-institution, single-arm trial being led at the University of Michigan. Tumors undergo profiling by the OncotypeDX 21-gene recurrence assay to similarly identify putatively low-risk tumors. Patients that have a low risk score on the OncotypeDX assay may then forego adjuvant RT.

Thus, randomized data support the omission of RT among low-risk older-age patients, and ongoing efforts using molecular profiling are designed to identify younger cohorts who may safely be spared the risks and toxicity of therapy.

REFERENCES

1. Fisher B, Jeong JH, Anderson S, et al. Twenty-five-year follow-up of a randomized trial comparing radical mastectomy, total mastectomy, and total mastectomy followed by irradiation. N Engl J Med 2002;347(8):567–75.
2. Whelan TJ, Olivotto IA, Parulekar WR, et al, 20 Study Investigators. Regional nodal irradiation in early-stage breast cancer. N Engl J Med 2015;373(4):307–16.
3. Poortmans PM, Collette S, Kirkove C, et al. Internal mammary and medial supraclavicular irradiation in breast cancer. N Engl J Med 2015;373(4):317–27.
4. Hughes KS, Schnaper LA, Bellon JR, et al. Lumpectomy plus tamoxifen with or without irradiation in women age 70 years or older with early breast cancer: long-term follow-up of CALGB 9343. J Clin Oncol 2013;31(19):2382–7.
5. Smith BD, Arthur DW, Buchholz TA, et al. Accelerated partial breast irradiation consensus statement from the American Society for Radiation Oncology (ASTRO). Int J Radiat Oncol Biol Phys 2009;74(4):987–1001.
6. Chandra RA, Miller CL, Skolny MN, et al. Radiation therapy risk factors for development of lymphedema in patients treated with regional lymph node irradiation for breast cancer. Int J Radiat Oncol Biol Phys 2015;91(4):760–4.
7. Krag DN, Anderson SJ, Julian TB, et al. Sentinel-lymph-node resection compared with conventional axillary-lymph-node dissection in clinically node-negative patients with breast cancer: overall survival findings from the NSABP B-32randomised phase 3 trial. Lancet Oncol 2010;11(10):927–33.
8. Giuliano AE, Hunt KK, Ballman KV, et al. Axillary dissection vs no axillary dissection in women with invasive breast cancer and sentinel node metastasis: a randomized clinical trial. JAMA 2011;305(6):569–75.
9. Giuliano AE, Ballman KV, McCall L, et al. Effect of axillary dissection vs no axillary dissection on 10-year overall survival among women with invasive breast cancer and sentinel node metastasis: the ACOSOG Z0011 (Alliance) randomized clinical trial. JAMA 2017;318(10):918–26.
10. Galimberti V, Cole BF, Viale G, et al. International Breast Cancer Study Group Trial 23-01. Axillary dissection versus no axillary dissection in patients with breast cancer and sentinel-node micrometastases (IBCSG 23-01): 10-year follow-up of a randomised, controlled phase 3 trial. Lancet Oncol 2018;19(10):1385–93.
11. Rutgers EJ, Donker M, Poncet C, et al. Radiotherapy or surgery of the axilla after a positive sentinel node in breast cancer patients: 10 year follow up results of the EORTC AMAROS trial (EORTC 10981/22023). San Antonio Breast Cancer Symposium. 2018. Abstract. December 4, 2018.
12. Morrow M, Van Zee KJ, Patil S, et al. Axillary dissection and nodal irradiation can be avoided for most node-positive Z0011-eligible breast cancers: a prospective validation study of 793 patients. Ann Surg 2017;266(3):457–62.
13. Savolt A, Peley G, Polgar C, et al. Eight-year follow up result of the OTOASOR trial: the optimal treatment of the axilla – surgery or radiotherapy after positive

sentinel lymph node biopsy in early-stage breast cancer: a randomized single centre, phase III, non-inferiority trial. Eur J Surg Oncol 2017;43:672–9.

14. Krishnan MS, Recht A, Bellon JR, et al. Trade-offs associated with axillary lymph node dissection with breast irradiation versus breast irradiation alone in patients with a positive sentinel node in relation to the risk of non-sentinel node involvement: implications of ACOSOG Z0011. Breast Cancer Res Treat 2013;138(1): 205–13.

15. Warren LE, Miller CL, Horick N, et al. The impact of radiation therapy on the risk of lymphedema after treatment for breast cancer: a prospective cohort study. Int J Radiat Oncol Biol Phys 2014;88(3):565–71.

16. Jagsi R, Chadha M, Moni J, et al. Radiation field design in the ACOSOG Z0011 (Alliance) trial. J Clin Oncol 2014;32(32):3600–6.

17. Poortmans P, Collette S, Struikmans H, et al. Fifteen-year results of the randomised EORTC trial 22922/10925 investigating internal mammary and medial supraclavicular (IM-MS) lymph node irradiation in stage I-III breast cancer. Abstract. American Society of Clinical Oncology Annual Meeting. December 4, 2018.

18. Hennequin C, Bossard N, Servagi-Vernat S, et al. Ten-year survival results of a randomized trial of irradiation of internal mammary nodes after mastectomy. Int J Radiat Oncol Biol Phys 2013;86(5):860–6.

19. Thorsen LB, Offersen BV, Danø H, et al. DBCG-IMN: a population-based cohort study on the effect of internal mammary node irradiation in early node-positive breast cancer. J Clin Oncol 2016;34(4):314–20.

20. Sartor CI, Peterson BL, Woolf S, et al. Effect of addition of adjuvant paclitaxel on radiotherapy delivery and locoregional control of node-positive breast cancer: cancer and leukemia group B 9344. J Clin Oncol 2005;23(1):30–40.

21. Anderson SJ, Wapnir I, Dignam JJ, et al. Prognosis after ipsilateral breast tumor recurrence and locoregional recurrences in patients treated by breast-conserving therapy in five National Surgical Adjuvant Breast and Bowel Project protocols of node-negative breast cancer. J Clin Oncol 2009;27(15):2466–73.

22. von Minckwitz G, Huang CS, Mano MS, et al, KATHERINEInvestigators. Trastuzumab emtansine for residual invasive her2-positive breast cancer. N Engl J Med 2019;380(7):617–28.

23. Romond EH, Perez EA, Bryant J, et al. Trastuzumab plus adjuvant chemotherapy for operable HER2-positive breast cancer. N Engl J Med 2005;353(16):1673–84.

24. Kyndi M, Sørensen FB, Knudsen H, et al, Danish Breast Cancer Cooperative Group. Estrogen receptor, progesterone receptor, HER-2, and response to post-mastectomy radiotherapy in high-risk breast cancer: the Danish Breast Cancer Cooperative Group. J Clin Oncol 2008;26(9):1419–26.

25. Woodward WA, Barlow WE, R. Jagsi R, et al. The 21-gene recurrence score and locoregional recurrence rates in patients with node-positive breast cancer treated on SWOG S8814. [Abstract]. Int J Radiat Oncol Biol Phys 2016;96(2, Supplement):S146.

26. Mamounas EP, Liu Q, Paik S, et al. 21-gene recurrence score and locoregional recurrence in node-positive/ER-positive breast cancer treated with chemo-endocrine therapy. J Natl Cancer Inst 2017;109(4). https://doi.org/10.1093/jnci/djw259.

27. Morrow M, White J, Moughan J, et al. Factors predicting the use of breast-conserving therapy in stage I and II breast carcinoma. J Clin Oncol 2001;19(8): 2254–62.

28. Whelan TJ, Pignol J-P, Levine MN, et al. Long-term results of hypofractionated radiation therapy for breast cancer. N Engl J Med 2010;362(6):513–20.
29. Haviland JS, Owen JR, Dewar JA, et al. The UK Standardisation of Breast Radiotherapy (START) trials of radiotherapy hypofractionation for treatment of early breast cancer: 10-year follow-up results of two randomised controlled trials. Lancet Oncol 2013;14(11):1086–94.
30. Recht A, Houlihan MJ. Conservative surgery without radiotherapy in the treatment of patients with early-stage invasive breast cancer. A review. Ann Surg 1995; 222(1):9.
31. Solin LJ, Fowble B, Martz K, et al. Results of re-excisional biopsy of the primary tumor in preparation for definitive irradiation of patients with early stage breast cancer. Int J Radiat Oncol Biol Phys 1986;12(5):721–5.
32. Holland R, Connolly JL, Gelman R, et al. The presence of an extensive intraductal component following a limited excision correlates with prominent residual disease in the remainder of the breast. J Clin Oncol 1990;8(1):113–8.
33. Vicini F, Kini VR, Chen P, et al. Irradiation of the tumor bed alone after lumpectomy in selected patients with early-stage breast cancer treated with breast conserving therapy. J Surg Oncol 1999;70(1):33–40.
34. King TA, Bolton JS, Kuske RR, et al. Long-term results of wide-field brachytherapy as the sole method of radiation therapy after segmental mastectomy for Tis, 1, 2 breast cancer. Am J Surg 2000;180(4):299–304.
35. Fentiman I, Poole C, Tong D, et al. Iridium implant treatment without external radiotherapy for operable breast cancer: a pilot study. Eur J Cancer Clin Oncol 1991;27(4):447–50.
36. Vaidya JS, Wenz F, Bulsara M, et al. Risk-adapted targeted intraoperative radiotherapy versus whole-breast radiotherapy for breast cancer: 5-year results for local control and overall survival from the TARGIT-A randomised trial. Lancet 2014;383(9917):603–13.
37. Formenti SC. External-beam partial-breast irradiation. Paper presented at: Seminars in radiation oncology. 2005. December 4, 2018.
38. Vicini F. Primary results of NSABP B-39/RTOG 0413 (NRG Oncology): a randomized phase III study of conventional whole breast irradiation (WBI) versus partial breast irradiation (PBI) for women with stage 0, I, or II breast cancer. SABCS 2018. San Antonio, TX, December 4, 2018.
39. Whelan T, Julian J, Levine M, et al. RAPID: a randomized trial of accelerated partial breast irradiation using 3-dimensional conformal radiotherapy (3D-CRT). SABCS 2018. San Antonio, TX, December 4, 2018.
40. Coles CE, Griffin CL, Kirby AM, et al. Partial-breast radiotherapy after breast conservation surgery for patients with early breast cancer (UK IMPORT LOW trial): 5-year results from a multicentre, randomised, controlled, phase 3, non-inferiority trial. Lancet 2017;390(10099):1048–60.
41. Braunstein LZ, Thor M, Flynn J, et al. Daily fractionation of external beam accelerated partial breast irradiation to 40 Gy is well tolerated and locally effective. Int J Radiat Oncol Biol Phys 2019;104(4):859–66.
42. Correa C, Harris EE, Leonardi MC, et al. Accelerated partial breast irradiation: executive summary for the update of an ASTRO evidence-based consensus statement. Pract Radiat Oncol 2017;7(2):73–9.
43. Fisher B, Anderson S, Bryant J, et al. Twenty-year follow-up of a randomized trial comparing total mastectomy, lumpectomy, and lumpectomy plus irradiation for the treatment of invasive breast cancer. N Engl J Med 2002;347(16):1233–41.

44. Fyles AW, McCready DR, Manchul LA, et al. Tamoxifen with or without breast irradiation in women 50 years of age or older with early breast cancer. N Engl J Med 2004;351(10):963–70.
45. Early Breast Cancer Trialists' Collaborative Group (EBCTCG), Darby S, McGale P, Correa C, et al. Effect of radiotherapy after breast-conserving surgery on 10-year recurrence and 15-year breast cancer death: meta-analysis of individual patient data for 10,801 women in 17 randomised trials. Lancet 2011;378(9804):1707–16.
46. Schnitt SJ, Hayman J, Gelman R, et al. A prospective study of conservative surgery alone in the treatment of selected patients with stage I breast cancer. Cancer 1996;77(6):1094–100.
47. Lim M, Bellon JR, Gelman R, et al. A prospective study of conservative surgery without radiation therapy in select patients with Stage I breast cancer. Int J Radiat Oncol Biol Phys 2006;65(4):1149–54.
48. Holli K, Hietanen P, Saaristo R, et al. Radiotherapy after segmental resection of breast cancer with favorable prognostic features: 12-year follow-up results of a randomized trial. J Clin Oncol 2009;27(6):927–32.
49. Winzer KJ, Sauerbrei W, Braun M, et al. Radiation therapy and tamoxifen after breast-conserving surgery: updated results of a 2 x 2 randomised clinical trial in patients with low risk of recurrence. Eur J Cancer 2010;46(1):95–101.
50. Veronesi U, Marubini E, Mariani L, et al. Radiotherapy after breast-conserving surgery in small breast carcinoma: long-term results of a randomized trial. Ann Oncol 2001;12(7):997–1003.
51. Hughes KS, Schnaper LA, Berry D, et al. Lumpectomy plus tamoxifen with or without irradiation in women 70 years of age or older with early breast cancer. N Engl J Med 2004;351(10):971–7.
52. Arvold ND, Taghian AG, Niemierko A, et al. Age, breast cancer subtype approximation, and local recurrence after breast-conserving therapy. J Clin Oncol 2011; 29(29):3885–91.
53. Miles RC, Gullerud RE, Lohse CM, et al. Local recurrence after breast-conserving surgery: multivariable analysis of risk factors and the impact of young age. Ann Surg Oncol 2012;19(4):1153–9.
54. Canavan J, Truong PT, Smith SL, et al. Local recurrence in women with stage I breast cancer: declining rates over time in a large, population-based cohort. Int J Radiat Oncol Biol Phys 2014;88(1):80–6.
55. Smith SL, Truong PT, Lu L, et al. Identification of patients at very low risk of local recurrence after breast-conserving surgery. Int J Radiat Oncol Biol Phys 2014; 89(3):556–62.
56. Perou CM, Sorlie T, Eisen MB, et al. Molecular portraits of human breast tumours. Nature 2000;406(6797):747–52.
57. Sorlie T, Perou CM, Tibshirani R, et al. Gene expression patterns of breast carcinomas distinguish tumor subclasses with clinical implications. Proc Natl Acad Sci U S A 2001;98(19):10869–74.
58. Sorlie T, Tibshirani R, Parker J, et al. Repeated observation of breast tumor subtypes in independent gene expression data sets. Proc Natl Acad Sci U S A 2003; 100(14):8418–23.
59. Fan C, Oh DS, Wessels L, et al. Concordance among gene-expression-based predictors for breast cancer. N Engl J Med 2006;355(6):560–9.
60. Nguyen PL, Taghian AG, Katz MS, et al. Breast cancer subtype approximated by estrogen receptor, progesterone receptor, and HER-2 is associated with local and distant recurrence after breast-conserving therapy. J Clin Oncol 2008; 26(14):2373–8.

61. Voduc KD, Cheang MC, Tyldesley S, et al. Breast cancer subtypes and the risk of local and regional relapse. J Clin Oncol 2010;28(10):1684–91.
62. Dowsett M, Sestak I, Lopez-Knowles E, et al. Comparison of PAM50 risk of recurrence score with oncotype DX and IHC4 for predicting risk of distant recurrence after endocrine therapy. J Clin Oncol 2013;31(22):2783–90.
63. Gnant M, Filipits M, Greil R, et al. Predicting distant recurrence in receptor-positive breast cancer patients with limited clinicopathological risk: using the PAM50 Risk of Recurrence score in 1478 postmenopausal patients of the ABCSG-8 trial treated with adjuvant endocrine therapy alone. Ann Oncol 2014; 25(2):339–45.
64. Filipits M, Nielsen TO, Rudas M, et al. The PAM50 risk-of-recurrence score predicts risk for late distant recurrence after endocrine therapy in postmenopausal women with endocrine-responsive early breast cancer. Clin Cancer Res 2014; 20(5):1298–305.

Current Role of Radiation Therapy in the Management of Malignant Central Nervous System Tumors

Ahsan Farooqi, MD, PhD[a], Jing Li, MD, PhD[a], John de Groot, MD[b],
Debra Nana Yeboa, MD[a,c],*

KEYWORDS

- Central nervous system brain tumors • Radiation therapy • Glioma • Meningioma
- Brain metastases • Clinical review

KEY POINTS

- The 2016 World Health Organization classification now classifies gliomas according to both molecular and histologic parameters, which is evolving the treatment management.
- Meningiomas can be managed similar to the guidelines of cooperative group trials, which report good progression-free survival with radiation; studies are ongoing regarding atypical meningiomas.
- The management of brain metastases is changing because of increased use of stereotactic radiosurgery, hippocampal-sparing whole-brain irradiation, and the introduction of immunotherapy/targeted therapy for intracranial disease.

GLIOMAS

Overview

Gliomas include astrocytomas and oligodendrogliomas, and make up 20% to 30% of central nervous system (CNS) tumors.[1] There are an estimated 2000 to 3000 cases of low-grade glioma (LGG) and 20,000 cases of high-grade glioma (HGG) diagnosed every year in the United States.

Clinical Presentation

Initial clinical presentation depends largely on the location and size of the tumor. The most common presenting symptom for LGG are seizures, whereas patients

Disclosure: The authors have no disclosures related to this article.
[a] Radiation Oncology Department, University of Texas MD Anderson Cancer Center, 1515 Holcombe Boulevard, Unit 97, Houston, TX 77030, USA; [b] Neuro-Oncology Department, University of Texas MD Anderson Cancer Center, 1515 Holcombe Boulevard, Unit 431, Houston, TX 77030, USA; [c] Health Services Research Department, University of Texas MD Anderson Cancer Center, 1515 Holcombe Boulevard, Houston, TX 77030, USA
* Corresponding author. 1515 Holcombe Boulevard, Unit 97, Houston, TX 77030.
E-mail address: dnyeboa@mdanderson.org

Hematol Oncol Clin N Am 34 (2020) 13–28
https://doi.org/10.1016/j.hoc.2019.08.015
0889-8588/20/© 2019 Elsevier Inc. All rights reserved.

with HGG typically present with focal neurologic symptoms, including cognitive, sensory, aphasic, and motor deficits.[2,3] Along with a history of headaches, patients may also present with additional signs of increased intracranial pressure, including nausea, vomiting, confusion, or papilledema.

Diagnostic Evaluation and Imaging

A complete history and physical examination with a detailed neurologic examination is necessary to establish the baseline functional performance status of the patient. LGG classically are non–contrast enhancing on MRI compared with HGG, which typically show strong enhancement with contrast. In addition, both LGGs and HGGs can present with a significant edematous component best seen as a hyperintense signal on the T2 fluid-attenuated inversion recovery (FLAIR) sequence.

Classification Systems

Historically, gliomas were classified according to histologic examination of the cell of origin and degree of differentiation on hematoxylin-eosin–stained sections evaluating the presence or absence of nuclear atypia, mitotic rate, necrosis, and angiogenesis.[4] In recent years there has been a recognition that molecular classification factors may allow improved tumor classification in addition to histology. Consequently, this system underwent a significant restructuring in the 2016 World Health Organization (WHO) classification of CNS tumors, and for the first time gliomas are classified according to both molecular and histologic parameters.[5] The updated WHO classification for gliomas is shown in **Fig. 1**.[5] Management paradigms are rapidly evolving to include molecular factors. Moreover, because prior clinical trials have been based primarily on histologic parameters, this article focuses on how that literature informs current practice, with an eye toward future strategies incorporating molecular information.

Management of Low-Grade Gliomas

Optimal management of LGG requires a careful multidisciplinary discussion between the treating physicians, including radiation oncology, neuro-oncology, neurosurgery, as well as neuropathology and neuroradiology consultants. Following maximal safe surgical resection, a variety of factors must be considered before recommending postoperative radiation treatment (RT). In the randomized European Organisation for Research and Treatment of Cancer (EORTC) 22845 trial, adjuvant RT to 54 Gy improved progression-free survival (PFS) (5.3 years vs 3.4 years) and seizure control at 1 year (41% vs 25%) compared with salvage delayed RT, although without a long-term overall survival (OS) benefit. Thus benefits of early RT must be weighed against potential neurocognitive toxicities of treatment.[6] Both the EORTC and the Intergroup North Central Cancer Treatment Group (NCCTG)/Radiation Therapy Oncology Group (RTOG)/Eastern Cooperative Oncology Group (ECOG) trials showed that between a lower dose (45–50.4 Gy) and higher dose (59.4–64.8 Gy), OS and PFS were nonsignificant but increased toxicity.[7,8] As a result, the most common dose regimens for adjuvant RT in LGG are 50.4 to 54 Gy in 28 to 30 once-daily fractions (fx) of 1.8 Gy per fraction.

Regarding chemotherapy, RTOG 9802 randomized patients with LGG with high-risk features (≥40 years or age <40 years of age with subtotal resection) to RT versus RT followed by 6 cycles of adjuvant procarbazine, lomustine, and vincristine (PCV). Median OS (13.3 years vs 7.8 years) and PFS (10.4 years vs 4.0 years) were improved with the addition of chemotherapy driven primarily by oligodendroglioma histology and gliomas with 1p19q codeletion on subset analysis.[9,10] Next, the phase II RTOG 0424 trial delivered concurrent temozolomide (TMZ) with 54 Gy to high-risk patients

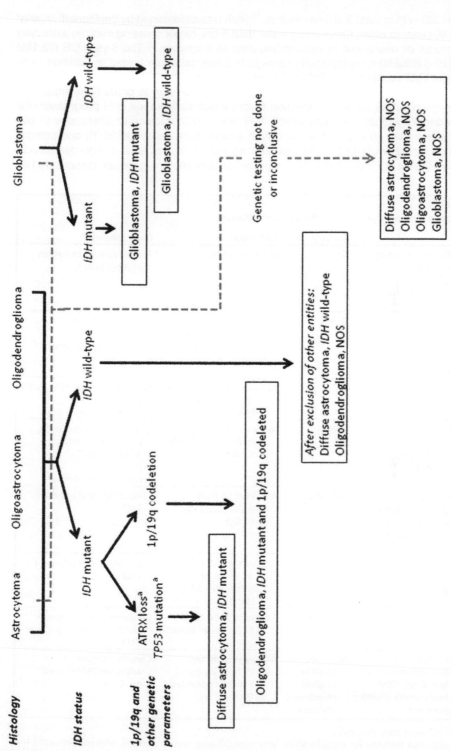

Fig. 1. The 2016 WHO classification of tumors of the central nervous system. NOS, not otherwise specified. [a] Characteristic but not required for diagnosis. (*From* Louis DN, Perry A, Reifenberger G, et al. The 2016 World Health Organization Classification of Tumors of the Central Nervous System: a summary. Acta Neuropathol 2016;131(6):809; with permission.)

with LGG with at least 3 of 5 risk factors.[11] Risk was determined by the Pignatti criteria: age 40 years or older, tumor size greater than 5 cm, tumor crossing midline, astrocytic histology, or neurologic symptoms/seizures at diagnosis.[12] The 3-year OS (73.1%) and PFS (59.2%) were reported improved to historical control rates. In addition, concurrent TMZ versus sequential PCV is being tested in the CODEL (NCT00887146) trial, which began enrolling high-risk grade II gliomas in addition to grade III gliomas.

In practice, the authors' institution favors initial surveillance until progression for oligodendrogliomas with concurrent IDH and 1p19q molecular alterations in patients less than 40 years of age and with a gross total resection (GTR) and consideration for early upfront RT for patients with LGG with at least 1 high-risk clinical factor (**Table 1**). For grade II and grade III IDH mutant gliomas without 1p19q

Table 1
Options for management of primary brain gliomas

	Surgery	Radiation	Chemotherapy
IDH mut or 1p19q codeleted, oligodendroglioma, or grade II, and <40 y age	GTR	At progression	As adjuvant to radiation at progression
IDH mut or 1p19q codeleted glioma, or grade II, and at least 1 high-risk feature[a]	GTR	Consider early adjuvant RT 50.4–54 Gy (can consider BN005)	Adjuvant TMZ or PCV (PCV for oligodendroglioma)
IDH mut, grade II glioma, and >40 y age	STR	Adjuvant to 50.4–54 Gy in 28–30 fx or consider BN005	Adjuvant TMZ or PCV (PCV for oligodendroglioma)
IDH mut, grade III, or 1p19q noncodeleted glioma	GTR/STR	Adjuvant to 59.4 Gy in 33 fx (consider BN005 or 57 Gy in 30 fx)	Can consider concurrent but must include adjuvant TMZ or PCV (PCV for oligodendroglioma)
IDH wild-type glioma, grade II or grade II with multiple (3) high-risk features[a]	GTR/STR	Adjuvant 54 (can consider doses up to 60 Gy)	Concurrent and adjuvant TMZ
IDH wild-type astrocytoma, grade III	GTR/STR	Adjuvant to 59.4–60 Gy in 33–30 fx (can consider 57 Gy in 30 fx)	Concurrent and adjuvant TMZ
Histologic GBM	GTR/STR	Adjuvant to 60 Gy in 30 fx (consider BN001)	Concurrent and adjuvant TMZ (consider adjuvant TTF)
IDH wild-type astrocytoma or histologic GBM and age>65 y with poor PFS	Maximal feasible surgical resection if operable	Adjuvant to 40 Gy in 15 fx or 25 Gy in 5 fx (can consider 50 Gy in 20 fx)	Consider concurrent or adjuvant TMZ (based on KPS)

Abbreviation: mut, mutation.
[a] High-risk features for consideration: large size (>5 cm), tumor crossing midline, astrocytic histology, and/or neurologic symptoms/seizures at diagnosis (Pignatti criteria).

codeletion or with subtotal resection (STR), our institution favors sequential RT followed by chemotherapy or consideration for enrollment on clinical trials such as NRG-BN005 offering RT and sequential TMZ. Specifically, for patients with 1p19q codeletion, our neuro-oncology group practice presently is to offer PCV when tolerated.

Management of High-Grade Gliomas

Grade III/anaplastic gliomas

For patients presenting with HGG, maximal feasible surgical resection, radiation, and chemotherapy are standard of care. EORTC 26951 randomized both anaplastic astrocytomas and oligodendrogliomas after surgical resection and adjuvant RT (59.4 Gy/33 fx) to either observation or treatment with 6 cycles of PCV.

The RT plus PCV arm had significantly improved OS (42.3 v 30.6 months in the RT arm, hazard ratio [HR], 0.75; $P = .018$).[13] The HR reduction of the addition of PCV was more pronounced in the 25% of patients with 1p/19q-codeleted tumors, which would now be classified molecularly to behave more akin to lower-grade gliomas. The median OS was not reached in the RT plus PCV group versus 112 months in the RT group (HR, 0.56; $P = .059$). In the patients with noncodeleted tumors, which better reflects the grade III glioma population, the risk reduction was significantly less (OS of 25 vs 21 months; HR, 0.83; $P = .185$). Because use of TMZ has increased for glioma management because of the more favorable toxicity profile, use of PCV is supported specifically for oligodendrogliomas at our institution when tolerated.

Similar to the CODEL trial, the CATNON (EORTC study 26053–22054) trial was designed to test the role of TMZ chemotherapy in newly diagnosed 1p/19q noncodeleted anaplastic gliomas. Patients were randomized to treatment with RT (59.4 Gy/33 fx) alone, RT plus adjuvant TMZ, concurrent chemoradiation treatment (CRT), or CRT plus adjuvant TMZ. Initial results from a planned interim analysis showed improved OS at 5 years with use of adjuvant TMZ (55.9% vs 44.1%; HR, 0.65).[14] Grade 3 to 4 adverse events were seen in 8% to 12% of patients assigned TMZ, which is significantly less than the historical rates seen with PCV. The report of CATNON is awaited, and management for grade III gliomas or *IDH* wild-type gliomas can vary from use of sequential to concurrent chemotherapy based on both molecular and clinical features (see **Table 1**). Based on available data, the authors favor adjuvant RT treatment of *IDH* mutant, 1p19q noncodeleted grade III gliomas followed by adjuvant treatment with TMZ (concurrent TMZ treatment optional). However, if the tumor is histologically a grade III but is *IDH* wild-type, concurrent and adjuvant TMZ treatment is reasonable because these tumors are expected to behave more aggressively.

Glioblastoma

For WHO Grade IV glioblastoma, the role of postoperative CRT with TMZ was defined by the seminal EORTC 26981/22981-NCIC trial, which prospectively randomized patients after surgical resection to RT alone (60 Gy/30 fx) versus CRT plus adjuvant TMZ. The 2-year OS was significantly improved with the addition of TMZ at 10% (RT alone) versus 26% (CRT), (HR, 0.63; $P<.001$).[15] This study was followed by the EF-14 NovoTTF trial, which randomized patients after surgery and CRT to maintenance therapy with TMZ alone or TMZ plus tumor-treating fields (TTFs). Median OS was significantly improved with the addition of TTF (20.5 months vs 15.6 months; HR, 0.64; $P = .004$).[16] Although there is ongoing discussion regarding the role of TTF, presently TTF has been incorporated into National Comprehensive Cancer Network (NCCN) guidelines.[17]

For elderly patients or those with poor Karnofsky performance status (KPS), hypofractionated RT with a shorter overall treatment time may be preferred to 6 weeks of RT. Trials showed that 3 weeks (40 Gy in 15 fx) compared with 6 weeks of RT alone or even 1 week (25 Gy in 5 fx) compared with 3 weeks of RT had noninferior OS in patients more than 50 years old with low KPS of 50 to 70 or who were older than 60 to 65 years, frail, and not candidates for chemotherapy.[18,19] Our institution has also adopted an intermediate hypofractionated regimen between 60 Gy and 40 Gy of 50 Gy in 20 fractions.

Future Radiation Studies

Proton beam therapy may reduce doses to normal tissue relative to intensity-modulated radiation therapy (IMRT), which could potentially translate into clinical benefit. The randomized phase II clinical trial NRG-BN005, comparing proton radiation therapy versus IMRT among patients with *IDH* mutant grade II or grade III glioma, will evaluate cognition as the primary end point.[20,21] Treatment entails 54 Gy with adjuvant TMZ. Few agents have shown new efficacy in glioblastoma multiforme (GBM), and thus studies are ongoing. NRG-BN001, a phase III randomized controlled trial (RCT) of IMRT versus intensity-modulated proton therapy, evaluates 60 Gy versus dose-escalation to 75 Gy with concurrent and adjuvant TMZ.[22] Although therapy for gliomas is evolving to include management primarily by molecular and histology features, prior clinical risk factors can be incorporated to assist in guiding management if needed. Recent publications regarding molecular classification are informing a moving neuro-oncology field. An outline describing options of management representing current practices at our institution is provided in **Table 1**. We anticipate there will be changes over the next few years as the field evolves, and acknowledge there are institutional variations in management.

Radiation Treatment Techniques for Gliomas

At simulation, patients are immobilized using an Aquaplast mask. Fusing the planning computed tomography (CT) scan with the T1 contrasted and T2-FLAIR pre-operative and postoperative high-resolution MRI scans should be used for target delineation. For LGG, the gross tumor volume (GTV) is defined as the surgical cavity with hyperintense signal on the T2-FLAIR sequence with a 1-cm clinical target volume (CTV1). Care must be taken to limit CTV expansions to anatomic boundaries of disease spread (eg, bones, falx, tentorium, and ventricles). Our intuition recommends postoperative MRI within 72 hours to 2 weeks of surgery and starting RT within 4 weeks of surgery for HGG provided the patient is well healed. A repeat MRI scan for treatment planning is encouraged if more than 3 weeks have passed from surgery to RT planning, consistent with current open protocols such as BN001.

For grade III gliomas and GBM, a cone-down technique or simultaneous-integrated boost (SIB) is used to dose escalate the center of the tumor bed. For anaplastic astrocytoma (AA), the GTV is the surgical cavity and any areas of residual T1 contrast enhancement (T1+C) and T2-FLAIR gross tumor abnormality with an expansion of 2 cm (or 1.5 cm) to form the CTV1, which is prescribed 50.4 Gy in 28 fx. For 2-cm CTV (CTV2), the GTV is expanded 1 cm and receives an additional 9 Gy in 5 fx for a total of 59.4 Gy in 33 fx with some similarity to RTOG 9402.[23] For nonenhancing AA, these may be treated to the entire FLAIR GTV with a 1.5-cm to 2-cm expansion to 59.4 Gy similar to CATNON.[14] The authors have adopted an SIB technique using 50 Gy in 1.67 Gy per fx to the low-risk CTV and 57 Gy in 1.9 Gy per fx to the high-risk boost CTV in a total of 30 fx as an alternative to the sequential cone-down boost technique at our institution.

For GBM, the RTOG describes the CTV1 with 2-cm expansion from a GTV that includes both T1+C and T2-FLAIR abnormality to 46 Gy in 23 fx. It is followed by a cone-down to the CTV2 with 2 cm expansion from GTV including primarily cavity and T1+C, which receives an additional 14 Gy for a total of 60 Gy. One alternative with tighter volumes for HGGs used at MD Anderson Cancer Center is shown in **Fig. 2**. It is an SIB technique in which the CTV (GTV + 2 cm) receives 50 Gy in 30 fx (at 1.66 Gy/fx) and the GTV (cavity plus residual contrast enhancement) receives 60 Gy in 30 fx (at 2 Gy/fx). The high-dose cone-down includes a direct expansion from GTV (cavity and T1+C) plus 3 to 5 mm planning tumor volume (PTV) to PTV60. The CTV50 Gy includes a 2-cm expansion from GTV cavity, which encompasses all FLAIR abnormality rather than an expansion from FLAIR abnormality. A PTV margin on CTV50 of 3 to 5 mm becomes PTV50 and allows smaller overall treatment volumes because of smaller expansions, and is a reasonable strategy, especially if dose constraints are not met with the larger expansion volumes. Similar volume expansions using a 1.5-cm CTV are used for AA at our institution.

MENINGIOMAS
Overview

Meningiomas are the most common primary brain tumors, with an estimated 25,000 to 30,000 cases seen per year in the United States, and comprising approximately 37% of CNS tumors.[1] Most of these tumors are low grade (~85%). There is an increased incidence for women relative to men (2:1), and the incidence peaks in the sixth to seventh decades of life.[24] The leading acquired risk factor for the development of meningioma is exposure to ionizing radiation.[25] The most common genetic alteration seen is mutation of the *NF2* tumor-suppressor gene on chromosome 22.[26] Although the median recurrence-free survival is 12.5 years for grade I meningiomas, for grade II it is less than 7 years and for grade III less than 2.5 years.[27] Although grade I meningiomas may be considered benign, it is of note that, for higher-grade meningiomas, the median OS for grade II

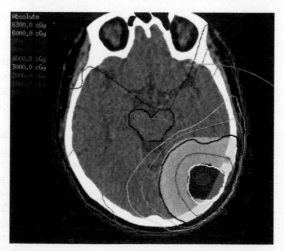

Fig. 2. RT isodose plan in axial view for glioblastoma. An SIB technique was used to dose escalate the GTV (*red*) with planning tumor volume (*blue*) to 60 Gy in 30 fractions, whereas the CTV (*tan*) received 50 Gy within the same number of fractions with PTV expansion (*aqua*). The 50-Gy isodose line is in blue, and the 60 Gy isodose line is in white.

meningiomas is less than 12 years and for anaplastic meningiomas is 4.7 years with a 5-year OS of 41%.[28]

Clinical Presentation

Meningiomas are commonly found incidentally on imaging with patients relatively asymptomatic at the time of diagnosis. With tumor progression, mass effect may cause local deficits, including seizures, weakness, or cognitive changes.

Diagnostic Evaluation and Imaging

On CT scan, an isodense extra-axial dural mass may be seen displacing normal brain tissue, and some show prominent calcification. On MRI, meningiomas can be contrast enhancing on T1+C and hyperintense on the T2 sequences. Classically meningiomas extend along the dura, which is seen as a co-called dural tail on the T1+C sequence. Most occur within the skull at the sites of dural reflection (falx, tentorium, venous sinuses), but they also present less commonly in the optic nerve sheath.

Grading Systems

Meningiomas are classified according to the WHO schema, which divides them into 3 groups based on mitotic activity: grade I, tumors with fewer than 4 mitoses per 10 high-powered fields (HPF), grade II show 4 or more mitoses per HPF, and grade III is defined as 20 or more mitoses per HPF.[5] The Simpson grading system is also used frequently for meningioma because it estimates risk of 10-year recurrence based on extent of surgical resection (Table 2).[29] Unlike gliomas, molecular information is not currently integrated into the risk stratification for meningiomas. However, recurrent mutations in the gene encoding the telomerase reverse-transcriptase enzyme (TERT) and methylation profiling have identified distinct classes of meningiomas that predict for increased risk of recurrence and prognosis compared with the WHO classification.[30,31] Another marker being explored in the current NRG-BN003 trial is histone H3 phosphorylated at serine 10 (pHH3), which has been found to be a strong mitotic marker for proliferation.[27] It is possible that these will inform future WHO classification schema for meningioma.

Table 2		
Simpson grading system for meningioma		
Grade	Description	10-y Recurrence (%)
1	GTR, including dural attachment and any abnormal bone	9
2	GTR, with coagulation instead of resection of dural attachment	19
3	GTR of meningioma without resection or coagulation of dural attachment	29
4	Subtotal resection	44
5	Tumor debulking or decompression only	NA

Abbreviation: NA, not available.

Data from Nanda A, Bir SC, Maiti TK, et al. Relevance of Simpson grading system and recurrence-free survival after surgery for World Health Organization Grade I meningioma. J Neurosurg 2017;126(1):201-211.

Management of Meningiomas

Meningiomas found incidentally can be observed serially with repeat MRI at 3, 6, and 12 months during the first year to monitor progression. Close to 70% remain stable because there is a much higher likelihood for these to be indolent, slow-growing grade I meningiomas compared with grade II or grade III. If meningiomas are progressive or are causing local symptoms because of mass effect, then maximal safe resection is the initial treatment of choice.

RTOG 0539, a phase II trial that risk stratified meningiomas based on pathologic grade and extent of resection, outlines options of postoperative management.[32] Low-risk tumors are pathologically grade I and grossly resected or subtotally resected. Intermediate-risk meningiomas are recurrent grade I tumors or any grade II after GTR. Higher-risk tumors are subtotally resected or recurrent grade II tumors as well as all grade III meningioma. Adjuvant RT dosing and expansions for conventional external beam radiation therapy are dictated by the risk stratification and are outlined in **Table 3**. On this trial, low-risk tumors were observed after surgical resection, intermediate-risk tumors were treated adjuvantly to 54 Gy, and high-risk tumors were treated to a maximal dose of 60 Gy. An interim analysis for patients treated on RTOG 0539 showed low-risk patients that were observed had a 3-year PFS of 92%. Intermediate-risk patients treated to 54 Gy had a 3-year PFS of 94%, significantly higher than historical control rates. High-risk patients treated to 60 Gy had a 3-year PFS of 59%. Although practice patterns favor observation for grade I meningioma in noneloquent locations and immediate adjuvant treatment to 60 Gy for grade III meningiomas, the role of adjutant radiation for grade II meningiomas remains variable. Thus,

Table 3			
Radiation treatment of meningioma per Radiation Therapy Oncology Group 0539			
Risk	**Definition**	**RT and Dose**	**CTV Expansions**
Low	Newly diagnosed WHO grade I, GTR or STR	Observe after resection	NA
Intermediate	Recurrent WHO grade I, GTR or STR Newly diagnosed WHO grade II, GTR	54 Gy in 30 fx	Tumor/resection cavity + 1 cm (CTV expansions vary by institution. Our institution uses 0.5 cm for intermediate risk along dura not extending into brain parenchyma unless there is brain invasion)
High	WHO grade III, GTR or STR Recurrent WHO grade II, GTR or STR Newly diagnosed WHO Grade II, STR	CTV1: 60 Gy in 30 fx CTV2: 54 Gy in 30 fx Alternatively: 50.4 Gy with CD to 59.4 Gy is used at some institutions Our institution uses SIB 60 Gy PTV1 and 50 Gy PTV2	CTV1: tumor/resection cavity + 1 cm CTV2: tumor/resection cavity + 2 cm Our institution uses the SIB with tight margins similar to GBM PTV1: GTV/T1c + 0.3 cm directly from GTV to PTV with daily KV PTV2: CTV 2 cm from T1c GTV + 0.3 cm with daily KV setup

Abbreviations: CD, cone-down; kv, kilovoltage.

presently NRG-BN003 is a randomized trial of grade II meningioma after GTR randomizing patients to adjuvant radiation to 59.4 Gy versus initial observation with a primary end point of PFS.[33]

Treatment with stereotactic radiosurgery (SRS) is also a viable option for low-grade meningiomas with sufficient distance from critical structures such as the optic apparatus. SRS is increasingly used for treating skull-based meningiomas not amenable to surgical resection.[34,35] Doses for Gamma Knife single fractions can range from 14 to 16 Gy, and at our institution 14 Gy is most commonly used with highly conformal planning. SRS provides greater than 90% actuarial local tumor control at 5 and 10 years for benign meningiomas of appropriate size.[36,37] SRS may also be indicated for recurrent meningiomas that have previously received fractionated RT as a salvage option that limits surrounding radiation dose and improves PFS.[38]

Management for fractionated RT by RTOG 0539 is shown in **Table 3**. Coverage of the dural tail is controversial. The dural tail is composed of hypervascular dura in many cases, and although microscopic clusters of meningioma cells may be found on sectioned pathology, it has also been noted that these may be identified in other parts of the dura. Overall, there has not been conclusive evidence for coverage of the dural tail.[39] In practice at our institution, although it is not overtly covered in SRS, for fractionated RT it tends to be within the CTV/PTV expansions. Our institution also reserves expansion into brain parenchyma primarily for high-risk meningiomas, grade III meningiomas, or grade II meningiomas with brain invasion.

BRAIN METASTASES
Overview

Brain metastases are the most common intracranial tumor, with approximately 200,000 cancer cases annually. Historically, the prognosis of patients after developing brain metastases was extremely poor, with a median survival of 1 month with observation, which was improved to 2 months with steroids. The median survival after whole-brain RT (WBRT) was estimated to be ~6 months.[40] The treatment of brain metastases has evolved considerably over the past decades with increased use of SRS, advanced surgical techniques, and novel targeted systemic therapy agents that have variable penetration of the blood-brain barrier (BBB).

Clinical Presentation

The most common histologies seen are lung, breast, and melanoma. Common presenting symptoms include headaches, nausea, vomiting, seizures, vision changes, and focal neurologic deficits.

Diagnostic Evaluation and Imaging

MRI with and without contrast is the standard imaging modality for evaluating brain metastases. For patients presenting to the emergency department with acute worsening neurologic deficits, a CT scan should be done first to rule out hemorrhage. Brain metastases present as ring-enhancing lesions on the T1+C MRI sequences, with surrounding vasogenic edema best seen on the T2-FLAIR sequence, and occur commonly in the grey-white matter junctions. Prognostic factors associated with survival include age, KPS score, cancer type and histology, and severity of the presenting symptoms. Recursive partitioning analysis from 3 RTOG brain metastases trials identified factors that predicted median survival and this was further expanded with the graded prognostic assessment.[41,42]

Management of Brain Metastases

The management of brain metastases is guided by numerous factors. If symptomatic at diagnosis, consider urgent treatment with steroids. Antiepileptic drugs (AEDs) are given only if patients are actively having seizures because a meta-analysis found no benefit for routine use of AEDs for seizure prophylaxis.[43]

If a lesion is symptomatic and large (>3 cm), surgical resection is the preferred treatment. If unresectable or if the patient is asymptomatic with a smaller lesion (or multiple lesions), then RT is the preferred treatment option. Following surgical resection, postoperative RT to the surgical cavity with SRS was compared with adjuvant WBRT in a large phase III multicenter RCT (NCCTG N107C/CEC.3).[44] Cognitive deterioration–free survival was improved in the SRS arm (HR, 0.47; $P<.0001$) with equivalent median OS (12.2 months for SRS vs 11.6 moths for WBRT; $P = .70$). Another RCT conducted in patients with 1 to 3 brain metastases confirmed improved local control with SRS compared with observation (72% vs 43% at 12 months; $P = .015$).[45] Based on these data, postoperative SRS has become the standard care for resection cavities in patients with limited intracranial disease burden. Studies to evaluate the role of preoperative SRS to decrease the risk of leptomeningeal disease and improve target delineation are being conducted, including a phase III randomized trial of preoperative versus postoperative SRS at authors' institution (NCT03741673).

Dosing for single-fraction SRS from RTOG 9005 was based on maximal tumor diameter: 24 Gy for tumors less than or equal to 2 cm, 18 Gy for tumors between 2 to 3 cm, and 15 Gy for tumors between 3 and 4 cm.[46] Importantly, this trial did not include resection cavities. Dosing by volume for all brain metastases as an extrapolation from N107C is used at some institutions rather than diameter. SRS can be delivered through any of several stereotactic techniques, including Gamma Knife radiosurgery, which uses conformal cobalt-60 sources, Cyberknife, or standard external beam linear accelerators with thin multileaf collimators with stereotactic technology. Typically, no CTV expansions are used, with PTV expansions varying depending on RT treatment modality (typically 0–2 mm).

WBRT remains standard of care for patients with numerous brain metastatic lesions (often at least 10). WBRT is commonly delivered using opposed lateral beams to a total dose of 30 to 35 Gy in 10 to 12 fx. Patients undergoing WBRT should be considered to receive memantine based on RTOG 0614, an RCT that showed improvement in time to cognitive failure in the WBRT plus memantine arm compared with the WBRT-only arm.[47] An IMRT-based WBRT technique may be used in select cases for avoidance of the hippocampus because of emerging data from a single-arm phase II study (RTOG 0933) that showed improved preservation of memory and cognitive function relative to historical control rates with conformal avoidance of the hippocampus.[48] The preliminary analysis of the phase III trial (NRG-CC001) evaluating neurocognitive toxicities and outcomes of WBRT plus memantine with or without hippocampal avoidance suggests similar neurocognitive benefits in abstract form.[49]

For patients presenting with 4 to 10 lesions or fewer than 4 but with a large cumulative intracranial tumor volume, the decision of WBRT versus SRS can be determined on a case-to-case basis. Discussion between the radiation oncologist, neurosurgeon, and medical oncologist is necessary, with a focus on treatment goals, expected outcomes, and disease burden. The JLGK0901 prospective observational study evaluated survival of patients with 2 to 4 versus 5 to 10 brain metastases with good performance status treated with SRS alone. The primary end point was OS and was similar between both groups (median 10.8 months for both), suggesting that SRS may be a viable treatment strategy for patients with 5 to 10 brain metastases with less severe cognitive side effects relative to WBRT.[50] Based on these data, it is reasonable to use SRS to treat patients with multiple brain lesions and good performance status, limited disease burden well controlled on systemic therapy, or radioresistant histologies such as melanoma and renal cell.

With the rapidly growing availability of targeted systemic therapies such as tyrosine kinase inhibitors and immune checkpoint inhibitors, many patients with metastatic disease to the brain are living longer. Although surgery and radiation were historically considered the only treatment options for brain metastases, newer-generation targeted and immunologic therapies such as epidermal growth factor receptor (EGFR), programmed death (PD), programmed death-ligand 1 (PD-L1) and BRAF inhibitors have shown increased penetration of the BBB. For example, a Japanese phase II study recently evaluated use of gefitinib alone in 41 patients with EGFR mutant lung adenocarcinoma and brain metastases, with an overall response rate of 86.8% and median OS of 21.9 months.[51] Additional agents, such as erlotinib and afatinib, are also being studied. These results have led to increasing delayed use of radiation for patients with brain metastases. However, a multiinstitutional retrospective analysis in patients with non–small cell lung cancer with EGFR mutation who developed brain metastases showed compromised survival when radiation, either WBRT or SRS, was delayed, bringing such change of practice into question. The OS at 2 years for upfront SRS, WBRT, and EGFR-TKI (tyrosine kinase inhibitor) groups was 78%, 62%, and 51% respectively. After controlling for significant demographic and clinical factors in a multivariable model, upfront SRS was independently associated with improved OS relative to EGFR-TKI.[52] A phase III study is needed to better delineate the timing of radiation. Similarly, nivolumab combined with ipilimumab or dabrafenib with or without trametinib have shown intracranial efficacy in melanoma[53,54] and is being considered in other histologies. In a study of 94 patients receiving nivolumab combined with ipilimumab with 14-month median follow-up, there was a 57% intracranial benefit with 26% complete response.[53] This finding has changed the paradigm for select patients with brain metastasis to allow systemic management with observation for patients with low intracranial brain metastases burden, thus reserving treatment with SRS to only progressive lesions. At this time, it is unclear how to identify patients who will or will not respond intracranially, and whether addition of SRS increases local control and distant brain control through abscopal effects.

As the role of systemic therapy continues to evolve, the role of radiation to both primary and metastatic brain lesions will also continue to evolve in the coming years. Trials assessing the efficacy of RT among differing molecular classes of CNS neoplasms will inform future treatment strategies. In addition, combining RT with systemic agents that penetrate the BBB, including agents that inhibit DNA repair and cell signaling pathways, along with immunotherapy may show potential for improving outcomes in these patients.

REFERENCES

1. Ostrom QT, Gittleman H, Truitt G, et al. CBTRUS statistical report: primary brain and other central nervous system tumors diagnosed in the United States in 2011-2015. Neuro Oncol 2018;20(suppl_4):iv1–86.
2. Chang SM, Parney IF, Huang W, et al. Patterns of care for adults with newly diagnosed malignant glioma. JAMA 2005;293(5):557–64.
3. Ruda R, Bello L, Duffau H, et al. Seizures in low-grade gliomas: natural history, pathogenesis, and outcome after treatments. Neuro Oncol 2012;14(Suppl 4): iv55–64.

4. Louis DN, Ohgaki H, Wiestler OD, et al. The 2007 WHO classification of tumours of the central nervous system. Acta Neuropathol 2007;114(2):97–109.
5. Louis DN, Perry A, Reifenberger G, et al. The 2016 World Health Organization classification of tumors of the central nervous system: a summary. Acta Neuropathol 2016;131(6):803–20.
6. Brown PD, Buckner JC, O'Fallon JR, et al. Effects of radiotherapy on cognitive function in patients with low-grade glioma measured by the folstein mini-mental state examination. J Clin Oncol 2003;21(13):2519–24.
7. Shaw E, Arusell R, Scheithauer B, et al. Prospective randomized trial of low-versus high-dose radiation therapy in adults with supratentorial low-grade glioma: initial report of a North Central Cancer Treatment Group/Radiation Therapy Oncology Group/Eastern Cooperative Oncology Group study. J Clin Oncol 2002; 20(9):2267–76.
8. van den Bent MJ, Afra D, de Witte O, et al. Long-term efficacy of early versus delayed radiotherapy for low-grade astrocytoma and oligodendroglioma in adults: the EORTC 22845 randomised trial. Lancet 2005;366(9490):985–90.
9. Shaw EG, Wang M, Coons SW, et al. Randomized trial of radiation therapy plus procarbazine, lomustine, and vincristine chemotherapy for supratentorial adult low-grade glioma: initial results of RTOG 9802. J Clin Oncol 2012;30(25): 3065–70.
10. Buckner JC, Shaw EG, Pugh SL, et al. Radiation plus procarbazine, CCNU, and vincristine in low-grade glioma. N Engl J Med 2016;374(14):1344–55.
11. Fisher BJ, Hu C, Macdonald DR, et al. Phase 2 study of temozolomide-based chemoradiation therapy for high-risk low-grade gliomas: preliminary results of Radiation Therapy Oncology Group 0424. Int J Radiat Oncol Biol Phys 2015;91(3): 497–504.
12. Pignatti F, van den Bent M, Curran D, et al. Prognostic factors for survival in adult patients with cerebral low-grade glioma. J Clin Oncol 2002;20(8):2076–84.
13. van den Bent MJ, Brandes AA, Taphoorn MJ, et al. Adjuvant procarbazine, lomustine, and vincristine chemotherapy in newly diagnosed anaplastic oligodendroglioma: long-term follow-up of EORTC brain tumor group study 26951. J Clin Oncol 2013;31(3):344–50.
14. van den Bent MJ, Baumert B, Erridge SC, et al. Interim results from the CATNON trial (EORTC study 26053-22054) of treatment with concurrent and adjuvant temozolomide for 1p/19q non-co-deleted anaplastic glioma: a phase 3, randomised, open-label intergroup study. Lancet 2017;390(10103):1645–53.
15. Stupp R, Hegi ME, Mason WP, et al. Effects of radiotherapy with concomitant and adjuvant temozolomide versus radiotherapy alone on survival in glioblastoma in a randomised phase III study: 5-year analysis of the EORTC-NCIC trial. Lancet Oncol 2009;10(5):459–66.
16. Stupp R, Taillibert S, Kanner A, et al. Effect of tumor-treating fields plus maintenance temozolomide vs maintenance temozolomide alone on survival in patients with glioblastoma: a randomized clinical trial. JAMA 2017;318(23):2306–16.
17. NCCN. National Comprehensive cancer Network clinical practice guidelines in oncology: central nervous system cancers. 2016; Version 1. 2016. Available at: https://www.nccn.org/professionals/physician_gls/PDF/cns.pdf. Accessed October 29, 2016.
18. Roa W, Brasher PM, Bauman G, et al. Abbreviated course of radiation therapy in older patients with glioblastoma multiforme: a prospective randomized clinical trial. J Clin Oncol 2004;22(9):1583–8.

19. Roa W, Kepka L, Kumar N, et al. International atomic energy agency randomized phase III study of radiation therapy in elderly and/or frail patients with newly diagnosed glioblastoma multiforme. J Clin Oncol 2015;33(35):4145–50.

20. ClinicalTrials.gov. NRG BN005 A Phase II Randomized Trial of Proton Vs. Photon Therapy (IMRT) for Cognitive Preservation in Patients With IDH Mutant, Low to Intermediate Grade Gliomas. 2018. Available at: https://clinicaltrials.gov/ct2/show/NCT03180502. Accessed September 12, 2018.

21. ClinicalTrials.gov. BN005: Proton Beam or Intensity-Modulated Radiation Therapy in Preserving Brain Function in Patients With IDH Mutant Grade II or III Glioma. 2019. Available at: https://clinicaltrials.gov/ct2/show/NCT03180502. Accessed April 30, 2019.

22. ClinicalTrials.gov. BN001: dose-Escalated Photon IMRT or proton beam radiation therapy versus standard-dose radiation therapy and temozolomide in treating patients with newly diagnosed glioblastoma. 2019. Available at: https://clinicaltrials.gov/ct2/show/study/NCT02179086?show_desc=Y#desc. Accessed April 30, 2019.

23. Cairncross G, Wang M, Shaw E, et al. Phase III trial of chemoradiotherapy for anaplastic oligodendroglioma: long-term results of RTOG 9402. J Clin Oncol 2013;31(3):337–43.

24. Claus EB, Bondy ML, Schildkraut JM, et al. Epidemiology of intracranial meningioma. Neurosurgery 2005;57(6):1088–95 [discussion: 1088–5].

25. Braganza MZ, Kitahara CM, Berrington de Gonzalez A, et al. Ionizing radiation and the risk of brain and central nervous system tumors: a systematic review. Neuro Oncol 2012;14(11):1316–24.

26. Abedalthagafi M, Bi WL, Aizer AA, et al. Oncogenic PI3K mutations are as common as AKT1 and SMO mutations in meningioma. Neuro Oncol 2016;18(5): 649–55.

27. Olar A, Wani KM, Sulman EP, et al. Mitotic index is an independent predictor of recurrence-free survival in meningioma. Brain Pathol 2015;25(3):266–75.

28. Orton A, Frandsen J, Jensen R, et al. Anaplastic meningioma: an analysis of the National Cancer Database from 2004 to 2012. J Neurosurg 2018;128(6):1684–9.

29. Nanda A, Bir SC, Maiti TK, et al. Relevance of Simpson grading system and recurrence-free survival after surgery for World Health Organization Grade I meningioma. J Neurosurg 2017;126(1):201–11.

30. Sahm F, Schrimpf D, Olar A, et al. TERT promoter mutations and risk of recurrence in meningioma. J Natl Cancer Inst 2016;108(5). djv377.

31. Sahm F, Schrimpf D, Stichel D, et al. DNA methylation-based classification and grading system for meningioma: a multicentre, retrospective analysis. Lancet Oncol 2017;18(5):682–94.

32. Rogers L, Zhang P, Vogelbaum MA, et al. Intermediate-risk meningioma: initial outcomes from NRG Oncology RTOG 0539. J Neurosurg 2018;129(1):35–47.

33. ClinicalTrials.gov. BN003: observation or radiation therapy in treating patients with newly diagnosed grade II meningioma that has been completely removed by surgery. 2019. Available at: https://clinicaltrials.gov/ct2/show/NCT03180268. Accessed April 30, 2019.

34. Lee JY, Niranjan A, McInerney J, et al. Stereotactic radiosurgery providing long-term tumor control of cavernous sinus meningiomas. J Neurosurg 2002;97(1): 65–72.

35. Nicolato A, Foroni R, Alessandrini F, et al. Radiosurgical treatment of cavernous sinus meningiomas: experience with 122 treated patients. Neurosurgery 2002; 51(5):1153–9 [discussion: 1159–1].

36. Kondziolka D, Flickinger JC, Perez B. Judicious resection and/or radiosurgery for parasagittal meningiomas: outcomes from a multicenter review. Gamma Knife Meningioma Study Group. Neurosurgery 1998;43(3):405–13 [discussion: 413–4].

37. Pollock BE, Stafford SL, Link MJ, et al. Single-fraction radiosurgery for presumed intracranial meningiomas: efficacy and complications from a 22-year experience. Int J Radiat Oncol Biol Phys 2012;83(5):1414–8.

38. Wojcieszynski AP, Ohri N, Andrews DW, et al. Reirradiation of recurrent meningioma. J Clin Neurosci 2012;19(9):1261–4.

39. Rogers L, Jensen R, Perry A. Chasing your dural tail: Factors predicting local tumor control after gamma knife stereotactic radiosurgery for benign intracranial meningiomas: In regard to DiBiase et al. (Int J Radiat Oncol Biol Phys 2004;60:1515-1519). Int J Radiat Oncol Biol Phys 2005;62(2):616–8 [author reply: 618–9].

40. Borgelt B, Gelber R, Kramer S, et al. The palliation of brain metastases: final results of the first two studies by the Radiation Therapy Oncology Group. Int J Radiat Oncol Biol Phys 1980;6(1):1–9.

41. Gaspar L, Scott C, Rotman M, et al. Recursive partitioning analysis (RPA) of prognostic factors in three Radiation Therapy Oncology Group (RTOG) brain metastases trials. Int J Radiat Oncol Biol Phys 1997;37(4):745–51.

42. Sperduto PW, Kased N, Roberge D, et al. Summary report on the graded prognostic assessment: an accurate and facile diagnosis-specific tool to estimate survival for patients with brain metastases. J Clin Oncol 2012;30(4):419–25.

43. Sirven JI, Wingerchuk DM, Drazkowski JF, et al. Seizure prophylaxis in patients with brain tumors: a meta-analysis. Mayo Clin Proc 2004;79(12):1489–94.

44. Brown PD, Ballman KV, Cerhan JH, et al. Postoperative stereotactic radiosurgery compared with whole brain radiotherapy for resected metastatic brain disease (NCCTG N107C/CEC.3): a multicentre, randomised, controlled, phase 3 trial. Lancet Oncol 2017;18(8):1049–60.

45. Mahajan A, Ahmed S, McAleer MF, et al. Post-operative stereotactic radiosurgery versus observation for completely resected brain metastases: a single-centre, randomised, controlled, phase 3 trial. Lancet Oncol 2017;18(8):1040–8.

46. Shaw E, Scott C, Souhami L, et al. Single dose radiosurgical treatment of recurrent previously irradiated primary brain tumors and brain metastases: final report of RTOG protocol 90-05. Int J Radiat Oncol Biol Phys 2000;47(2):291–8.

47. Brown PD, Pugh S, Laack NN, et al. Memantine for the prevention of cognitive dysfunction in patients receiving whole-brain radiotherapy: a randomized, double-blind, placebo-controlled trial. Neuro Oncol 2013;15(10):1429–37.

48. Gondi V, Pugh SL, Tome WA, et al. Preservation of memory with conformal avoidance of the hippocampal neural stem-cell compartment during whole-brain radiotherapy for brain metastases (RTOG 0933): a phase II multi-institutional trial. J Clin Oncol 2014;32(34):3810–6.

49. Gondi V, Deshmukh S, Brown PD, et al. Preservation of neurocognitive function (NCF) with conformal avoidance of the hippocampus during whole-brain radiotherapy (HA-WBRT) for brain metastases: preliminary results of phase III trial NRG oncology CC001. Int J Radiat Oncol Biol Phys 2018;102(5):1607.

50. Yamamoto M, Serizawa T, Shuto T, et al. Stereotactic radiosurgery for patients with multiple brain metastases (JLGK0901): a multi-institutional prospective observational study. Lancet Oncol 2014;15(4):387–95.

51. Iuchi T, Shingyoji M, Sakaida T, et al. Phase II trial of gefitinib alone without radiation therapy for Japanese patients with brain metastases from EGFR-mutant lung adenocarcinoma. Lung Cancer 2013;82(2):282–7.

52. Magnuson WJ, Lester-Coll NH, Wu AJ, et al. Management of brain metastases in tyrosine kinase inhibitor-naive epidermal growth factor receptor-mutant non-small-cell lung cancer: a retrospective multi-institutional analysis. J Clin Oncol 2017;35(10):1070–7.
53. Tawbi HA, Forsyth PA, Algazi A, et al. Combined nivolumab and ipilimumab in melanoma metastatic to the brain. N Engl J Med 2018;379(8):722–30.
54. Davies MA, Saiag P, Robert C, et al. Dabrafenib plus trametinib in patients with BRAF(V600)-mutant melanoma brain metastases (COMBI-MB): a multicentre, multicohort, open-label, phase 2 trial. Lancet Oncol 2017;18(7):863–73.

Novel Radiotherapy Technologies in the Treatment of Gastrointestinal Malignancies

Shraddha Mahesh Dalwadi, MD, MBA[a],
Joseph M. Herman, MD, MSc, MSHCM[b], Prajnan Das, MD, MS, MPH[b],
Emma B. Holliday, MD[b],*

KEYWORDS

- Radiotherapy • Image guidance • SBRT • Proton therapy

KEY POINTS

- Radiation therapy is playing an increasing role in the treatment of gastrointestinal malignancies.
- This paradigm shift was paved by improvements in target delineation, immobilization, treatment planning, and image-guided treatment delivery.
- Modern techniques are better able to localize individual at-risk volumes and thereby avoid unnecessary dose to normal tissue in gastrointestinal malignancy.

INTRODUCTION

Historically, radiation therapy has been relegated to the palliative, preoperative or postoperative settings in the treatment of gastrointestinal (GI) malignancies. This is largely because of the inherent radiosensitivity of the GI organs, which makes curative doses unachievable without unacceptable risk of serious normal tissue toxicity. However, in the past 2 decades, advances have made it possible to deliver a higher dose to select high-risk volumes. This paradigm shift was paved by improvements in target

Disclosure Statement: Dr J.M. Herman has received research funding from Oncosil, Galera, and Augmenix. He has acted as a scientific advisor for Boston Scientific Corp., Bristol-Myers-Squibb, Astra-Zeneca, Medtronic, and Augmenix. Dr P. Das has received an honorarium from Adlai Nortye. Dr E.B. Holliday receives research support from Merck unrelated to the article. The rest of the authors have no relevant financial or commercial disclosures.
[a] Department of Radiation Oncology, Baylor College of Medicine, 1 Baylor Plaza, Houston, TX 77004, USA; [b] Department of Radiation Oncology, MD Anderson Cancer Center, 1515 Holcombe Boulevard, Unit 1422, Houston, TX 77030, USA
* Corresponding author.
E-mail address: ebholliday@mdanderson.org

Hematol Oncol Clin N Am 34 (2020) 29–43
https://doi.org/10.1016/j.hoc.2019.08.016
0889-8588/20/© 2019 Elsevier Inc. All rights reserved.

delineation, immobilization, and image guidance and treatment delivery, such as intensity-modulated radiation therapy (IMRT), stereotactic body radiotherapy (SBRT), and proton therapy.

ESOPHAGEAL AND GASTRIC CANCERS
Esophageal Cancer

Radiation therapy for esophageal cancer is most commonly administered in the preoperative setting as a component of combined modality therapy. The CROSS trial showed carboplatin and paclitaxel-based chemoradiation (CRT) to a total dose of 41.4 Gy in 23 fractions improved overall survival (OS) and disease-free survival (DFS) compared with surgery alone.[1] Given that pathologic complete response (pCR) rates for patients on the CROSS trial were 49% for squamous cell carcinoma and 23% for adenocarcinoma, definitive CRT is an option for patients who either refuse surgery or who have tumors in the cervical esophagus where surgery would be especially morbid. Dose escalation is not typically recommended above 50.4 Gy in standard 1.8 to 2.0-Gy fractions based on results of INT-0123, which showed no difference in locoregional failure or OS between 50.4 Gy and 64.8 Gy.[2] However, National Comprehensive Cancer Network (NCCN) guidelines state doses higher than 50.4 Gy may be appropriate for tumors in the cervical esophagus, particularly if no subsequent surgery is planned.[3]

Gastric Cancer

Postoperative radiotherapy for gastric cancer was the standard of care based on the Intergroup 0116 study showing the survival benefit of adjuvant fluorouracil-based CRT to 45 Gy in 25 fractions compared with surgery alone.[4] However, most patients treated in Western countries are now more likely to receive perioperative chemotherapy based on the MAGIC trial results.[5,6] The CRITICS study showed no survival benefit to CRT given after adequate preoperative chemotherapy and at least a D1 nodal dissection.[7] In Eastern countries, the practice is to routinely perform a more extensive (D2) nodal dissection, and chemotherapy is the preferred adjuvant treatment.[8] The ARTIST study showed no benefit to adding adjuvant CRT to adjuvant chemotherapy.[9] ARTIST II recently reported no survival advantage for a higher-risk population of patients with positive lymph nodes at the time of surgery.[10] Toxicity limits completion rates for both CRT and chemotherapy given in the postoperative setting.[4,8] The CRITICS II study aims to ascertain the optimal preoperative treatment: chemotherapy, chemotherapy followed by CRT, or CRT.[11]

Novel Technologies for Esophagogastric Cancers

Esophagogastric tumors can move substantially during the respiratory cycle due to their proximity to the diaphragm. There are several ways to quantify and plan for internal motion due to respiration. So-called "4-dimensional computed tomography (CT)-simulation" is the use of multiphase CT-simulation conducted throughout the different points in the respiratory cycle and allows for more accurate expansion of target volumes to account for demonstrated patient-specific respiratory motion.[12] Depending on the planning target volumes used, kilovoltage (KV) imaging may be sufficient for daily alignment to bony landmarks. However, cone-beam CT (CBCT) can be used to align to soft tissue targets as well.

With regard to treatment delivery, IMRT has been widely adopted for the treatment of upper GI tract malignancies. Although doses used to treat gastric and esophageal cancers are relatively low in the perioperative setting, retrospective data suggest that

IMRT may minimize cardiotoxicity risk.[13,14] Consensus guidelines have been developed for the safe and effective use of IMRT in esophageal and gastric malignancies.[15] There is ongoing study of proton therapy in the upper abdomen. The rationales for proton therapy include escalating dose for definitive CRT and reducing postoperative cardiopulmonary toxicities for preoperative CRT. One study of passive scatter proton therapy for esophageal cancer at MD Anderson showed high rates of local control with very few severe toxicities using 50.4-Gy equivalents (GyE).[16] Intensity-modulated proton therapy (IMPT) has the potential to further decrease dose to organs at risk (OARs)[17] and is associated with decreased rates of lymphopenia as well as lower rates of postoperative cardiopulmonary complications when given preoperatively (Fig. 1).[18,19] A retrospective review at the University of Tsukuba and 2 case reports substantiate similar safety and efficacy in the definitive setting for esophageal and gastric cancers.[20,21] However, a randomized multicenter study will be necessary to examine longer-term toxicity benefits, survival, and cost-effectiveness over photon IMRT.

PANCREATIC AND HEPATOBILIARY CANCERS
Pancreatic Cancer

Surgical resection is the mainstay of treatment for patients with resectable pancreatic cancer, but the median survival with surgery alone is only 20 months.[22] After oncologic resection with pancreaticoduodenectomy, systemic therapy has been shown to improve DFS,[23,24] but the use of postoperative CRT is controversial.[25,26] A randomized trial, RTOG 0848, is currently evaluating this.[27] Because of low completion rates of planned postoperative therapy, there is also a growing interest in preoperative treatment for resectable or borderline resectable disease.[28] The goals of preoperative CRT are to sterilize the tumor-vessel interface and increase the likelihood of a margin-negative resection.[29] The PREOPANC trial randomized patients with resectable or borderline resectable disease either to 36 Gy in 15 fractions with concurrent

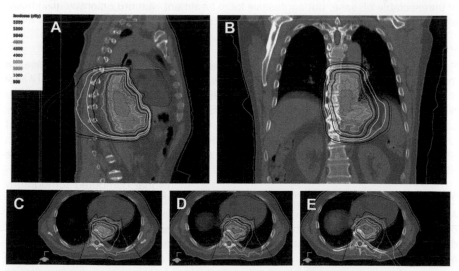

Fig. 1. Representative (A) sagittal, (B) coronal, and (C–E) axial images from an IMPT plan for a patient with esophageal adenocarcinoma. He received 50.4 Gy (Relative Biological Effectiveness) with concurrent chemotherapy in the preoperative setting. This plan shows sharp dose fall-off and sparing of cardiopulmonary organs-at-risk.

gemcitabine followed by surgery or to surgery alone. Postoperative chemotherapy was given in both arms.[30] Results presented in abstract form showed a higher 2-year OS rate (42% vs 30%) for those receiving preoperative CRT.[31] SBRT has emerged as an alternative to standard fractionated radiotherapy, although the NCCN currently recommends this be performed at a high-volume center, preferably in the context of a clinical trial.[32,33] Five fraction total doses of 25 to 33 Gy have been used with 4-dimensional planning and motion management (see later in this article). The role of definitive CRT for patients with unresectable, locally advanced disease is in question due to the lack of an OS benefit demonstrated in the LAP07 trial evaluating consolidative CRT given after 4 months of induction chemotherapy; however, CRT did result in improved local control.[34] As systemic therapy continues to improve, local progression may become a more pressing issue for patients with locally advanced disease, and local treatment modalities such as CRT or SBRT may have a bigger role to play.[35]

Primary Liver Tumors

Similar to pancreatic cancer, definitive surgical management is the only widely accepted curative option for patients with hepatocellular carcinoma (HCC),[36] but most patients are not eligible for resection or transplant at diagnosis.[37] NCCN guidelines list radiotherapy as a 2B category for locoregional therapy.[38] Ablation and arterially directed therapies are also listed as options for disease that is too advanced for surgical resection but still confined to the liver. Although prospective studies have shown local control rates of approximately 80% with standard fractionation radiotherapy,[39,40] it seems that dose matters, as studies have shown higher survival rates with a biologic equivalent dose (BED) greater than 75 Gy.[41] Intrahepatic cholangiocarcinoma is a less common primary liver malignancy with a worse overall prognosis and a higher propensity of distant metastases.[42] The mainstay of curative treatment is also surgical resection, with no conclusive data to guide adjuvant therapy recommendations.[43] Cisplatin and gemcitabine are most commonly recommended in the treatment of unresectable disease, but aggressive local treatment with radiotherapy has shown to be successful, particularly if a BED greater than 80 Gy is achieved.[44]

Liver Metastases

Recently, studies have shown that aggressive treatment of oligometastatic disease may be beneficial.[45] Specifically for patients with colorectal cancer, resection of liver metastases in combination with more effective chemotherapy has increased the median survival to 20 months and the 10-year OS to 20% to 25%.[46] However, as many patients are not surgical candidates, there has been growing interest in the use of radiotherapy in the treatment of liver metastases. Dose escalation, particularly with SBRT, is of particular interest given studies showing a correlation between higher BED prolonged survival.[47,48]

Novel Technologies for Pancreatic and Hepatobiliary Cancers

Advances in motion management and image guidance have opened the door for curative treatment approaches to pancreatic and hepatobiliary malignancies. Two validated strategies for the management of respiratory motion of pancreatic and hepatobiliary tumors include motion compensating and motion control. Motion compensating techniques (such as gating and tumor tracking) allow for free motion and only treat when motion is within certain parameters[49] (Fig. 2). Tumor gating involves the use of reflective markers mounted on the abdominal skin surface, which are, in turn, monitored using camera systems. Tumor tracking is a similar concept,

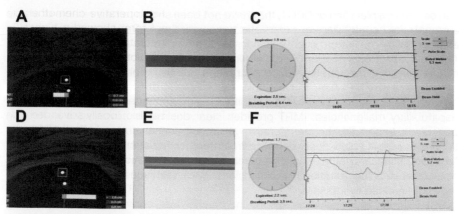

Fig. 2. (*A–C*) Patient during normal respiration. (*D–F*) The same patient performing a deep inspiratory breath hold. (*A* and *D*) The detector box positioned on the patient's abdomen. (*B* and *E*) The real-time visual feedback seen by the patient using a pair of goggles. The yellow line represents the breath and the blue bar represents the goal breath hold window. When the breath is held within the goal bar, the yellow line turns green. (*C* and *F*) The breath hold output on a monitor evaluated by radiation therapists, physicists, and physicians during stereotactic body radiotherapy treatments.

except with radiopaque markers placed intratumorally or paratumorally and monitored using fluoroscopic real-time imaging.[50] Motion control techniques such as abdominal compression and active breath control decrease internal motion.[51] Active breath control uses a feedback system in which the patient is able to monitor the variability of his or her breathing and thereby autoregulate.[52]

The advance of volumetric imaging such as with CBCT and CT on-rails helps to ensure accurate and reproducible alignment to the tumor itself. If the tumor target cannot be reliably visualized, radiopaque fiducial markers can be placed in or adjacent to the tumor target. Fiducials are commonly placed within liver or pancreatic tumors for this purpose (**Fig. 3**). Although patients may have existing bile duct stents that

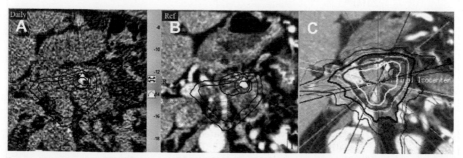

Fig. 3. (*A–C*) Representative axial images from a pancreatic stereotactic body radiation therapy plan for a patient with unresectable pancreatic adenocarcinoma. The radiopaque gold fiducials used for daily alignment can be seen. Fiducials were placed by interventional radiology under endoscopic ultrasound guidance. (*A*) Axial image from the CT-on-rails obtained daily before treatment. (*B*) Reference image from the plan. Daily alignment was performed using the fiducials, but shifts were made based on soft tissue anatomy if needed to avoid high dose in radiosensitive organs-at-risk because of daily anatomic variation in bowel gas or contents. (*C*) Plan isodose lines in full color.

can be seen on plain film or CBCT, they have not been shown to be a reliable or stable surrogate for hepatobiliary or pancreatic tumor position.[53] Daily volumetric imaging also can allow for interfraction changes so large as to require adaptive planning. Although most forms of adaptive radiotherapy use resimulation and replanning, techniques involving the real-time dose adaptation are being developed, especially in combination with MRI-based image guidance.[54]

Advances in treatment delivery have shifted the therapeutic ratio for pancreatic and hepatobiliary malignancies. IMRT provides clear dosimetric advantages in treating pancreatic tumors in the preoperative or postoperative setting.[55,56] In addition, IMRT has enabled high-dose, definitive treatment for hepatobiliary cancers, such as hepatocellular carcinoma, cholangiocarcinoma, and liver metastases, which were not possible using traditional 3-dimensional (3D) techniques due to the risk of radiation-induced liver disease.[57,58]

SBRT further decreases this risk by increasing dose conformality when treating pancreatic and hepatobiliary malignancies (**Table 1**). Successful implementation requires experienced physics support as well as robust motion management and image guidance strategies. Although data comparing efficacy of local therapies for hepatocellular cancer are limited, SBRT is one of many ablative therapies available for primary and secondary liver tumors (**Fig. 4**). For locally advanced pancreatic adenocarcinoma, SBRT after chemotherapy for locally advanced and borderline resectable tumors has yielded low rates of toxicity and encouraging rates of complete successful surgical resection.[59] Optimal dose constraints have yet to be established and prospective trials are ongoing.[33] Dose constraints

Table 1
Select studies of stereotactic body radiation therapy in gastrointestinal malignancy

Site	Author	Conclusion	Comments
Liver	Bujold (JCO, 2013)[85]	Pooled prospective I/II trial: 87% 1-y LC, 30% G3 toxicity	Tumor vascular thrombosis portends worse OS
	Sanuki (Acta Oncol, 2014)[86]	91% 3-y LC and 70% 3-y OS in a cohort of 277 pts	13% with G3 toxicity
	Yoon (PLoS One, 2013)[87]	92.1% LC and 53% OS at 3 y	Toxicity a concern, especially in higher-risk patients
Pancreas	Chang (Cancer, 2009)[88]	25 Gy/1fx with CyberKnife = good local control in unresectable cases	High duodenal toxicity (29%)
	Pollom (IJROBP, 2014)[89]	5fx SBRT LC = 1fx SBRT LC with reduced GI toxicity when fractionated	Heterogeneous cohort
	Mahadevan (IJROBP, 2011)[90]	Candidates for SBRT can be selected by response to induction chemotherapy	No disruption in systemic therapy
	Moningi et al,[59] 2015	SBRT after chemotherapy for locally advanced and unresectable pancreatic cancer has low rates of toxicity	Most patients achieved resection without radiographic response

Abbreviations: GI, gastrointestinal; OS, overall survival; SBRT, stereotactic body radiotherapy.

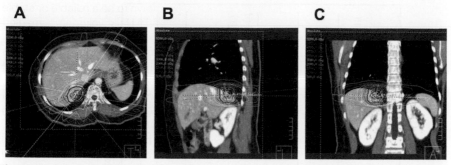

Fig. 4. Representative (A) axial, (B) sagittal, and (C) coronal images from a stereotactic body radiation therapy plan for a patient with a solitary liver lesion biopsy proven to be oligometastatic breast cancer. She received 50 Gy in 4 fractions using IMRT delivered using a deep inspiratory breath hold technique and daily CT-on-rails for image guidance. LC, local control; fx, fractions.

currently used for normal tissues at various dose/fractionation regimens are listed in **Table 2**.

Proton therapy allows for further normal liver sparing while treating hepatobiliary cancers. Investigators at the University of Tsukuba have published multiple studies substantiating safe and effective use of protons in hepatocellular cancer, with no reported cases of radiation-induced liver disease and very few reports of serious toxicity.[60] In the United States, Loma Linda conducted a phase II study of proton radiotherapy in the context of inoperable hepatocellular carcinoma and cirrhosis, and 33% of patients who ultimately underwent transplant had achieved pCR.[61] Other multi-institutional prospective phase II studies have shown comparable results, and a randomized trial for proton radiotherapy in hepatocellular cancer is currently under way under the NRG Oncology Cooperative Group.[62,63] For pancreatic cancer, Massachusetts General Hospital has published on the successful delivery of proton-based radiation therapy in the preoperative setting with excellent local control and survival rivaling that of currently published photon-based SBRT series.[64,65] Proton therapy has also been explored in the treatment of unresectable disease. Proton therapy using standard fractionation was associated with 69% 2-year freedom from local progression, no grade 2 or greater acute toxicity[66]; however, high toxicity rates in patients who received 67.5 GyE in 25 fractions with concurrent gemcitabine raise concerns regarding dose escalation.[67]

RECTAL AND ANAL CANCERS
Rectal Cancer

For patients with T3, T4, or node-positive rectal adenocarcinoma, the most common treatment in the United States is to administer neoadjuvant CRT to a total dose of 45.0 to 50.4 Gy in 25 to 28 fractions before total mesorectal surgical excision followed by adjuvant chemotherapy as per the German rectal cancer trial.[68] However, the latest version of the NCCN guidelines outlines additional options, including neoadjuvant chemotherapy before preoperative radiation in a total neoadjuvant therapy (TNT) approach as well as an alternative radiation schedule known as short course radiation (SCRT) (5 Gy × 5 fractions).[69] SCRT has been favored in Northern Europe for decades, with several randomized trials showing similar efficacy, toxicity, and postoperative complications when compared with standard long-course preoperative CRT.[70–72] Results from the RAPIDO study are much anticipated.[73] TNT has been shown to increase completion rates of chemotherapy and increase pCR rates.[74] Omission of

Table 2
Dose constraints for SBRT, standard fractionation and hypofractionation regimens for hepatobiliary tumors

Organ at Risk	Pancreas SBRT (5 fxns)	Pancreas Standard Fractionation (28 fxns)	Liver SBRT (5 fxns)	Liver Hypofractionation (15 fxns)
Stomach	V35 Gy <1 cc[a], Dmax <40 Gy[a]	Max ≤58 Gy[b], <10% receiving 50-56 Gy[b], <15% receiving 45-52 Gy[b]	D0.5 cc ≤30 Gy[c]	D0.5 cc ≤40 Gy[c]
Duodenum/Small bowel	V35 Gy <1 cc[a], Dmax <40 Gy[a]	Max ≤58 Gy[b], <10% receiving 50-56 Gy[b], <15% receiving 45-52 Gy[b]	D0.5 cc ≤30 Gy[c]	D0.5 cc ≤40 Gy[c]
Liver	V12 Gy <50%[a]	Mean <30 Gy[b]	Liver-GTV mean ≤13 Gy[c] (if 50 Gy prescription dose)	Liver-GTV mean ≤20.5 Gy[c] (if 67.5 Gy prescription dose)
Kidney	V12 Gy <25% (each)[a]	The equivalent of 1 functioning kidney should receive mean ≤18 Gy[b]	D33% <15 Gy, Mean <10 Gy (combined)[c]	V18 Gy <30% (combined), V10 Gy <60% (if only one functional kidney)
Spinal cord[a], spinal canal[b] or cord +5 mm[c]	V20 Gy <1 cc[a]	Max ≤50 Gy	D0.5 cc ≤25 Gy[c]	D0.5 cc ≤30 Gy[c]
Chest wall	N/A	N/A	D2 cc <35 Gy[c]	D2 cc <40 Gy[c]
Heart	N/A	N/A	D0.5 cc <20 Gy[c]	D0.5 cc <30 Gy[c]

Abbreviations: Dmax, the maximum dose; Dx ≤ y, the dose to x volume does not exceed y dose; fxs, fractions; Gy, Gray; SBRT, stereotactic body radiotherapy; N/A, not applicable; Vx ≤ y, the volume receiving x Gy does not exceed volume or percentage of the organ at risk.
[a] Alliance Trial A021501.
[b] RTOG 0484.
[c] NRG-GI003.

preoperative CRT,[75] as well as omission of surgery with a "watch and wait" approach after CRT[76] have been the topic of recent investigation, but are not yet considered standard of care off-trial at most US institutions.

Anal Cancer

The current standard of care for squamous cell carcinoma of the anal canal was solidified by RTOG 9811 and includes definitive CRT with 5-fluorouracil (5FU) and mitomycin-C (MMC).[77] However, subsequent studies have shown equivalent results with 5FU with cisplatin as concurrent treatment,[78] so that regimen is also used at some centers.[79] IMRT emerged as the new standard of care in the treatment of anal cancer when RTOG 0529 showed decreased grade 2 + hematologic and grade 3 + dermatologic toxicity.[80] Not much has changed in the treatment of anal cancer over the past 2 decades, but current and upcoming trials seek to better understand which early-stage patients for whom we may deescalate or omit CRT after local excision and which locally advanced patients may benefit from escalated therapy.[81]

Applications of New Technology in the Treatment of Anorectal Cancers

With regard to the use of IMRT in the lower GI tract, clinical practice is mixed. Many institutions still use IMRT sparingly in the treatment of rectal cancer, as the large target volumes overlapping with normal bowel mean its benefit over conventional techniques is often nominal. RTOG 0822 evaluated preoperative IMRT and failed to show decreased toxicity; however, this trial was difficult to evaluate, as concurrent oxaliplatin was used with the IMRT.[82] As such, many physicians treat standard preoperative fields with 3D conformal radiation. NCCN guidelines support this, recommending IMRT only in the setting of reirradiation or "highly unique anatomic situations."[69] In contrast, IMRT is the clear standard of care for patients with anal squamous cell carcinoma. RTOG 0529 established IMRT as standard of care for anal cancer after showing a reduction in hematologic, GI, and dermatologic toxicity when compared with historic controls.[80] However, data from this study illustrate how IMRT delivery requires expertise and particular attention to target volumes to avoid marginal misses; 81% of patients treated on RTOG 0529 required replanning on central review, most notably because of inconsistencies in delineating elective nodal volumes. Similarly, proton beam therapy has shown mixed success in the treatment of recurrent rectal cancer, where previous irradiation limits the ability to treat recurrence safety with photon-based radiation alone. Of 7 patients treated at the University of Pennsylvania, only 1 achieved complete response with high rates of significant toxicity.[83] Ongoing trials are investigating the use of proton beam therapy in anal cancer.[84]

SUMMARY

Recent advances in radiation therapy planning and delivery have served to improve the therapeutic ratio for patients with GI malignancies. Advances in imaging, motion management, and image guidance have allowed for tighter margins and smaller target volumes with less exposure to nontarget normal tissues. More conformal techniques, such as SBRT and proton therapy can allow for a more favorable dose distribution. Undoubtedly, these advances have expanded the role of radiation in the treatment of gastroesophageal, pancreatic, hepatobiliary, and anorectal cancers. With the potential for safer dose escalation with reduced toxicities, the indications are likely to continue to increase.

REFERENCES

1. Shapiro J, van Lanschot JJB, Hulshof MCCM, et al. Neoadjuvant chemoradiotherapy plus surgery versus surgery alone for oesophageal or junctional cancer (CROSS): long-term results of a randomised controlled trial. Lancet Oncol 2015;16(9):1090–8.
2. Minsky BD, Pajak TF, Ginsberg RJ, et al. INT 0123 (Radiation Therapy Oncology Group 94-05) phase III trial of combined-modality therapy for esophageal cancer: high-dose versus standard-dose radiation therapy. J Clin Oncol 2002;20(5): 1167–74.
3. NCCN. National Comprehensive Cancer Network Guidelines Version 1.2019 Esophageal and Esophagogastric Junction Cancers. National Comprehensive Cancer Network. Available at: https://www.nccn.org/professionals/physician_gls/pdf/esophageal.pdf. Accessed May 22, 2019.
4. Macdonald JS, Smalley SR, Benedetti J, et al. Chemoradiotherapy after surgery compared with surgery alone for adenocarcinoma of the stomach or gastroesophageal junction. N Engl J Med 2001;345(10):725–30.
5. Cunningham D, Allum WH, Stenning SP, et al. Perioperative chemotherapy versus surgery alone for resectable gastroesophageal cancer. N Engl J Med 2006; 355(1):11–20.
6. Al-Batran S-E, Homann N, Pauligk C, et al. Perioperative chemotherapy with fluorouracil plus leucovorin, oxaliplatin, and docetaxel versus fluorouracil or capecitabine plus cisplatin and epirubicin for locally advanced, resectable gastric or gastro-oesophageal junction adenocarcinoma (FLOT4): a randomised, phase 2/3 trial. Lancet 2019;393(10184):1948–57.
7. Cats A, Jansen EPM, van Grieken NCT, et al. Chemotherapy versus chemoradiotherapy after surgery and preoperative chemotherapy for resectable gastric cancer (CRITICS): an international, open-label, randomised phase 3 trial. Lancet Oncol 2018;19(5):616–28.
8. Bang Y-J, Kim Y-W, Yang H-K, et al. Adjuvant capecitabine and oxaliplatin for gastric cancer after D2 gastrectomy (CLASSIC): a phase 3 open-label, randomised controlled trial. Lancet 2012;379(9813):315–21.
9. Lee J, Lim DH, Kim S, et al. Phase III trial comparing capecitabine plus cisplatin versus capecitabine plus cisplatin with concurrent capecitabine radiotherapy in completely resected gastric cancer with D2 lymph node dissection: the ARTIST trial. J Clin Oncol 2012;30(3):268–73.
10. Park SH, Zang DY, Han B, et al. ARTIST 2: Interim results of a phase III trial involving adjuvant chemotherapy and/or chemoradiotherapy after D2-gastrectomy in stage II/III gastric cancer (GC). J Clin Oncol 2019;37(suppl) [abstract 4001].
11. Slagter AE, Jansen EPM, van Laarhoven HWM, et al. CRITICS-II: a multicentre randomised phase II trial of neo-adjuvant chemotherapy followed by surgery versus neo-adjuvant chemotherapy and subsequent chemoradiotherapy followed by surgery versus neo-adjuvant chemoradiotherapy followed by surgery in resectable gastric cancer. BMC Cancer 2018;18(1):877.
12. Kwong Y, Mel AO, Wheeler G, et al. Four-dimensional computed tomography (4DCT): A review of the current status and applications. J Med Imaging Radiat Oncol 2015;59(5):545–54.
13. Lin SH, Wang L, Myles B, et al. Propensity score-based comparison of long-term outcomes with 3-dimensional conformal radiotherapy vs intensity-modulated

radiotherapy for esophageal cancer. Int J Radiat Oncol Biol Phys 2012;84(5): 1078–85.

14. Chakravarty T, Crane CH, Ajani JA, et al. Intensity-modulated radiation therapy with concurrent chemotherapy as preoperative treatment for localized gastric adenocarcinoma. Int J Radiat Oncol Biol Phys 2012;83(2):581–6.

15. Wu AJ, Bosch WR, Chang DT, et al. Expert consensus contouring guidelines for intensity modulated radiation therapy in esophageal and gastroesophageal junction cancer. Int J Radiat Oncol Biol Phys 2015;92(4):911–20.

16. Lin SH, Komaki R, Liao Z, et al. Proton beam therapy and concurrent chemotherapy for esophageal cancer. Int J Radiat Oncol Biol Phys 2012;83(3):e345–51.

17. Prayongrat A, Xu C, Li H, et al. Clinical outcomes of intensity modulated proton therapy and concurrent chemotherapy in esophageal carcinoma: a single institutional experience. Adv Radiat Oncol 2017;2(3):301–7.

18. Lin SH, Merrell KW, Shen J, et al. Multi-institutional analysis of radiation modality use and postoperative outcomes of neoadjuvant chemoradiation for esophageal cancer. Radiother Oncol 2017;123(3):376–81.

19. Fang P, Shiraishi Y, Verma V, et al. Lymphocyte-sparing effect of proton therapy in patients with esophageal cancer treated with definitive chemoradiation. Int J Part Ther 2018;4(3):23–32.

20. Koyama S, Kawanishi N, Fukutomi H, et al. Advanced carcinoma of the stomach treated with definitive proton therapy. Am J Gastroenterol 1990;85(4):443–7.

21. Shibuya S, Takase Y, Aoyagi H, et al. Definitive proton beam radiation therapy for inoperable gastric cancer: a report of two cases. Radiat Med 1991;9(1):35–40.

22. Sohn TA, Yeo CJ, Cameron JL, et al. Resected adenocarcinoma of the pancreas—616 patients: results, outcomes, and prognostic indicators. J Gastrointest Surg 2000;4(6):567–79.

23. Oettle H, Post S, Neuhaus P, et al. Adjuvant chemotherapy with gemcitabine vs observation in patients undergoing curative-intent resection of pancreatic cancer: a randomized controlled trial. JAMA 2007;297(3):267–77.

24. Neoptolemos JP, Stocken DD, Bassi C, et al. Adjuvant chemotherapy with fluorouracil plus folinic acid vs gemcitabine following pancreatic cancer resection: a randomized controlled trial. JAMA 2010;304(10):1073–81.

25. Neoptolemos JP, Dunn JA, Stocken DD, et al. Adjuvant chemoradiotherapy and chemotherapy in resectable pancreatic cancer: a randomised controlled trial. Lancet 2001;358(9293):1576–85.

26. Abrams RA, Lillemoe KD, Piantadosi S. Continuing controversy over adjuvant therapy of pancreatic cancer. Lancet 2001;358(9293):1565–6.

27. Radiation Therapy Oncology Group. RTOG 0848 Protocol Information. Available at: https://www.rtog.org/ClinicalTrials/ProtocolTable/StudyDetails.aspx?study=0848. Accessed May 28, 2019.

28. Katz MHG, Shi Q, Ahmad SA, et al. Preoperative modified FOLFIRINOX treatment followed by capecitabine-based chemoradiation for borderline resectable pancreatic cancer: Alliance for Clinical Trials in Oncology Trial A021101. JAMA Surg 2016;151(8):e161137.

29. Varadhachary GR, Wolff RA, Crane CH, et al. Preoperative gemcitabine and cisplatin followed by gemcitabine-based chemoradiation for resectable adenocarcinoma of the pancreatic head. J Clin Oncol 2008;26(21):3487–95.

30. Versteijne E, van Eijck CHJ, Punt CJA, et al. Preoperative radiochemotherapy versus immediate surgery for resectable and borderline resectable pancreatic cancer (PREOPANC trial): study protocol for a multicentre randomized controlled trial. Trials 2016;17(1):127.

31. Van Tienhoven G, Versteijne E, Suker M, et al. Preoperative chemoradiotherapy versus immediate surgery for resectable and borderline resectable pancreatic cancer (PREOPANC-1): A randomized, controlled, multicenter phase III trial. J Clin Oncol 2018;36(18_suppl):LBA4002.
32. NCCN. National Comprehensive Cancer Network guidelines version 2.2019 pancreatic adenocarcinoma. Available at: https://www.nccn.org/professionals/physician_gls/pdf/pancreatic.pdf. Accessed May 28, 2019.
33. Katz MHG, Ou F-S, Herman JM, et al. Alliance for clinical trials in oncology (ALLIANCE) trial A021501: preoperative extended chemotherapy vs. chemotherapy plus hypofractionated radiation therapy for borderline resectable adenocarcinoma of the head of the pancreas. BMC Cancer 2017;17(1):505.
34. Hammel P, Huguet F, van Laethem J-L, et al. Effect of chemoradiotherapy vs chemotherapy on survival in patients with locally advanced pancreatic cancer controlled after 4 months of gemcitabine with or without erlotinib: the LAP07 randomized clinical trial. JAMA 2016;315(17):1844–53.
35. Crane CH, Varadhachary GR, Yordy JS, et al. Phase II trial of cetuximab, gemcitabine, and oxaliplatin followed by chemoradiation with cetuximab for locally advanced (T4) pancreatic adenocarcinoma: correlation of Smad4(Dpc4) immunostaining with pattern of disease progression. J Clin Oncol 2011;29(22):3037–43.
36. Poon RT, Fan ST, Lo CM, et al. Improving survival results after resection of hepatocellular carcinoma: a prospective study of 377 patients over 10 years. Ann Surg 2001;234(1):63–70.
37. Bruix J, Llovet JM. Prognostic prediction and treatment strategy in hepatocellular carcinoma. Hepatology 2002;35(3):519–24.
38. NCCN. National Comprehensive Cancer Network Guidelines: Hepatobiliary Cancers Version 2.2019. Available at: https://www.nccn.org/professionals/physician_gls/pdf/hepatobiliary.pdf. Accessed May 28, 2019.
39. Mornex F, Girard N, Beziat C, et al. Feasibility and efficacy of high-dose three-dimensional-conformal radiotherapy in cirrhotic patients with small-size hepatocellular carcinoma non-eligible for curative therapies–mature results of the French Phase II RTF-1 trial. Int J Radiat Oncol Biol Phys 2006;66(4):1152–8.
40. Ben-Josef E, Normolle D, Ensminger WD, et al. Phase II trial of high-dose conformal radiation therapy with concurrent hepatic artery floxuridine for unresectable intrahepatic malignancies. J Clin Oncol 2005;23(34):8739–47.
41. Skinner HD, Sharp HJ, Kaseb AO, et al. Radiation treatment outcomes for unresectable hepatocellular carcinoma. Acta Oncol 2011;50(8):1191–8.
42. Rahnemai-Azar AA, Weisbrod A, Dillhoff M, et al. Intrahepatic cholangiocarcinoma: molecular markers for diagnosis and prognosis. Surg Oncol 2017;26(2):125–37.
43. Weber SM, Ribero D, O'Reilly EM, et al. Intrahepatic cholangiocarcinoma: expert consensus statement. HPB (Oxford) 2015;17(8):669–80.
44. Tao R, Krishnan S, Bhosale PR, et al. Ablative radiotherapy doses lead to a substantial prolongation of survival in patients with inoperable intrahepatic cholangiocarcinoma: a retrospective dose response analysis. J Clin Oncol 2016;34(3):219–26.
45. Gomez DR, Blumenschein GR, Lee JJ, et al. Local consolidative therapy versus maintenance therapy or observation for patients with oligometastatic non-small-cell lung cancer without progression after first-line systemic therapy: a multicentre, randomised, controlled, phase 2 study. Lancet Oncol 2016;17(12):1672–82.

46. Kopetz S, Chang GJ, Overman MJ, et al. Improved survival in metastatic colorectal cancer is associated with adoption of hepatic resection and improved chemotherapy. J Clin Oncol 2009;27(22):3677–83.

47. Hong TS, Wo JY, Borger DR, et al. Phase II study of proton-based stereotactic body radiation therapy for liver metastases: importance of tumor genotype. J Natl Cancer Inst 2017;109(9). https://doi.org/10.1093/jnci/djx031.

48. McPartlin A, Swaminath A, Wang R, et al. Long-term outcomes of phase 1 and 2 studies of SBRT for hepatic colorectal metastases. Int J Radiat Oncol Biol Phys 2017;99(2):388–95.

49. Wagman R, Yorke E, Ford E, et al. Respiratory gating for liver tumors: use in dose escalation. Int J Radiat Oncol Biol Phys 2003;55(3):659–68.

50. Shirato H, Shimizu S, Kitamura K, et al. Four-dimensional treatment planning and fluoroscopic real-time tumor tracking radiotherapy for moving tumor. Int J Radiat Oncol Biol Phys 2000;48(2):435–42.

51. Eccles CL, Dawson LA, Moseley JL, et al. Interfraction liver shape variability and impact on GTV position during liver stereotactic radiotherapy using abdominal compression. Int J Radiat Oncol Biol Phys 2011;80(3):938–46.

52. Eccles C, Brock KK, Bissonnette J-P, et al. Reproducibility of liver position using active breathing coordinator for liver cancer radiotherapy. Int J Radiat Oncol Biol Phys 2006;64(3):751–9.

53. van der Horst A, Lens E, Wognum S, et al. Limited role for biliary stent as surrogate fiducial marker in pancreatic cancer: stent and intratumoral fiducials compared. Int J Radiat Oncol Biol Phys 2014;89(3):641–8.

54. Rosenberg SA, Henke LE, Shaverdian N, et al. A multi-institutional experience of MR-guided liver stereotactic body radiation therapy. Adv Radiat Oncol 2019;4(1):142–9.

55. Yovino S, Poppe M, Jabbour S, et al. Intensity-modulated radiation therapy significantly improves acute gastrointestinal toxicity in pancreatic and ampullary cancers. Int J Radiat Oncol Biol Phys 2011;79(1):158–62.

56. Colbert LE, Moningi S, Chadha A, et al. Dose escalation with an IMRT technique in 15 to 28 fractions is better tolerated than standard doses of 3DCRT for LAPC. Adv Radiat Oncol 2017;2(3):403–15.

57. Goodman KA, Regine WF, Dawson LA, et al. Radiation Therapy Oncology Group consensus panel guidelines for the delineation of the clinical target volume in the postoperative treatment of pancreatic head cancer. Int J Radiat Oncol Biol Phys 2012;83(3):901–8.

58. Bae SH, Jang WI, Park HC. Intensity-modulated radiotherapy for hepatocellular carcinoma: dosimetric and clinical results. Oncotarget 2017;8(35):59965–76.

59. Moningi S, Dholakia AS, Raman SP, et al. The role of stereotactic body radiation therapy for pancreatic cancer: a single-institution experience. Ann Surg Oncol 2015;22(7):2352–8.

60. Nakayama H, Sugahara S, Tokita M, et al. Proton beam therapy for hepatocellular carcinoma: the University of Tsukuba experience. Cancer 2009;115(23):5499–506.

61. Bush DA, Kayali Z, Grove R, et al. The safety and efficacy of high-dose proton beam radiotherapy for hepatocellular carcinoma: a phase 2 prospective trial. Cancer 2011;117(13):3053–9.

62. Hong TS, Wo JY, Yeap BY, et al. Multi-institutional phase II study of high-dose hypofractionated proton beam therapy in patients with localized, unresectable hepatocellular carcinoma and intrahepatic cholangiocarcinoma. J Clin Oncol 2016;34(5):460–8.

63. NRG. Clinical Trials.Gov. National Radiotherapy Group (NRG) GI003. Available at: https://clinicaltrials.gov/ct2/show/NCT03186898. Accessed May 21, 2019.

64. Hong TS, Ryan DP, Blaszkowsky LS, et al. Phase I study of preoperative short-course chemoradiation with proton beam therapy and capecitabine for resectable pancreatic ductal adenocarcinoma of the head. Int J Radiat Oncol Biol Phys 2011;79(1):151–7.

65. Hong TS, Ryan DP, Borger DR, et al. A phase 1/2 and biomarker study of preoperative short course chemoradiation with proton beam therapy and capecitabine followed by early surgery for resectable pancreatic ductal adenocarcinoma. Int J Radiat Oncol Biol Phys 2014;89(4):830–8.

66. Nichols RC, George TJ, Zaiden RA, et al. Proton therapy with concomitant capecitabine for pancreatic and ampullary cancers is associated with a low incidence of gastrointestinal toxicity. Acta Oncol 2013;52(3):498–505.

67. Takatori K, Terashima K, Yoshida R, et al. Upper gastrointestinal complications associated with gemcitabine-concurrent proton radiotherapy for inoperable pancreatic cancer. J Gastroenterol 2014;49(6):1074–80.

68. Sauer R, Liersch T, Merkel S, et al. Preoperative versus postoperative chemoradiotherapy for locally advanced rectal cancer: results of the German CAO/ARO/AIO-94 randomized phase III trial after a median follow-up of 11 years. J Clin Oncol 2012;30(16):1926–33.

69. NCCN. National Comprehensive Cancer Network guidelines version 1.2019 rectal cancer. National Comprehensive Cancer Network. 2019. Available at: https://www.nccn.org/professionals/physician_gls/pdf/rectal.pdf. Accessed April 18, 2019.

70. Ngan SY, Burmeister B, Fisher RJ, et al. Randomized trial of short-course radiotherapy versus long-course chemoradiation comparing rates of local recurrence in patients with T3 rectal cancer: Trans-Tasman Radiation Oncology Group trial 01.04. J Clin Oncol 2012;30(31):3827–33.

71. Bujko K, Nowacki MP, Nasierowska-Guttmejer A, et al. Long-term results of a randomized trial comparing preoperative short-course radiotherapy with preoperative conventionally fractionated chemoradiation for rectal cancer. Br J Surg 2006;93(10):1215–23.

72. Erlandsson J, Holm T, Pettersson D, et al. Optimal fractionation of preoperative radiotherapy and timing to surgery for rectal cancer (Stockholm III): a multicentre, randomised, non-blinded, phase 3, non-inferiority trial. Lancet Oncol 2017;18(3):336–46.

73. Nilsson PJ, van Etten B, Hospers GAP, et al. Short-course radiotherapy followed by neo-adjuvant chemotherapy in locally advanced rectal cancer–the RAPIDO trial. BMC Cancer 2013;13:279.

74. Garcia-Aguilar J, Chow OS, Smith DD, et al. Effect of adding mFOLFOX6 after neoadjuvant chemoradiation in locally advanced rectal cancer: a multicentre, phase 2 trial. Lancet Oncol 2015;16(8):957–66.

75. Schrag D, Weiser MR, Goodman KA, et al. Neoadjuvant chemotherapy without routine use of radiation therapy for patients with locally advanced rectal cancer: a pilot trial. J Clin Oncol 2014;32(6):513–8.

76. van der Valk MJM, Hilling DE, Bastiaannet E, et al. Long-term outcomes of clinical complete responders after neoadjuvant treatment for rectal cancer in the International Watch & Wait Database (IWWD): an international multicentre registry study. Lancet 2018;391(10139):2537–45.

77. Ajani JA, Winter KA, Gunderson LL, et al. Fluorouracil, mitomycin, and radiotherapy vs fluorouracil, cisplatin, and radiotherapy for carcinoma of the anal canal: a randomized controlled trial. JAMA 2008;299(16):1914–21.
78. Glynne-Jones R, Kadalayil L, Meadows HM, et al. Tumour- and treatment-related colostomy rates following mitomycin C or cisplatin chemoradiation with or without maintenance chemotherapy in squamous cell carcinoma of the anus in the ACT II trial. Ann Oncol 2014;25(8):1616–22.
79. Eng C, Chang GJ, You YN, et al. Long-term results of weekly/daily cisplatin-based chemoradiation for locally advanced squamous cell carcinoma of the anal canal. Cancer 2013;119(21):3769–75.
80. Kachnic LA, Winter K, Myerson RJ, et al. RTOG 0529: a phase 2 evaluation of dose-painted intensity modulated radiation therapy in combination with 5-fluorouracil and mitomycin-C for the reduction of acute morbidity in carcinoma of the anal canal. Int J Radiat Oncol Biol Phys 2013;86(1):27–33.
81. PLATO. International Standard Randomised Controlled Trials Number (ISRCTN) Registry. PLATO—Personalising anal cancer radiotherapy dose. Available at: http://www.isrctn.com/ISRCTN88455282. Accessed May 21, 2019.
82. Hong TS, Moughan J, Garofalo MC, et al. NRG Oncology Radiation Therapy Oncology Group 0822: a phase 2 study of preoperative chemoradiation therapy using intensity modulated radiation therapy in combination with capecitabine and oxaliplatin for patients with locally advanced rectal cancer. Int J Radiat Oncol Biol Phys 2015;93(1):29–36.
83. Berman A, Both S, Sharkoski T. Proton reirradiation of recurrent rectal cancer: dosimetric comparison, toxicities, and preliminary outcomes. Int J Part Ther 2014;1:2–13.
84. Grandhi N, Mohiuddin J, Plastaras J. Outcomes of pencil beam scanning proton therapy for anal cancer: a single institution study. Int J Radiat Oncol Biol Phys 2019;103(5 supplement):E9.
85. Available at: https://ascopubs.org/doi/full/10.1200/jco.2012.44.1659.
86. Available at: https://www.tandfonline.com/doi/full/10.3109/0284186X.2013.820342.
87. Yoon SM, Lim YS, Park MJ, et al. Stereotactic body radiation therapy as an alternative treatment for small hepatocellular carcinoma. PLoS One 2013;8(11):e79854.
88. Available at: https://onlinelibrary.wiley.com/doi/full/10.1002/cncr.24059.
89. Available at: https://linkinghub.elsevier.com/retrieve/pii/S0360-3016(14)03457-9.
90. Available at: https://www.ncbi.nlm.nih.gov/pubmed/21658854.

Radiation Therapy for Prostate Cancer

Sophia C. Kamran, MD[a],*, Anthony V. D'Amico, MD, PhD[b]

KEYWORDS

- Localized prostate cancer • Radiation therapy • Brachytherapy
- Oligometastatic prostate cancer • Postprostatectomy adjuvant and salvage therapy
- Androgen deprivation therapy • Hypofractionation

KEY POINTS

- Men with very low-risk or low-risk prostate cancer (PC) should be considered for active surveillance; however, notable exceptions are discussed.
- Favorable intermediate-risk PC may be best treated with monotherapies, whereas unfavorable intermediate-risk PC may be best treated with high-dose radiation therapy (RT) + short-course androgen deprivation therapy (ADT) (4–6 months).
- High-risk PC should be treated with a multimodality approach. Radiotherapeutic treatment of the prostate in men with limited oligometastatic PC should be discussed.
- Indications for adjuvant postoperative radiation are pT3a, pT3b, and R1. Whether adjuvant is superior to salvage therapy is unknown. Salvage treatment includes RT + ADT.
- Given disparate results, predictive markers are needed to define the role of docetaxel in managing high-risk PC. Abiraterone may be indicated in N1M0 PC.

INTRODUCTION

There are estimated to be 174,650 new cases and 31,620 deaths from prostate cancer (PC) in 2019.[1] PC is the most common noncutaneous malignancy in men in the United States. Most PCs are now diagnosed while clinically localized because of the introduction and adoption of prostate-specific antigen (PSA) screening. Localized PC is treated based on risk group. Risk stratification is based on clinical staging by digital rectal examination (DRE), pretreatment PSA, Gleason score on biopsy, and the number of biopsy cores involved with cancer.[2,3]

Disclosure Statement: The authors have nothing to disclose.
[a] Department of Radiation Oncology, Massachusetts General Hospital, Harvard Medical School, 55 Fruit Street-Cox 3, Boston, MA 02114, USA; [b] Department of Radiation Oncology, Brigham and Women's Hospital/Dana-Farber Cancer Institute, Harvard Medical School, 75 Francis Street, ASB1 L2, Boston, MA 02215, USA
* Corresponding author.
E-mail address: skamran@partners.org
twitter: @sophia_kamran (S.C.K.)

Hematol Oncol Clin N Am 34 (2020) 45–69
https://doi.org/10.1016/j.hoc.2019.08.017
0889-8588/20/© 2019 Elsevier Inc. All rights reserved.

NEWLY DIAGNOSED NONMETASTATIC PROSTATE CANCER
Low-Risk Disease

Standard management approaches for very-low- to low-risk PC include active surveillance, radical prostatectomy (RP), and radiation (brachytherapy or external beam radiation therapy [EBRT]). In general, active surveillance is the preferred approach unless life expectancy is limited, in which case men are observed and only treated for symptomatic progression (ie, watchful waiting). In men with adverse histologic or high-risk gene expression profiles, definitive management may be offered given these men have a high risk for progression.[4,5]

Active surveillance

Active surveillance is the endorsed treatment for men with very-low- to low-risk PC because it allows for the postponement of therapy (and its associated side effects).[2,4,5] When screening is detected early, it may not become clinically significant during a patient's lifetime. Hence, for many men, low-risk PC may never require treatment or treatment can be postponed without losing the opportunity to cure.[6] The indolent nature of low-risk PC has been demonstrated in several studies. For example, autopsy studies performed on men who died without a known PC indicate that there is a high incidence of occult low-grade PC.[7] In the Prostate Cancer Prevention trial,[8] among men who received placebo (vs finasteride) and without an elevated PSA or abnormal DRE, 15% were found to have PC.

Active surveillance differs from watchful waiting in that it entails close follow-up, including PSA, DRE, and repeat prostate biopsy. Several practitioners also use multiparametric MRI (mpMRI) of the prostate gland during surveillance as well. There are no defined appropriate testing intervals. **Table 1** describes a suggested active surveillance schedule. Upstaging or upgrading reflected in the presence of a new nodule on DRE or grade 4 PC on repeat biopsy are triggers for treatment consideration. Watchful waiting is preferred for men with an estimated life expectancy less than 10 years. This watchful waiting involves monitoring the disease with the plan to deliver therapy for palliation if symptoms develop.

Evidence from several single-institution trials demonstrates the indolent clinical course from patients managed with active surveillance, as shown in **Table 2**.[9] The best evidence for active surveillance comes from the large, randomized Prostate Testing for Cancer and Treatment (ProtecT) trial conducted in the United Kingdom.[9] In the trial, 1643 patients were randomly assigned to either (1) active monitoring, (2) RP, or (3) EBRT (74 Gy/37 fractions) with neoadjuvant and concurrent androgen deprivation therapy (ADT) for 3 to 6 months. The active monitoring arm included PSA levels every 3 months for 1 year and every 6 to 12 months thereafter. The trigger to consider intervention was driven by PSA; biopsies were not routinely performed. Most men with low-risk disease were included (77% of men had Gleason 6 disease). After a median follow-up of 10 years, 10-year cancer-specific survival was 98.8%, 99%, and 99.6% for active monitoring, RP, and EBRT, respectively. There were no significant differences in all-cause mortality between the 3 groups. A secondary endpoint, metastases, was significantly more frequent in patients managed with active monitoring (33 men, or 6.3 per 1000 person-years). The metastasis rate differed from those managed with RP (13 men, or 2.4 per 1000 person-years) or radiation (16 men, or 3.0 per 1000 person-years). Forty percent of men assigned to active monitoring underwent treatment within 5 years and nearly two-thirds by 10 years. There are several limitations to this trial, including lack of screening prostate biopsies, prostate mpMRI, and genomic testing for those on the "active monitoring" arm as well as the lack of diversity within the cohort (men of African or Caribbean ethnicity only made up 1% of the cohort).

Table 1
Recommended schedule for active surveillance

	At Time of Diagnosis	Every 3–6 mo	Every 12–24 mo
DRE	X	X	
PSA test	X	X	
Prostate biopsy	X		X

Nevertheless, this is the only prospective randomized trial and therefore the most robust evidence to date regarding the clinical course of PSA monitoring for men who are candidates for such an option.

Active treatment

For men with low-risk disease who are interested in pursuing definitive treatment, 2 established options are available. One option, RP, can be performed using an open

Table 2
Single-institution active surveillance trials in prostate cancer

Trial	N	Patient Characteristics	Median Follow-Up (y)	Surveillance Schedule	Results
Klotz et al	933	Low- or intermediate-risk PC	6.4	PSA every 3 mo for 2 y, then every 6 mo. Confirmatory bx within 12 mo of initial bx	Actuarial cause specific survival: 98.1% at 5 y, 94.3% at 10 y
Tosoian et al	1298	Very low-risk disease or older men with low-risk disease	5	PSA and DRE every 6 mo and annual bx	OS: 93% at 10 y, 69% at 15 y; Cancer-specific survival: 99.9% at 10 y, 99.9% at 15 y; Metastasis-free survival: 99.4% at 10 y, 99.4% at 15 y; Median treatment-free survival: 8.5 y; 10-y estimate for definitive treatment: 50%; 15-y estimate for definitive treatment: 57%
Welty et al	810	Low-risk PC	5	PSA every 3 mo, semiannual transrectal ultrasound and annual bx	5-y OS of 98%; Treatment-free survival: 60%; Biopsy reclassification-free survival: 40%

Abbreviation: bx, biopsy.
Modified from Litwin MS, Tan HJ. The Diagnosis and Treatment of Prostate Cancer: A Review. JAMA 2017;317(24):2535; with permission.

or robotic technique. The latter technique is associated with less blood loss and a shorter hospital stay but is operator dependent.[10,11] The other option is EBRT. Both offer equal chance for cure, based on results from the ProtecT trial. Longer follow-up of the ProtecT trial is needed to elucidate differences in outcomes, if any, between the 2 treatment modalities.

Radiation therapy (RT) can be delivered via EBRT or brachytherapy. Improved treatment techniques, including intensity-modulated RT, have allowed radiation oncologists to escalate dose up to 79.2 Gy safely via EBRT. This dose has been compared with 70.2 Gy in a randomized trial using modern techniques (Radiation Therapy Oncology Group [RTOG] 0126, NCT00033631) and was found to significantly improve biochemical control and rates of distant metastases; it is now generally accepted as standard dose.[12] Brachytherapy is an alternative to EBRT. Brachytherapy involves the use of implanting a radioactive source directly into the prostate gland. Brachytherapy can either be low-dose-rate, which involves the use of permanently implanted radioactive seeds, or high-dose-rate, using a temporary radiation source, which is inserted into the prostate via hollow catheters or needles that have been positioned and later removed.

Intermediate-Risk Disease

Intermediate-risk PC is a heterogeneous disease with regards to clinical outcomes, including PSA progression, recurrence, and prostate cancer–specific mortality (PCSM). To further refine this heterogeneity, intermediate-risk disease has been sub-classified into favorable or unfavorable disease based on a study[13] that reviewed 1024 patients with intermediate-risk PC treated with definitive EBRT with or without neoadjuvant and concurrent ADT. It was found that men with unfavorable intermediate-risk PC had significantly worse PC control outcomes compared with men with favorable intermediate-risk disease. Separately, an evaluation of a cohort of 2510 intermediate-risk PC patients treated with brachytherapy with or without neoadjuvant ADT in men with favorable disease and brachytherapy with neoadjuvant EBRT or ADT in men with unfavorable disease found that neoadjuvant ADT followed by brachytherapy was associated with a reduction in PCSM risk compared with neoadjuvant EBRT followed by brachytherapy in unfavorable intermediate-risk disease.[14] There was no significant difference, however, in the risk of PCSM with or without the addition of neoadjuvant ADT to brachytherapy in favorable intermediate-risk PC patients. This finding highlights the heterogeneous nature of intermediate-risk disease and the potential to recommend or exclude ADT based on this subcategorization.

Favorable intermediate-risk disease

Per the NCCN guidelines, treatment options and cancer control outcomes for men with favorable intermediate-risk disease are similar to patients with low-risk disease.[2] However, this is mostly derived from retrospective data. Brachytherapy or high-dose RT as monotherapy are accepted, but may not be appropriate for all men with favorable intermediate PC, particularly those with high-volume disease as represented by the percent positive biopsies or palpable extent of the disease based on DRE, or in those with a PSA velocity greater than 2 ng/mL/y.[14] Careful identification and selection of these patients are crucial to ensure optimal cancer control outcomes.

Hypofractionation in intermediate-risk disease

Recently, there has been increasing interest and accumulating data demonstrating that PC harbors a lower α/β (a metric characterizing tissue and/or tumor sensitivity to radiation dose per treatment) compared with the normal surrounding tissues, indicating that hypofractionated RT, a method that delivers a higher biologic dose to the prostate gland per treatment in fewer total treatments, may improve cancer control outcomes for PC. As shown in **Table 3**, 3 recent noninferiority trials[8,15] were published comparing conventional fractionation with hypofractionated RT in localized PC; these studies were sufficiently powered and were able to demonstrate noninferiority of 70 Gy in 28 fractions compared with 73.8 Gy in 41 fractions (RTOG 0415) and 60 Gy in 20 fractions (CHHiP,[8] PROFIT[15]) compared with 74 Gy in 37 fractions and 78 Gy in 39 fractions, respectively. Hypofractionated RT was generally well tolerated; however, the median follow-up for the 3 trials currently does not exceed 6 years, and given that late genitourinary (GU) toxicity is often a delayed event happening beyond 5 and up to 10 years after RT,[15] there is a chance for late GU toxicity that has not yet been observed. A recent metaanalysis of the 3 randomized noninferiority trials demonstrated significant improvement in disease-free survival (DFS) in patients treated with hypofractionated radiotherapy compared with conventional fractionation treatment, but no significant difference in overall survival (OS).[15] A randomized superiority trial comparing 75.6 Gy in 1.8 Gy per fraction with 72 Gy in 2.4 Gy per fraction also demonstrated improved cancer control with moderately hypofractionated RT.[16] Taken together, these results provide evidence that hypofractionated RT may be a preferred approach for men with intermediate-risk PC given the potential for superior cancer control. Further investigation is needed to address the question of late GU toxicity, but this may be a good option for men with no risk factors for late GU toxicity, such as the use of anticoagulants, history of transurethral resection of prostate, or diabetes mellitus.

Unfavorable intermediate-risk disease

Three randomized trials have evaluated the optimal duration of ADT in men with intermediate-risk PC[8] (**Table 4**). From these studies, it was determined that 4 to 6 months of ADT with, by today's standards, low-dose RT (66–70 Gy) improves OS. The survival benefit appears to be most beneficial in intermediate-risk patients and in those with no or minimal comorbidity, although there was no prerandomization stratification by risk group or comorbidity status in these studies.

Based on this, the question of whether the addition of ADT imparts a survival benefit in the dose-escalated era for intermediate-risk patients is an important consideration. One trial, EORTC 22991,[9] evaluated various doses ± ADT, with an endpoint of biochemical DFS. It found that the addition of ADT improved clinical and DFS, but OS data are not mature at this time after a median follow-up of 7.2 years. Although there was no interaction observed between dose and biochemical DFS, 1 limitation of this study is that the treating physician selected the radiation dose as opposed to having it used as a prerandomization stratification factor. Another study presented in abstract form (GETUG 14)[17] compared 80 Gy of radiation ± 4 months of ADT. With a median follow-up of 6.8 years, an improvement in relapse-free survival is seen with the addition of ADT; additional follow-up is needed to determine the effect on OS (**Table 5**). Finally, the ongoing RTOG 0815 (Clinicaltrials.gov NCT00936390) with planned enrollment of 1520 men is evaluating treatment using modern RT dose regiments of 79.2 Gy delivered via EBRT alone or 45-Gy EBRT + brachytherapy boost, ± 6 months of ADT. Patients were stratified before randomization by the number of intermediate-risk factors (1 vs 2–3), ACE-27 comorbidity (no/mild vs moderate/severe), and radiation modality. Percent positive biopsy data were not collected, so a further stratification by favorable versus unfavorable intermediate-risk PC is not possible. The primary endpoint is OS. This study has the potential to identify in

Table 3
Hypofractionation trials for prostate cancer

Trial	Type	N	Median Follow-Up (y)	Trial Arms	Primary Endpoint	Results	Toxicities
RTOG 0415[15]	Noninferiority	1092	5.8	73.8 Gy/41 Fx 70 Gy/28 Fx	DFS Noninferiority 95% CI upper bound: <1.52	HR (95% CI): 0.85 (0.64–1.14)	Increased GI/GU late grade 2+ toxicity with hypoFx
CHHiP[8,15]	Noninferiority	3163	5.2	74 Gy/37 Fx 60 Gy/20 Fx 57 Gy/19 Fx + 3–6 mo ADT	PSA Noninferiority 95% CI upper bound: <1.208	HR (95% CI): 0.84 (0.68–1.03) 57 Gy/19 Fx inferior to 74 Gy/37 x	No significant differences but trend toward increased late grade 2+ GU toxicity (P = .07)
PROFIT[15]	Noninferiority	1206	6.0	78 Gy/39 Fx 60 Gy/20 Fx	DFS Noninferiority 95% CI upper bound: <1.32	HR (95% CI): 0.96 (0.74–1.25)	No significant difference in late toxicity
Hoffman et al,[16] 2018	Superiority	206	8.5	75.6 Gy/42 Fx 72 Gy/30 Fx	PSA failure	8-y failure rate 10.7% (95% CI: 5.8%–19.1%) for 72 Gy vs 15.4% (95% CI: 9.1%–25.4%) for 75.6 Gy, P = .036	Nonsignificant increase in late grade 2+ GI toxicity with hypoFx (P = .08)
Royce et al,[15] 2015	Metaanalysis	5484	5.2–6	60–70 Gy in 20–28 Fx vs 73.8–78 Gy in 39–41 Fx	DFS	HR (95% CI): 0.869 (0.757–0.998)	Nonsignificant increase in late-grade 2+ GU toxicity RR 1.18 (P = .08) with hypoFx

Abbreviations: Fx, fractions; GI, gastrointestinal; hypoFx, hypofractionation; RR, risk ratio.

whom 6 months of ADT is necessary to prolong OS with modern RT doses as well as validate or refute whether comorbidity interacts with ADT.

High-Risk Disease

Definition and historical perspective
High-risk PC is defined as PSA greater than 20 or Gleason score $\geq$8 or DRE defined as T3a–T4 disease. Historically, the EORTC 22863 trial[8] was the first evidence to suggest that the standard of care for high-risk disease was long-term ADT and 70 Gy of RT to the prostate and seminal vesicles (**Table 6**). This trial demonstrated a significant 10-year OS benefit for RT + ADT (39.8% RT alone vs 58.1% RT + ADT, hazard ratio [HR] 0.60, 95% confidence interval [CI] 0.45–0.80, P = .0004).[8] However, the question was raised as to whether radiation was necessary to confer the survival benefit, which led to the performance of both the SPCG-7/SFUO-3[8] and the Intergroup T94-0110[9] trials. These trials examined whether long-term ADT alone was sufficient treatment of high-risk disease. Both trials found inferior survival related to ADT alone; SPCG-7/SFUO-3 demonstrated relative risk of overall death to be 0.68 (95% CI 0.52–0.89, P = .004) in favor of ADT + RT, whereas Intergroup T94-0110 found improved OS (HR 0.70, 95% CI 0.57–0.85, P<.001) in the combination ADT + RT arm, thus establishing the necessity for the addition of radiotherapy (see **Table 6**) and making radiation and long-term ADT a standard of care for high-risk PC.

Duration of androgen deprivation therapy for high-risk prostate cancer
Several landmark trials then investigated the optimal duration of ADT in combination with RT in high-risk disease (see **Table 6**). RTOG 9202 investigated 4 months of ADT compared with 28 months of ADT.[8] With 11.3 years of follow-up, 10-year PC-specific survival was significantly improved with the longer duration of ADT (88.7% vs 83.9%, P = .0042; HR = 0.65, 95% CI 0.582–0.726, P<.0001); however, there was no statistically significant difference for OS (53.9% vs 51.6%, P = .359; HR 0.922, 95% CI 0.804–1.057, P = .2447). EORTC 22961 evaluated the duration of ADT as 6 months or 36 months,[8] demonstrating superiority on a postrandomization analysis of 36 months ADT (OS HR 1.42, upper 1-sided 95.71% CI 1.79, P = .65 for noninferiority) in men with high-risk disease. Finally, the PCS IV trial evaluated whether 36 months was superior to 18 months of ADT in men with high-risk disease,[18] finding that 36 months was not superior to 18 months (OS HR 1.02, 95% CI 0.81–1.29, P = .8); thus, 18 months of ADT may be a valid option for these patients (although the trial was not designed as noninferiority and so this remains hypothesis generating and therefore restricted to men who cannot tolerate 28–36 months of ADT and/or who have significant cardiometabolic comorbidity). However, critics of these trials[19,20] point out that modern prostate patients are treated to higher RT doses than what was used in these historic investigations, thus highlighting the question of whether the benefit of ADT persists in the era of high-dose RT.

Radiation therapy dose and technique for high-risk prostate cancer
Subsequently, the DART01/05 trial stratified men before randomization by intermediate versus high- risk and studied the benefit of either short-term (4 months) or long-term (28 months) ADT along with high-dose (78 Gy) radiation.[9] It was found that long-term ADT improved biochemical control and OS in men with high-risk disease (biochemical DFS HR 1.88, 95% CI 1.12–3.15, P = .01; OS HR 2.31, 95% CI 1.23–3.85, P = .01). The DART01/05 trial is the only trial that demonstrated a survival benefit with the use of 28 months of ADT in the setting of high-dose RT, making both high-dose RT and long-term ADT a standard of care for men with high-risk PC.

Table 4
Optimal duration of androgen deprivation therapy in intermediate-risk disease

Trial	N	Patient Characteristics	Trial Arms	Median Follow-Up (y)	Primary Endpoint	Results
RTOG 9408	1979	53% intrisk 51% T2 26% GS 7 8% GS 8–10	Arm 1: 4 mo ADT + RT (66.6 Gy in 37 Fx: 46.8 to pelvis, 19.8 prostate) ADT: NSAA + LHRH agonist Arm 2: RT (66.6 Gy in 37 Fx)	9.1	OS (DSM)	*OS (10 y) RT vs ADT/RT* • HR 1.17 95% CI 1.01–1.35 P = .03 • Int-risk HR 1.23 95% CI 1.02–1.49 P = .03 • High-risk HR 1.16 95% CI 0.78–1.71 P = NS *DSM (10 y)* • RT vs ADT/RT 1.87 P = .001 • Int-risk HR 2.49 95% CI 1.50–4.11 P = .004 • High-risk HR 1.53 95% CI 0.72–3.26 P = NS
DFCI 95096	206	27% T2b 76% no/low cormorbidity 57.6% GS 7 14.6% GS 8–10	Arm 1: 6 mo ADT/70.35 Gy in 36 Fx 3DCRT ADT: NSAA + LHRH agonist Arm 2: 70.35 Gy in 36 Fx 3DCRT	7.6	ACM (PCSM)	*ACM* • RT vs 6 mo ADT/RT HR 1.8 95% CI 1.1–2.9 P = .01 *ACM (none/min comorbidity)* • 6 mo ADT/RT vs RT HR 4.2 95% CI 2.1–8.5 P<.001 *ACM (mod/sev comorbidity)* • RT vs 6 mo ADT/RT HR 0.54 95% CI 0.27–1.10 P = NS *PCSM* • RT vs 6 mo ADT/RT HR 4.1 95% CI 1.4–12.1 P = .01

(continued on next page)

Table 4
(continued)

Trial	N	Patient Characteristics	Trial Arms	Median Follow-Up (y)	Primary Endpoint	Results
TROG 96.01	802	16.1% int risk 25.7% T2b 38% GS 7 17.1% GS 8–10	Arm 1: RT (66 Gy in 33 Fx) Arm 2: 3 mo ADT/RT Arm 3: 6 mo ADT/RT ADT: NSAA + LHRH agonist	10.6	PCSM, ACM	All compare ADT/RT vs RT: *PCSM* • 3 mo HR 0.86 95% CI 0.60–1.23 $P = .398$ 6 mo HR 0.49 95% CI 0.32–0.74 $P = .0008$ *ACM* • 3 mo HR 0.84 95% CI 0.65–1.08 $P = .180$ 6 mo HR 0.63 95% CI 0.48–0.83 $P = .0008$

Abbreviations: 3DCRT, 3-dimensional conformal radiotherapy; ACM, all-cause mortality; DSM, disease-specific mortality; GS, Gleason Score; int, intermediate; min, minimal; mod, moderate; NS, not significant; NSAA, nonsteroidal antiandrogen; sev, severe.

From Sathianathen NJ, Konety BR, Crook J, et al. Landmarks in prostate cancer. Nat Rev Urol 2018;15(10):627-642; with permission.

Last, the question of a benefit of adding a brachytherapy boost to EBRT in high-risk disease was addressed by the ASCENDE-RT trial.[21,22] Patients received 12 months total of ADT along with 46-Gy EBRT to the pelvic lymph nodes, prostate, and seminal vesicles. Patients were then randomized to 32-Gy boost with EBRT versus I-125 low-dose-rate brachytherapy boost to a minimum peripheral dose of 115 Gy. With a median follow-up of 6.5 years, the 78-Gy EBRT arm demonstrated a significant increase in biochemical relapse (HR 2.04 95% CI 1.25–3.33, $P = .004$), without any significant difference in OS (HR 1.13, 95% CI 0.69–1.84, $P = .62$) or PC-specific survival (HR 0.71, 95% CI 0.27–1.88, $P = .49$) between the 2 arms. Longer follow-up is needed to evaluate the impact of adding a brachytherapy boost on these later endpoints, which will be important because there was a significant increase in late GU toxicity in the combination EBRT + boost radiation treatment arm ($P<.001$). This finding necessitates the establishment of validated dose constraints for this technique to be safely and effectively implemented for men with high-risk PC. This trial also calls into question whether the use of 2 years of ADT would eliminate the benefit in DFS observed using a brachytherapy boost because 1 year of ADT may not be sufficient for these patients.

Very high-risk prostate cancer
A retrospective cohort study of pooled patients from 12 centers evaluated outcomes in men with Gleason 9 to 10 PC who were treated with RP, EBRT + ADT, or EBRT + brachytherapy boost + ADT.[23] It was found, using a propensity-score adjusted analysis accounting for age and known PC prognostic factors, that patients who received EBRT + brachytherapy boost + ADT had significantly improved PCSM

Table 5
Impact of androgen deprivation therapy in intermediate-risk disease in dose-escalated era

Trial	N	Patient Characteristics	Trial Arms	Median Follow-Up (y)	Primary Endpoint	Results
EORTC 22991[9]	819	Median PSA 10.4 50.9% T2a 40.9% GS 7 17.6% IMRT (58.4% 78 Gy)	All arms ± 6 mo ADT Arm 1: 70 Gy in 35 Fx Arm 2: 74 Gy in 37 Fx Arm 3: 78 Gy in 39 Fx ADT: NSAA + LHRH agonist	7.2	b-DFS	b-DFS RT/ADT vs RT HR 0.52 95% CI 0.41–0.66 P<.001 b-DFS 70 Gy ADT/RT vs RT HR 0.58 95% CI 0.39–0.86 74 Gy ADT/RT vs RT HR 0.52 95% CI 0.37–0.73 78 Gy ADT/RT vs RT HR 0.48 95% CI 0.29–0.77 Heterogeneity P = .79
GETUG 14[17]	370	Not yet reported	Arm 1: RT (80 Gy/40x) Arm 2: RT+4 mo ADT ADT: NSAA + LHRH agonist	6.8	RFS (OS)	RFS (5 y) RT 76% (95% CI 69%– 81%) vs RT/ADT 84% (78%–89%) (P = .02) OS (5 y) RT 94% (90%–97%) vs RT/ ADT 93% (88%– 96%) (P = NS)

Abbreviations: b-DFS, biochemical disease-free survival; IMRT, intensity-modulated radiation therapy; RFS, relapse-free survival.

as well as longer time to distant metastasis (DM) compared with men undergoing RP (adjusted PCSM HR 0.41, 95% CI 0.24–0.71, P = .002, adjusted DM HR 0.30, 95% CI 0.19–0.47, P<.001). There was no significant difference, however, when comparing to men who underwent at least 78-Gy RT and at least 2 years of ADT in the endpoint of death from PC (adjusted PCSM HR 1.24, 95% CI 0.45–3.40, P = .75).

Novel antiandrogens and docetaxel
Given the efficacy of docetaxel and abiraterone in the metastatic PC setting,[8,9] randomized studies have been conducted in the high-risk M0 setting. As shown in **Table 7**, RTOG 0521 evaluated the addition of adjuvant docetaxel and prednisone to standard EBRT + ADT and recently reported suggestion of a benefit in 4-year OS with the addition of docetaxel (HR 0.69, 90% CI 0.49–0.97, 1-sided P-value = .034)[24] but no reduction in death from PC (HR 0.65 95% CI: 0.34–1.24, 2-sided P-value = .18). GETUG-12 showed an improvement in relapse-free survival (0.71 95% CI: 0.54–0.94 P = .017),[9] whereas SPCG-13 showed no benefit in PSA failure-free survival (1.14 95% CI: 0.79–1.64 P = .49).[25] The STAMPEDE trial evaluated the addition of docetaxel or zoledronic acid or both to the standard of care (RT and long-term ADT) for men with PC, stratifying by metastatic status.[9] There was no survival benefit with the addition of docetaxel in men with high-risk N0 or N1 M0 PC (HR

Table 6
Trials in high-risk PC

Trial	N	Patient Characteristics	Trial Arms	Median Follow-Up (y)	Primary Endpoint	Results
EORTC 22863[8]	412	T1-2+ Grade 3 OR T3-4+ any grade	50 Gy pelvis + 20 Gy CD CAB 1 mo starting d1 RT → goserelin 36 mo vs observation	9.1	cDFS	10-y cDFS: RT + ADT HR 0.42 95% CI 0.33–0.55 $P \leq .0001$ 10-y OS: RT + ADT HR 0.60 95% CI 0.45–0.80 $P = .0004$
SPCG-7/ SFUO-3[8,39]	875	T1b-2+ Grade 2-3 or T3M0	ADT × 3 mo → indefinite flutamide ± 70-Gy EBRT	12	PCSM	ADT + RT: PCSM HR 0.42 95% CI 0.31–0.56 $P<.001$ OS HR 0.72 95% CI 0.60–0.86 $P = .003$
Intergroup T94-0110[9]	1205	T3/T4 or T2+ PSA >40 or T2+ PSA >20 + GS ≥8	Randomized to lifelong ADT (bilateral orchiectomy or 2 wk of CAB → goserelin) ± RT (64–69 Gy to prostate + SVs)	8	OS	10-y OS RT + ADT HR 0.70 95% CI 0.57–0.85 $P<.001$

(continued on next page)

Table 6
(continued)

Trial	N	Patient Characteristics	Trial Arms	Median Follow-Up (y)	Primary Endpoint	Results
RTOG 9202[8]	1521	cT2c-T4, PSA <150	45 Gy pelvis + 20–25 Gy CD 2 mo neoadjuvant CAB + 2 mo concurrent CAB (SC ADT) vs 2 mo neoadjuvant CAB + 2 mo concurrent CAB → goserelin 24 mo (LC ADT)	11.3	DFS	*10-y DFS:* LC ADT HR 0.65 95% CI 0.582–0.726 *P*<.0001 *10 y OS:* HR 0.922 95% CI 0.804–1.057 *P* = .2447
EORTC 22961[8]	1113	T1c-T2b pN1-N2 M0 or T2c-T4 N0-N2, PSA up to 40× upper limit of normal range	50 Gy/5 wk pelvis + 20 Gy/2 wk CD Prostate + SVs 6 mo of CAB (flutamide/bicalutamide + triptorelin) ± triptorelin for 2.5 y	6.4	OS	*5-y OS:* HR 1.42 Upper 1-sided 95.71% CI 1.79, *P*=0.65 for noninferiority
PCS IV[18]	630	T3-4, PSA >20 or GS >7. Must be N0	44 Gy/4.5 wk pelvis + 70 Gy/7 wk CD prostate 18 mo of neoadjuvant/concurrent/adjuvant ADT vs 36 mo	9.4	OS	*5-y OS:* HR 1.02 95% CI 0.81–1.29 *P* = .8
DART01/05[9]	355	T1c-T3bN0M0 w/intermediate- or high-risk features per NCCN (2005)	Median RT dose 78 Gy (range 76–82 Gy). Elective pelvic RT allowed but not required 4 mo of ADT (2 mo neoadjuvant, 2 mo concurrent CAB) vs 4 mo of CAB + 24 mo of adjuvant goserelin	5.3	bDFS	*5-y bDFS:* Long-term ADT HR 1.88 95% CI 1.12–3.15 *P* = .01 *5-y OS:* HR 2.31 95% CI 1.23–3.85 *P* = .01

Trial	N	Eligibility	Treatment	Median follow-up	Endpoint	Results
ASCENDE-RT[21,22]	398	Intermediate- and high-risk disease (NCCN criteria)	8 mo neoadjuvant ADT → 46-Gy EBRT (pelvis) Subsequently randomized to 32 Gy boost to prostate + SV vs I-125 LDR boost to minimum peripheral dose of 115 Gy. Total 12 mo ADT	6.5	bPFS	*5-y biochemical relapse:* Brachytherapy Boost HR 2.04 95% CI 1.25–3.33 P = .004 5 y OS: HR 1.13 95% CI 0.69–1.84 P = .62 PCSS: HR 0.71 95% CI 0.27–1.88 P = .49
STAMPEDE[8]	1917	At least 2 of: T3-T4, GS 8–10, and PSA ≥40; or relapse s/p RT or RP with high-risk features: PSA >4 + PSADT <6 mo, PSA >20, nodal or metastatic relapse, or <12 mo ADT with at least >12 mo w/o treatment	SOC (≥24 mo ADT) vs SOC + abiraterone 1000 mg every day and prednisolone 5 mg every day Local RT mandated for patients with N0M0 disease, encouraged for N+ disease Patients who received RT: treatment continued for 2 y or progression	3.3	OS	ADT + Abi vs ADT M0 HR 0.75 95% CI 0.48–1.18 P = .37

Abbreviations: Abi, abiraterone; CAB, combined androgen blockade; CD, cone down; cDFS, clinical disease-free survival; LC ADT, long-course ADT; PCSS, prostatecancer–specific survival; PSADT, PSA doubling time; SC ADT, short-course androgen deprivation therapy; SOC, standard of care; SVs, seminal vesicles.

Table 7
Trials investigating docetaxel in men with high-risk PC

Trial	N	Patient Characteristics	Trial Arms	Median Follow-Up (y)	Primary Endpoint	Results
RTOG 0521[24]	612	GS 7–8, any T stage, and PSA >20 OR GS 8, ≥T2, any PSA OR GS 9–10, any T stage, and PSA >20	EBRT to 75.6 Gy + long-term ADT ± docetaxel + prednisone	5.7	OS	Adjuvant docetaxel + prednisone: HR 0.69 90% CI 0.49–0.97 1-sided P = .034
STAMPEDE[9]	2962	At least 2 of: T3-T4, GS 8–10, and PSA ≥40; or relapse s/p RT or RP with high-risk features: PSA >4 + PSADT <6 mo, PSA >20, nodal or metastatic relapse, or <12 mo ADT with at least >12 mo w/o treatment	RT 6-9 mo postrandomization mandated for node-negative, nonmetastatic, encouraged for node-positive ≥24 mo ADT (SOC) vs SOC + ZA 4 mg 6, 21-d cycles → every 4 wk for 2 y (ZA) vs SOC + Doc 75 mg/m² 6, 21-d cycles (Doc) vs SOC + ZA + DOC	3.6	OS	SOC + CT subgroup: M0 (N0 or N1): HR 0.82 95% CI 0.48–1.40 P = .475
GETUG-12[9]	413	At least 1 of: T3-T4, GS ≥8, PSA >20, node-positive	ADT alone × 3 y vs ADT × 3 y + 4 cycles docetaxel and estramustine d1-5 every 3 wk Both arms received local treatment, which could consist of either RT or surgery	8.8	RFS	SOC + CT: RFS HR 0.71 95% CI 0.54–0.94 P = .0017
SPCG-13[25]	376	T2 disease with GS of 4 + 3, PSA >10; T2, GS 8–10 any PSA, or any T3 disease	All patients received neoadjuvant/adjuvant ADT along with RT Patients were then randomized to: Surveillance vs 6 cycles of adjuvant docetaxel every 3 wk	4.9	PSA failure	SOC + Docetaxel: HR 1.14 95% CI 0.79–1.64 P = .495

Abbreviations: CT, chemotherapy (docetaxel); Doc, docetaxel; RFS, relapse-free survival; SOC, standard of care; ZA, zoledronic acid.

0.82, 95% CI 0.48–1.40, $P = .475$). Separately, the evaluation of abiraterone in patients in the STAMPEDE trial found that there was no benefit among patients with nonmetastatic disease (OS HR nonmetastatic disease 0.75, 95% CI 0.48–1.18), although this was a small subset[8] and may have been underpowered. The ongoing DFCI 05043 trial is evaluating whether neoadjuvant docetaxel/prednisone along with weekly docetaxel during RT might provide any benefit in unfavorable intermediate- or high-risk patients. Given disparate results, predictive markers are needed to define the role of these agents in managing high-risk PC.

Role of pelvic nodal radiation therapy in high-risk prostate cancer

The use of pelvic RT in high-risk individuals is controversial, because many trials in men with high-risk PC[8,9,18,21,22] permitted pelvic RT based on the discretion of the treating physician (**Table 8**). One trial specifically compared whole-pelvic RT (WPRT) to prostate-only RT in patients with clinically localized PC.[26] This study found no benefit to WPRT when used along with ADT (neoadjuvant $P = .9629$ or adjuvant $P = .01$). However, there are many criticisms of this trial, because there were demonstrated interactions with hormonal therapy and the inconsistent size of the treatment field as well as unexplained findings, such as worse survival with the use of WPRT and adjuvant ADT yet improved progression-free survival (PFS) with the use of WPRT and neoadjuvant ADT. GETUG-01 also evaluated the role of pelvic radiotherapy in localized intermediate- and high-risk PC.[27] This study was also negative and did not find an improvement in PFS with WPRT (HR 0.96, 95% CI 0.64–1.43, $P = .821$) nor an effect on quality of life ($P =$ nonsignificant). Hence, at this time, WPRT can be considered for select young and very high-risk patients, but it is not a standard of care owing to the lack of level 1 evidence supporting its use. Nevertheless, with the introduction and increasing use of novel imaging markers, such as fluciclovine F-18 in PET for PC, men may be identified who might benefit from WPRT by detecting those who have microscopic disease in their pelvic nodes.[28] This novel indication requires further study but may provide an avenue for the use of WPRT in PC.

Node-Positive Prostate Cancer

Of all men who present with M0 PC, 12% will have evidence of clinically involved pelvic nodes based on imaging studies.[1] Men with evidence of a clinically involved node are classified as having stage IVA disease; however, having node-positive disease in the pelvis does not necessarily preclude definitive therapy. Although there are no randomized trials establishing the role of definitive RT in men with clinical lymph node involvement, extrapolations can be made from large, population-based studies (**Table 9**). In a large analysis from the National Cancer Database (NCDB) that identified 2967 men with clinically node positive PC without distant metastases,[29] 1987 men were treated with definitive local therapy (radiation ± ADT or RP ± ADT), and 980 received ADT alone. Receipt of definitive local therapy was associated with improved OS at 5 years compared with ADT alone (HR 0.31, 95% CI 0.13–0.74, $P = .007$). This difference remained significant on multivariable analysis after adjusting for baseline characteristics, including age, race, Charlson comorbidity index, median income of zip code, education status, insurance status, county category, facility type, region, year of diagnosis, PSA level at diagnosis, clinical T stage, and Gleason score (adjusted HR 0.51, 95% CI 0.44–0.60, $P<.001$).

A separate study evaluating 1107 patients who underwent RP and were found to have a pathologically involved lymph node and were then treated with adjuvant ADT ± RT[30] (35% of patients received radiation) disclosed an association with a lower risk of PCSM (HR 0.37, 95% CI 0.22–0.62, $P<.001$) with the receipt of adjuvant pelvic

Table 8
Pelvic nodal irradiation in high-risk disease

Trial	N	Patient Characteristics	Trial Arms	Median Follow-Up (y)	Primary Endpoint	Results
RTOG 9413[26]	1323	Clinically localized PC, PSA ≤100, LN risk >15% per Roach formula OR T2c-4 + GS ≥6 *Roach formula: PSA*2) 3+(GS-6)*10*	WPRT w/16 × 16 cm to 50.4 Gy + 19.8 Gy prostate + SV CD (11 × 11 cm) or 70.2 Gy to prostate Neoadjuvant ADT 2 mo pre-RT/ 2 mo concurrent, adjuvant ADT 4 mo post-RT *Randomization: 2 × 2 factorial design. PORT vs WPRT and neoadjuvant ADT vs adjuvant ADT*	6.6	PFS	No difference in PFS for WPRT vs PORT ($P = .99$) No difference in PFS for Neoadjuvant ADT vs adjuvant ADT ($P = .72$) Post hoc analysis: WPRT + neoadjuvant ADT led to improved PFS ($P = .066$) and bDFS ($P = .0098$) while WPRT + adjuvant ADT worsened OS ($P = .01$)
GETUG-01[27]	446	T1b-T3 N0 pNx M0. Any GS, any PSA. No lymphadenectomy patients	Pelvic 46 Gy, prostate dose (66 Gy-70 Gy). Seminal vesicles treated to 46 Gy or 60 Gy if involved. 6 mo neoadjuvant + concurrent CAB allowed for high-risk patients but not required *Randomization: WPRT vs PORT*	11.4	PFS	5-y PFS: WPRT vs PORT HR 0.96 95% CI 0.64 $P = .821$

Abbreviations: LN, lymph node; PORT, prostate only radiation therapy.

Table 9
Node-positive M0 disease

Study	N	Patient Characteristics	Trial Arms	Median Follow-Up (y)	Primary Endpoint	Results
NCDB[29]	2967	Patients with clinically involved nodes	Local therapy (RP vs RT) ± ADT	4.1	OS	Improved OS with RT: HR 0.31 95% CI 0.13–0.74 P = .007
Abdollah et al,[30] 2014	1107	Pathologic node-positive patients s/p RP	RP followed by ADT ± radiation	8.4 among those with RT + ADT vs 7.1 among those with ADT alone	CSM	Improved CSM among men who received RT: HR 0.37 95% CI 0.22–0.62 P<.001
STAMPEDE[9]	721	High-risk, hormone-naive patients with and without clinical node involvement Newly diagnosed N0M0 disease, newly diagnosed M1 or N+ disease, or disease previously treated with RT or RP presenting with relapse	LT ADT ± radiation	1.4	FFS, OS	Among node+ patients who received RT: HR 0.48 95% CI 0.29–0.79

Abbreviations: CSM, cancer-specific mortality; FFS, failure-free survival; LT ADT, long-term androgen deprivation therapy.

RT. When further stratifying men into risk groups, 2 groups appeared to be driving the benefit observed for adding adjuvant pelvic RT: (1) men with positive lymph node count ≤2, Gleason score 7–10, pT3b/pT4, or positive surgical margins; and (2) patients with positive lymph node count 3 to 4. Retrospective analyses such as this are limited because of the potential for confounding owing to potentially important unavailable clinical factors, such as comorbidity and whether the lymph node disease was identified using PET versus conventional MRI-based imaging and therefore are hypothesis generating.

Finally, in a postrandomization analysis of the control arm of the STAMPEDE trial evaluating men with N1M0 or N0M0 disease who were randomized to receive either long-term ADT or long-term ADT + RT to the primary, among the subset of men with N1M0 disease, pelvic lymph node radiation was delivered at the discretion of the treating physician.[9] A total of 721 men with newly diagnosed N1M0 disease were included, and DFS was improved in men who received pelvic RT among those with N+ disease (adjusted HR 0.48, 95% CI 0.29–0.79) after adjusting for initial Gleason sum score (≤7, >8, unknown), log-transformed pre-ADT PSA level, age at randomization (<60, 60–64, 65–69, ≥70 years), and World Health Organization performance status (0 vs 1–2). This study suggests that in carefully selected patients, local definitive RT may lead to a longer disease-free interval in those with node-positive disease. Taken together, these data suggest a possible benefit to adding pelvic lymph node RT to men with N1M0 PC, but prospective validation is needed.

NEWLY DIAGNOSED OLIGOMETASTATIC PROSTATE CANCER

Metastatic PC is a clinically and genetically heterogenous disease.[31,32] Moreover, a recently studied subgroup of metastatic PC is oligometastatic PC, which has various definitions that reflect a lower burden of metastatic disease. Per the recent CHAARTED study, oligometastatic PC was defined as having ≤3 bone metastases and no visceral metastases.[9] Low-volume oligometastatic PC may be biologically different than high-metastatic burden PC,[33] and it has been unclear as to whether local treatment has a role in the treatment of low burden oligometastatic PC.

Recently, the HORRAD trial was reported, which was a multicenter randomized control trial determining whether definitive local treatment to the primary prostate tumor with EBRT and ADT would confer a survival advantage.[33] After a median follow-up of 3.9 years and 432 patients recruited, there was no significant difference found in OS between those who received RT versus those who did not receive RT (HR 0.90, 95% CI 0.70–1.14). However, on subgroup analysis, in men with less than 5 metastases, there was a trend toward a benefit in OS with the addition of radiotherapy (HR 0.68, 95% CI 0.42–1.10), as shown in **Table 10**, whereas no benefit in men with a high metastatic burden (patients 5–15 metastases, HR 1.18, 95% CI 0.74–1.89; patients 15+ metastases, HR 0.93, 95% CI 0.66–1.32).

The recently published STAMPEDE trial also looked at the role of primary radiotherapy in metastatic PC patients, although in a larger cohort (n = 2061).[33] After a median follow-up of 3.1 years, it was found that the addition of radiation to the primary in men receiving the standard of care for metastatic disease (defined as lifelong ADT with upfront docetaxel) did not confer a survival advantage (HR 0.92, 95% CI 0.80–1.06, P = .266). However, on postrandomization analysis stratifying men by metastatic burden, defining men with low metastatic burden as ≤3 bone metastases and without visceral metastases, it was found that radiation to the primary disease in men with low metastatic burden improved survival (HR 0.68, 95% CI 0.52–0.90, P = .0098), which is strikingly similar to the result in the postrandomization analysis of the HORRAD study.

Table 10
Oligometastatic prostate cancer

Study	N	Patient Characteristics	Trial Arms	Median Follow-Up (y)	Primary Endpoint	Results
HORRAD[33]	432	Primary bone metastatic PC	ADT vs ADT + RT RT: 70 Gy in 35 fractions or 57.76 in 19 fractions to prostate only	3.9	OS	Overall OS with RT: HR 0.90 95% CI 0.70–1.14 $P = .4$ OS with RT: Low metastatic burden (<5) HR 0.68 95% CI 0.42–1.10 $P = $ NS High metastatic burden (≥5) HR 1.06 95% CI 0.80–1.39 $P = $ NS
STAMPEDE[33]	2061	Newly diagnosed metastatic PC (with no prior radical treatment)	Lifelong ADT + docetaxel ± RT to the primary RT: 36 Gy in 6 weekly fractions of 6 Gy or 55 Gy in 20 fractions to prostate only	3.1	OS	Overall OS with addition of RT: HR 0.92 95% CI 0.80–1.06 $P = .266$ Low metastatic burden: HR 0.68 95% CI 0.52–0.90 $P = .0098$ High metastatic burden: HR 1.07 95% CI 0.90–1.28 $P = $ NS
SABR-COMET[34]	99	Patients with a controlled primary and 1–5 metastatic lesions	Palliative SOC vs SBRT to all lesions SBRT dose/fractionation at discretion of treating physician	2.25	OS	Median OS in SOC arm 28 mo vs SBRT 41 mo, $P = .09$; PFS in SOC arm: 6 mo vs SBRT arm: 12 mo, $P = .001$

Again, the overall study was negative, and given that men were not stratified by metastatic burden before randomization in both the STAMPEDE and the HORRAD trial, prostate RT in men with a low metastatic burden remains hypothesis generating. However, given the possibility that a survival benefit may exist, a discussion of prostate RT in men with a low metastatic burden is indicated.

Finally, the recently presented SABR-COMET study evaluated the role of treatment of oligometastatic disease with high-dose stereotactic body radiation therapy (SBRT) in the setting of a controlled primary.[34] In this randomized phase 2 trial, 99 patients were enrolled with a controlled primary and 1 to 5 metastatic lesions. There were 16 prostate patients included. Patients were randomized to either palliative standard of care versus SBRT to all lesions. After a median follow-up of 2.25 years, median OS was 28 months in the palliative arm versus 41 months in the SBRT arm ($P = .09$). Median PFS was 6 months in the palliative arm versus 12 months in the SBRT arm ($P = .001$). Of note, the median number of oligometastatic sites was 3, reflecting a low burden of metastases. This trial has not yet been published, but given the low number of men with PC (N = 16) and the phase 2 nature of the study, more evidence will be needed before treatment of oligometastatic disease in men with PC with SBRT should be performed off study.

ADJUVANT AND SALVAGE THERAPY IN THE POSTOPERATIVE SETTING

PC that has been managed operatively is staged pathologically based on examination of the resection specimen (ie, prostate and seminal vesicles). Men may have pathologic extension beyond the prostate capsule (pT3a), extension into the seminal vesicles (pT3b), or invasion into rectum/bladder (pT4). Men may also be found to have positive margins (R1) on the resection specimen. Based on evidence from prospective randomized trials, men may either be managed with upfront adjuvant RT if they have pT3a/pT3b or R1 disease found at RP or salvage RT when evidence of PSA recurrence (defined per the American Urological Association guidelines as a serum PSA of ≥0.2 ng/mL, which is confirmed by a second determination with a PSA ≥0.2 ng/mL) presents.

There are 3 clinical trials that evaluated the impact of adjuvant RT on progression (Table 11), all of which show an approximate halving of progression with the use of adjuvant RT.[8,9] Despite this level 1 data, referrals for adjuvant RT in postprostatectomy patients have declined over time[35] for several reasons. For one, the SWOG study was the only trial that demonstrated an OS benefit with upfront adjuvant radiotherapy. In addition, the modern use of ultrasensitive PSA, which was not routinely available in the SWOG study given it was conducted during the pre-PSA to early PSA era, has changed the ability to detect a PSA recurrence earlier. In the observation arm of the SWOG study, most men did not have PSA monitoring, because many were watched until they were clinically symptomatic and/or had radiographic evidence of progression. Whether a survival benefit for upfront adjuvant RT in the modern era with ultrasensitive PSAs will be realized is being evaluated by the ongoing RADICALS (NCT00541047) and RAVES (NCT00860652) trials. The RADICALS trial is being performed in the United Kingdom and randomizes men with adverse pathologic features to upfront RT within 6 months after RP versus RT after either 2 rising PSAs and a PSA greater than 0.1 ng/mL or 3 consecutive rising PSAs. In addition, this trial is addressing the utility of hormonal therapy in addition to RT with a second randomization at the time of decision to initiate RT between no ADT, 6 months ADT, versus 2 years ADT. The RAVES trial is being performed in Australia, randomizing men to RT within 4 months of prostatectomy versus RT within 4 months after a documented PSA greater than 0.2; this trial is powered for its primary endpoint of biochemical PFS.

Table 11
Adjuvant and salvage therapy in the postoperative setting

Study	N	Patient Characteristics	Trial Arms	Median Follow-Up (y)	Primary Endpoint	Results
EORTC 22911[9]	1005	pT3 or positive margins	RT (60 Gy/30 fractions) vs observation	10.6	bPFS	bPFS: Adjuvant RT HR 0.49 95% CI 0.41–0.59 P<.0001
SWOG 8794[8]	431	pT3 or positive margins	RT (60–64 Gy/30–32 fractions) vs observation	12.6	Metastasis-free survival	Metastasis-free survival: Adjuvant RT HR 0.71 95% CI 0.54–0.94 P = .02 OS: HR 0.72 95% CI 0.55–0.96 P = .02
ARO 9602[8,9]	388	pT3 or positive margins	RT (60 Gy/30 fractions) vs observation	9.3	bPFS	bPFS: Adj RT HR 0.51 95% CI 0.37–0.70 P<.0001
RTOG 9601[36]	761	Elevated PSA postprostatectomy	RT 64.8 Gy/36 fractions ± 150 mg bicalutamide for 2 y	13	OS	OS: RT + ADT HR 0.77 95% CI 0.59–0.99 P = .04
GETUG-AFU 16[37]	743	Elevated PSA postprostatectomy	RT 66 Gy/37 fractions ± LHRH agonist for 6 mo	5.25	PFS	PFS: RT + ADT HR 0.50 95% CI 0.38–0.66 P<.0001

With respect to salvage radiotherapy, 2 recently published randomized trials address the utility of ADT along with radiation in this setting (see **Table 11**). The first is RTOG 9601,[36] which randomized 840 men with elevated PSA following prostatectomy to RT alone or RT plus ADT with bicalutamide (150 mg daily) for 2 years. Included in the final analysis were 761 men. At a median follow-up of 13 years, the actuarial OS rate at 12 years was improved in men receiving adjuvant bicalutamide (76% vs 71%, HR 0.77, 95% CI 0.59–0.99, $P = .04$). Death from PC was also improved at 12 years (5.8% vs 13.4%, HR 0.49, 95% CI 0.32–0.74, $P<.001$). However, the incidence of gynecomastia was increased compared with placebo (69.7% vs 10.9%, $P<.001$). The GETUG-AFU 16 trial randomized 743 men with elevated PSA postprostatectomy to RT alone versus RT and 6 months of Luteinizing hormone-releasing hormone (LHRH) agonist.[37] Median follow-up is 5.25 years and demonstrated a DFS benefit with the addition of the LHRH agonist (80% vs 62%, HR 0.50, 95% CI 0.38–0.66, $P<.0001$) but does not demonstrate an OS benefit (HR 0.66, $P = .18$); however, this may be due to the shorter follow-up time compared with RTOG 9601. In general, practice has thus evolved to the use of 6 months of an LHRH agonist along with RT in the salvage setting, particularly given the gynecomastia rate in the RTOG 9601 study and that it remains unknown as to whether 150 mg of bicalutamide daily for 2 years is noninferior to 6 months of an LHRH agonist with respect to DFS and OS.

Finally, the question remains with respect to the impact of pelvic lymph node radiation in the postoperative salvage setting. RTOG 0534 (NCT00567580) randomized 1736 men with pT2 or pT3, R0 or R1, N0 and Gleason score 9 or less to prostate bed RT alone, prostate bed RT + ADT (LHRH agonist injection for a total of 4–6 months), or prostate bed + nodal RT + ADT. The endpoint was failure-free survival. It has been presented in abstract form at ASTRO 2018 with a median follow-up of 5.4 years.[38] Among men who received 4 to 6 months of ADT, pelvic lymph node RT was superior to prostate bed RT with respect to PFS (ie, PSA nadir + 2 or local failure, regional failure or distant failure or death from any cause). Upon postrandomization analysis stratifying men based on PSA cutoffs, it was demonstrated that there may be a benefit to nodal irradiation in men with PSA greater than 0.34 ng/mL as compared with men with a PSA less than 0.34, which is hypothesis generating, given that men were stratified before randomization by a PSA level of 0.1 to 1.0 versus greater than 1.0 to less than 2.0 ng/mL. Before final recommendation for pelvic lymph node RT can be made, more follow-up will be needed to ascertain the impact on metastasis free and PCSM.

REFERENCES

1. Siegel RL, Miller KD, Jemal A. Cancer statistics, 2019. CA Cancer J Clin 2019; 69(1):7–34.

2. Network, N.C.C. Prostate cancer (version 1.2019). Available at: https://www.nccn.org/professionals/physician_gls/pdf/prostate.pdf. Accessed January 15, 2019.

3. Sanda MG, Cadeddu JA, Kirby E, et al. Clinically localized prostate cancer: AUA/ASTRO/SUO guideline. Part I: risk stratification, shared decision making, and care options. J Urol 2018;199(3):683–90.

4. Bekelman JE, Rumble RB, Chen RC, et al. Clinically localized prostate cancer: ASCO clinical practice guideline endorsement of an American Urological Association/American Society for Radiation Oncology/Society of Urologic Oncology Guideline. J Clin Oncol 2018. JCO1800606. [Epub ahead of print].

5. Sanda MG, Cadeddu JA, Kirby E, et al. Clinically localized prostate cancer: AUA/ASTRO/SUO guideline. Part II: recommended approaches and details of specific care options. J Urol 2018;199(4):990–7.
6. Dall'Era MA, Albertsen PC, Bangma C, et al. Active surveillance for prostate cancer: a systematic review of the literature. Eur Urol 2012;62(6):976–83.
7. Delongchamps NB, Singh A, Haas GP. The role of prevalence in the diagnosis of prostate cancer. Cancer Control 2006;13(3):158–68.
8. Sathianathen NJ, Konety BR, Crook J, et al. Landmarks in prostate cancer. Nat Rev Urol 2018;15(10):627–42.
9. Litwin MS, Tan HJ. The diagnosis and treatment of prostate cancer: a review. JAMA 2017;317(24):2532–42.
10. Hu JC, Gu X, Litsitz SR, et al. Comparative effectiveness of minimally invasive vs open radical prostatectomy. JAMA 2009;302(14):1557–64.
11. Trinh QD, Bjartell A, Freedland SJ, et al. A systematic review of the volume-outcome relationship for radical prostatectomy. Eur Urol 2013;64(5):786–98.
12. Michalski JM, Moughan J, Purdy J, et al. Effect of standard vs dose-escalated radiation therapy for patients with intermediate-risk prostate cancer: the NRG oncology RTOG 0126 randomized clinical trial. JAMA Oncol 2018;4(6):e180039.
13. Zumsteg ZS, Spratt DE, Pei I, et al. A new risk classification system for therapeutic decision making with intermediate-risk prostate cancer patients undergoing dose-escalated external-beam radiation therapy. Eur Urol 2013;64(6):895–902.
14. Keane FK, Chen MH, Zhang D, et al. Androgen deprivation therapy and the risk of death from prostate cancer among men with favorable or unfavorable intermediate-risk disease. Cancer 2015;121(16):2713–9.
15. Royce TJ, Lee DH, Keum N, et al. Conventional versus hypofractionated radiation therapy for localized prostate cancer: a meta-analysis of randomized noninferiority trials. Eur Urol Focus 2019;5(4):577–84.
16. Hoffman KE, Voong KR, Levy LB, et al. Randomized trial of hypofractionated, dose-escalated, intensity-modulated radiation therapy (IMRT) versus conventionally fractionated IMRT for localized prostate cancer. J Clin Oncol 2018;36(29):2943–9.
17. Dubray BM, Salleron J, Guerif SG, et al. Does short-term androgen depletion add to high dose radiotherapy (80 Gy) in localized intermediate risk prostate cancer? Final analysis of GETUG 14 randomized trial. J Clin Oncol 2016;34(Suppl 15).
18. Nabid A, Carrier N, Martin AG, et al. Duration of androgen deprivation therapy in high-risk prostate cancer: a randomized phase III trial. Eur Urol 2018;74(4):432–41.
19. Albertsen P. Androgen deprivation in prostate cancer–step by step. N Engl J Med 2009;360(24):2572–4.
20. Fang LC, Merrick GS, Wallner KE. Androgen deprivation therapy: a survival benefit or detriment in men with high-risk prostate cancer? Oncology (Williston Park) 2010;24(9):790–6, 798.
21. Morris WJ, Tyldesley S, Rodda S, et al. Androgen suppression combined with elective nodal and dose escalated radiation therapy (the ASCENDE-RT trial): an analysis of survival endpoints for a randomized trial comparing a low-dose-rate brachytherapy boost to a dose-escalated external beam boost for high- and intermediate-risk prostate cancer. Int J Radiat Oncol Biol Phys 2017;98(2):275–85.
22. Rodda S, Tyldesley S, Morris WJ, et al. ASCENDE-RT: an analysis of treatment-related morbidity for a randomized trial comparing a low-dose-rate brachytherapy boost with a dose-escalated external beam boost for high- and

intermediate-risk prostate cancer. Int J Radiat Oncol Biol Phys 2017;98(2): 286–95.

23. Kishan AU, Cook RR, Ciezki JP, et al. Radical prostatectomy, external beam radiotherapy, or external beam radiotherapy with brachytherapy boost and disease progression and mortality in patients with Gleason score 9-10 prostate cancer. JAMA 2018;319(9):896–905.

24. Rosenthan SA, Hu C, Sartor O, et al. Effect of chemotherapy with docetaxel with androgen suppression and radiotherapy for localized high-risk prostate cancer: the randomized phase III NRG oncology RTOG 0521 trial. J Clin Oncol 2019; 37(14):1159–68.

25. Kellokumpu-Lehtinen P-LI, Hjalm-Eriksson M, Astrom L, et al. A randomized phase III trial between adjuvant docetaxel and surveillance after radical radiotherapy for intermediate and high risk prostate cancer: results of SPCG-13 trial. J Clin Oncol 2018;36(15_suppl):5000.

26. Lawton CA, DeSilvio M, Roach M, et al. An update of the phase III trial comparing whole pelvic to prostate only radiotherapy and neoadjuvant to adjuvant total androgen suppression: updated analysis of RTOG 94-13, with emphasis on unexpected hormone/radiation interactions. Int J Radiat Oncol Biol Phys 2007; 69(3):646–55.

27. Pommier P, Chabaud S, Lagrange JL, et al. Is there a role for pelvic irradiation in localized prostate adenocarcinoma? Update of the long-term survival results of the GETUG-01 randomized study. Int J Radiat Oncol Biol Phys 2016;96(4): 759–69.

28. Schuster DM, Savir-Baruch B, Nieh PT, et al. Detection of recurrent prostate carcinoma with anti-1-amino-3-18F-fluorocyclobutane-1-carboxylic acid PET/CT and 111In-capromab pendetide SPECT/CT. Radiology 2011;259(3):852–61.

29. Seisen T, Vetterlein MW, Karabon P, et al. Efficacy of local treatment in prostate cancer patients with clinically pelvic lymph node-positive disease at initial diagnosis. Eur Urol 2017 [pii:S0302-2838(17)30697-8].

30. Abdollah F, Karnes RJ, Suardi N, et al. Impact of adjuvant radiotherapy on survival of patients with node-positive prostate cancer. J Clin Oncol 2014;32(35): 3939–47.

31. Attar RM, Takimoto CH, Gottardis MM. Castration-resistant prostate cancer: locking up the molecular escape routes. Clin Cancer Res 2009;15(10):3251–5.

32. Damodaran S, Kyriakopoulos CE, Jarrard DF. Newly diagnosed metastatic prostate cancer: has the paradigm changed? Urol Clin North Am 2017;44(4):611–21.

33. Slaoui A, Albisinni S, Aoun F, et al. A systematic review of contemporary management of oligometastatic prostate cancer: fighting a challenge or tilting at windmills? World J Urol 2019 [pii:S0302-2838(17)30697-8].

34. Palma DA, Olsen RA, Harrow S, et al. Stereotactic ablative radiation therapy for the comprehensive treatment of oligometastatic tumors (SABR-COMET): results of a randomized trial. Int J Radiat Oncol Biol Phys 2018;102(3):S3–4.

35. Sineshaw HM, Gray PJ, Efstathiou JA, et al. Declining use of radiotherapy for adverse features after radical prostatectomy: results from the National Cancer Data Base. Eur Urol 2015;68(5):768–74.

36. Shipley WU, Seiferheld W, Lukka HR, et al. Radiation with or without antiandrogen therapy in recurrent prostate cancer. N Engl J Med 2017;376(5):417–28.

37. Carrie C, Hasbini A, de Laroche G, et al. Salvage radiotherapy with or without short-term hormone therapy for rising prostate-specific antigen concentration after radical prostatectomy (GETUG-AFU 16): a randomised, multicentre, open-label phase 3 trial. Lancet Oncol 2016;17(6):747–56.

38. Pollack A, Karrison TG, Balogh AG Jr, et al. Short term androgen deprivation therapy without or with pelvic lymph node treatment added to prostate bed only salvage radiotherapy: the NRG oncology/RTOG 0534 SPPORT trial. Int J Radiat Oncol Biol Phys 2018;102(5):1605.
39. Fossa SD, Wiklund F, Klepp O, et al. Ten- and 15-yr prostate cancer-specific mortality in patients with nonmetastatic locally advanced or aggressive intermediate prostate cancer, randomized to lifelong endocrine treatment alone or combined with radiotherapy: final results of the Scandinavian Prostate Cancer Group-7. Eur Urol 2016;70(4):684–91.

Gynecologic Malignancies

Gita Suneja, MD, MSHP[a],*, Akila Viswanathan, MD, MPH, MSc[b]

KEYWORDS

- Uterine cancer • Cervical cancer • Vulvar cancer • Intensity modulated radiotherapy
- Image guidance • Brachytherapy

KEY POINTS

- Gynecologic malignancies are among the most prevalent cancers affecting women worldwide, but they are heterogeneous diseases with varying risk factors, management paradigms, and outcomes.
- Gynecologic cancers mediated by human papillomavirus (HPV) are preventable and curable with early detection and treatment. The public health importance of cancer prevention measures cannot be overstated, because dramatic reductions in cervical cancer incidence and mortality have been achieved through cancer screening and HPV vaccination.
- Radiotherapy plays a central role in the management of gynecologic malignancies. For some cancers, radiotherapy alone can be curative. More often, radiotherapy is used in conjunction with surgery and systemic therapy to improve locoregional control and extend overall survival.

INTRODUCTION

Gynecologic malignancies are among the most prevalent cancers affecting women worldwide, but they are heterogeneous diseases with varying risk factors, management paradigms, and outcomes.[1] Gynecologic cancers mediated by human papillomavirus (HPV) are preventable and curable with early detection and treatment. The public health importance of cancer prevention measures cannot be overstated, because dramatic reductions in cervical cancer incidence and mortality have been achieved through cancer screening and HPV vaccination.

Disclosure: G. Suneja is supported by grants K08CA228631 and P30AI064518 from the US National Institutes of Health. A. Viswanathan receives textbook royalties from Spring and is the National Cancer Institute Uterine Task Force Chair.

[a] Department of Radiation Oncology, University of Utah, 1950 Circle of Hope, Salt Lake City, UT 84112, USA; [b] Department of Radiation Oncology and Molecular Radiation Sciences, Johns Hopkins Medicine, Johns Hopkins Kimmel Cancer Center, The Weinberg Building, 401 North Broadway, Room 1454, Baltimore, MD 21287, USA
* Corresponding author.
E-mail address: Gita.suneja@icloud.com
twitter: @GitaSuneja (G.S.); anv@jhu.edu (A.V.)

Radiotherapy plays a central role in the management of gynecologic malignancies. For some cancers, radiotherapy alone can be curative. More often, radiotherapy is used in conjunction with surgery and systemic therapy to improve locoregional control and extend overall survival. Gynecologic radiation oncology has undergone major advances in treatment planning and delivery. This article reviews the most common gynecologic malignancies seen by radiation oncologists (uterine, cervix, and vulvar) and discusses innovative radiotherapy paradigms.

Uterine Cancer

Uterine cancer is the most common gynecologic malignancy in the United States, with more than 60,000 cases diagnosed per year (**Fig. 1**).[2] Risk factors for endometrial cancer include excess estrogen exposure, either endogenous (eg, obesity) or exogenous (eg, estrogen replacement).[3] In addition, women with hereditary nonpolyposis colorectal cancer syndrome (Lynch syndrome) have a significantly higher lifetime risk of developing uterine cancer, necessitating screening or other risk reduction strategies.[4] Most women with uterine cancer are diagnosed at an early stage because the classic symptom of postmenopausal bleeding develops early in the disease course. The most common histologic variant is endometrioid carcinoma, which has a favorable prognosis. Other histologies, such as carcinosarcoma, serous, and clear cell, have a worse prognosis.

Evaluation and staging

Evaluation for cancer should be performed for any woman with abnormal uterine bleeding.[5] Endometrial biopsy is the primary evaluation method. Transvaginal ultrasonography may be useful to characterize endometrial thickness, but is not an alternative to tissue sampling. The diagnosis is made histologically after evaluation of biopsy, curettage, or hysterectomy pathology. Uterine cancer is surgically staged with the International Federation of Gynecology and Obstetrics (FIGO) 2009 system or the American Joint Committee on Cancer (AJCC) 2017 system (**Table 1**).[6,7] Historically, the preferred staging procedure has been total hysterectomy, bilateral salpingo-oophorectomy, and lymphadenectomy, although more recently sentinel lymph node biopsy has gained favor for lymph node evaluation.[8,9] Additional surgical advances, including minimally invasive surgery (eg, laparoscopy, robotic), have decreased operative morbidity.[10,11]

Low risk

For endometrioid carcinoma, risk of recurrence is determined primarily by pathologic stage and histologic grade. Other factors contributing to recurrence risk include age, depth of invasion, and lymphovascular space invasion (LVSI). For women with endometrium-confined disease and low-grade tumors, surgery alone can be curative and adjuvant therapy is generally not indicated.[12]

Intermediate risk

Women with intermediate-risk disease (stage I with myometrial invasion or stage II with cervical stromal invasion) are candidates for adjuvant radiotherapy with external beam or vaginal brachytherapy, particularly if they have risk factors including older age, outer half myometrial invasion, grade 2 or 3 histology, or LVSI.[12] Chemotherapy is also considered for women at the highest end of the intermediate-risk spectrum. The optimal adjuvant management of early-stage, high-intermediate–risk, and high-risk disease is debated (**Fig. 2**). The authors recommend multidisciplinary discussion and sharing decision making taking patient preferences into account.

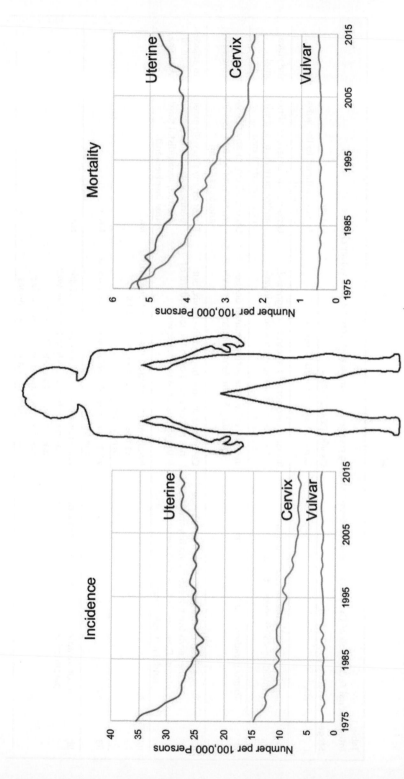

Fig. 1. United States incidence and mortality over time (*Data from* National Cancer Institute. Cancer Stat Facts 2016. Available at: https://seer.cancer.gov/statfacts/. Accessed May 3 2019.)

Table 1
International Federation of Gynecology and Obstetrics staging comparison for uterine, cervical, and vulvar cancers

Stage	Uterine (FIGO 2009)	Cervix (FIGO 2018)	Vulvar
I	NA	Carcinoma is confined to cervix	Tumor confined to the vulva and/or perineum
IA	Tumor limited to the endometrium or invading <50% myometrium	Invasive carcinoma that can be diagnosed only by microscopy, with a depth invasion of <5 mm	Lesions 2 cm or less, confined to the vulva and/or perineum, and with stromal invasion of ≤1 mm
IB	Tumor invading ≥50% myometrium	Invasive carcinoma with measured deepest invasion ≥5 mm, lesion limited to cervix	Lesions >2 cm, or any size with stromal invasion of >1 mm, confined to the vulva and/or perineum
II	Tumor invading the stromal connective tissue of the cervix but not extending beyond the uterus. Does not include endocervical glandular involvement	Carcinoma invades beyond the cervix, but has not extended onto the lower third of the vagina or to the pelvic wall	Tumor of any size with extension to adjacent perineal structures (lower/distal third of urethra, lower/distal third of the vagina, anal involvement)
IIA	NA	Involvement limited to the upper two-thirds of the vagina without parametrial involvement	NA
IIB	NA	With parametrial involvement but not up to the pelvic wall	NA
III	Tumor invading serosa, adnexa, vagina, or parametrium	Carcinoma involves the lower third of the vagina and/or extends to the pelvic wall and/or causes hydronephrosis or nonfunctioning kidney and/or involves pelvic and/or para-aortic lymph nodes	NA

Stage			
IIIA	Tumor involving the serosa and/or adnexa (direct extension or metastasis)	Carcinoma involves the lower third of the vagina, with no extension to the pelvic wall	Regional lymph node metastasis with 1 or 2 lymph node metastases each <5 mm, or 1 lymph node metastasis ≥5 mm, or lymph nodes with extranodal extension
IIIB	Vaginal involvement (direct extension or metastasis) or parametrial involvement	Extension to the pelvic wall and/or hydronephrosis or nonfunctioning kidney	Three or more lymph node metastases each <5 mm or 2 or more lymph node metastases ≥5 mm
IIIC	Regional lymph node metastasis to pelvic lymph nodes or to para-aortic lymph nodes	Involvement of pelvic and/or para-aortic lymph nodes, irrespective of tumor size and extent	Lymph nodes with extranodal extension
IV	NA	The carcinoma has extended beyond the true pelvis or has involved (biopsy proven) the mucosa or the bladder or rectum	Tumor of any size with extension to any of the following: upper/proximal two-thirds of the urethra, upper/proximal two-thirds of the vagina, bladder mucosa, or rectal mucosa; or fixed to the pelvic bone
IVA	Tumor invading the bladder mucosa and/or bowel mucosa (bullous edema is not sufficient to classify a tumor as T4)	Spread to adjacent pelvic organs	Tumor of any size with extension to any of the following: upper/proximal two-thirds of the urethra, upper/proximal two-thirds of the vagina, bladder mucosa, or rectal mucosa; or fixed to the pelvic bone
IVB	Distant metastasis	Spread to distant organs	Distant metastasis (including pelvic lymph node metastasis)

This table was generated using the FIGO 2009 and FIGO 2018 systems.

Abbreviation: NA, not available.

Adapted from Creasman W. Revised FIGO staging for carcinoma of the endometrium. Int J Gynaecol Obstet 2009;105(2):109-109; and Bhatla N, Aoki D, Sharma DN, et al. Cancer of the cervix uteri. Int J Gynaecol Obstet 2018;143 Suppl 2:24; with permission.

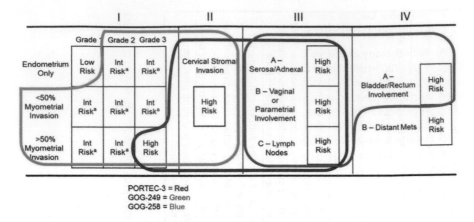

PORTEC-3 = Red
GOG-249 = Green
GOG-258 = Blue

Based on inclusion criteria for PORTEC-3, GOG-249and GOG-258.

Fig. 2. Uterine cancer risk groups and modern clinical trials landscape. [a] May be high-intermediate risk based on other risk factors, including age, LVSI, and tumor size. GOG, Gynecologic Oncology Group; HR, high risk; IR, intermediate risk; LR, low risk; PORTEC, Post Operative Radiation Therapy in Endometrial Carcinoma. (*Data from* Refs.[13–17])

Vaginal brachytherapy plus chemotherapy versus pelvic radiotherapy The Gynecologic Oncology Group (GOG)-249 study randomized 601 women posthysterectomy to vaginal brachytherapy followed by 3 cycles of chemotherapy or pelvic radiotherapy alone.[13,14] Recently published results show that 5-year recurrence-free survival and overall survival are comparable between study arms. Nodal recurrences and adverse events (mainly hematologic) were more common in the vaginal brachytherapy plus chemotherapy group, but late toxicities were comparable.

Chemotherapy versus no adjuvant therapy The European Network for Gynaecological Oncological Trials- EN2-Danish Gynecological Cancer Group (ENGOT-EN2-DGCG) study is currently enrolling women with stage I serous, clear cell, or grade 3 tumors with negative nodes following hysterectomy. Patients are randomized to 6 cycles of carboplatin and paclitaxel or no adjuvant therapy. Vaginal brachytherapy is optional on either arm, but pelvic radiotherapy is not allowed.

Molecular risk stratification There is substantial enthusiasm for tumor-specific molecular testing as a predictor of locoregional recurrence in addition to clinical-pathologic features. Post Operative Radiation Therapy in Endometrial Carcinoma - 4 (PORTEC-4) is currently randomizing women with early-stage, high-intermediate–risk disease to either adjuvant vaginal brachytherapy or treatment based on a validated molecular profile (low risk, observation; intermediate risk, vaginal brachytherapy; unfavorable risk, pelvic external beam radiotherapy [EBRT]). The primary end point is vaginal recurrence at 5 years.

High risk
Women with high-risk endometrial cancer, including stage III/IV or any stage serous/clear cell histology, are generally treated with adjuvant chemotherapy plus or minus radiotherapy. The role of radiotherapy in this high-risk population is being evaluated in ongoing clinical trials (see **Fig. 2**). Given the rapidly evolving landscape with imminent publications of ongoing trials, the authors recommend referencing the National

Comprehensive Cancer Network (NCCN; https://www.nccn.org/) guidelines for the most up-to-date management approaches.

Pelvic radiotherapy alone versus chemoradiation The PORTEC-3 study enrolled 686 women with high-risk stage I (defined as 1B grade 3 and/or LVSI), stage II, or stage III disease, or tumors with serous/clear cell histology.[15,16] Women were randomized to chemoradiation (concurrent cisplatin for 2 cycles during radiotherapy, followed by carboplatin/paclitaxel for 4 cycles) or pelvic radiotherapy alone. Five-year failure-free survival was higher in the chemoradiotherapy group, with greater benefit among those with stage III disease. No significant difference in overall survival was observed. Grade 3 adverse events, mostly hematologic, were more common in the chemoradiation group.

Chemoradiation versus chemotherapy alone The GOG-258 study enrolled more than 700 women with stage III to IVA or stage I/II serous or clear cell uterine cancers following surgery.[17] They were randomized to chemoradiation (concurrent cisplatin followed by 4 cycles of carboplatin and paclitaxel) or chemotherapy alone (carboplatin/paclitaxel for 6 cycles). Recently published results show no difference in relapse-free survival or overall survival between the two groups at 5-year follow-up. In the chemoradiotherapy arm, there were fewer vaginal recurrence and nodal relapses, as well more distant recurrences. Rates of toxicities were similar, but quality of life was inferior in the chemoradiotherapy group.[18]

Optimal sequencing of chemotherapy and radiotherapy
With new data emerging and practice paradigms evolving, the optimal sequencing of chemotherapy and radiotherapy is not known. Substantial practice variation exists and reasonable options include chemotherapy first followed by radiotherapy, concurrent chemoradiotherapy, or a sandwich approach with radiotherapy administered between cycle 3 and 4 of chemotherapy. A recent analysis of national tumor registry data shows that most women receiving chemoradiotherapy initiate chemotherapy before radiotherapy.[19]

Outcomes
Survival for endometrial carcinoma varies from 80% to 90% for stage I disease to 20% to 40% for stage IV disease.[3] Prognosis is determined by disease stage, grade, and histology. Following treatment, regular clinical examination is indicated. No routine surveillance imaging or blood work, including cancer antigen 125, has been found to improve outcomes.

Cervical Cancer

Cervical cancer is the third most common gynecologic malignancy in the United States (see **Fig. 1**).[2] Globally, cervical cancer is the second most common type of cancer and cause of death in women.[1,2] Cervical cancer disproportionately affects younger women, leading to significant social and economic impact on individuals, families, and communities. Most cervical cancer is attributable to HPV, primarily subtypes 16 and 18.[20] Risk factors include early-onset sexual activity, multiple sexual partners, history of sexually transmitted infection, and impaired HPV clearance caused by an immunocompromised state (eg, human immunodeficiency virus infection, transplants). Most cervical cancers are of squamous cell histology, and the second most common type is adenocarcinoma. Cervical cancer can be detected in asymptomatic women with appropriate screening; however, as tumors enlarge and spread, they can cause pain, bleeding, and discharge.

Evaluation and staging

Cervical cancer has historically been staged clinically using the FIGO system. Under the new FIGO 2018 system, advanced radiographic imaging (eg, PET/computed tomography [CT] and MRI) and pathology from biopsies are now used to determine stage (see **Table 1**).[21] FIGO 2018 also incorporates nodal status, which is important to optimize management and determine prognosis. MRI is useful to assess local spread of tumor to the adjacent organs, including vagina or parametria.[22] PET/CT is used to evaluate spread to lymph nodes or distant organs.[23]

Early stage

Women with early-stage cervical cancer have less than or equal to 4-cm lesions involving the cervix or upper vagina and no involved lymph nodes. Although both surgery and chemoradiotherapy are treatment options, young women with early-stage disease typically undergo modified radical hysterectomy.[24] A subset of women with early-stage, low-risk disease may be candidates for less extensive surgery, including cone biopsy or extrafascial hysterectomy. Minimally invasive surgery (MIS) and sentinel lymph node biopsy are currently under investigation, with recently published data suggesting survival detriment to MIS.[25,26]

For women with intermediate risk factors following hysterectomy, including tumor greater than or equal to 4 cm, lymphovascular invasion, or cervical stromal invasion, adjuvant radiotherapy is recommended.[24] For women with high-risk features following hysterectomy, including positive nodes, parametrial involvement, or positive margins, adjuvant chemoradiation improves overall survival.[24] Concurrent cisplatin is commonly used, but other chemotherapy options may be used in low-resource settings depending on availability. GOG-263 is an ongoing study examining the role of adjuvant radiation alone versus adjuvant chemoradiotherapy for high-risk, node-negative disease.

Locally advanced

Women with locally advanced cancer have lesions greater than 4 cm on examination, disease extending beyond the cervix and upper vagina (eg, pelvic sidewall, lower third vagina, rectum, bladder), or nodal involvement detected preoperatively. Primary chemoradiotherapy is recommended, including external beam radiation with concurrent cisplatin, followed by brachytherapy.[24] Some clinicians may offer hysterectomy following chemoradiotherapy for patients with initially large tumor or high posttreatment residual disease burden, but this approach does not improve survival. Other approaches for high-volume or residual disease include additional adjuvant chemotherapy. The Gynecologic Cancer Intergroup is currently assessing adjuvant carboplatin/paclitaxel following completion of concurrent chemoradiotherapy in the international phase III OUTBACK study. Immunotherapy for women with persistent, recurrent, or metastatic disease is an area of active investigation. The immune checkpoint inhibitor pembrolizumab has been approved for use in women with disease progression in the setting of advanced-stage cervical cancer.[27] Based on the favorable results of the KEYNOTE-158[28] and CheckMate 358[29] studies, the EMPOWER-Cervical1 study is a randomized phase III study enrolling women with progression or recurrence within 6 months of initial therapy to standard systemic therapy or immunotherapy.

Outcomes

The most important prognostic factor is stage, with survival ranging from 80% to 95% for stage I disease to 16% for stage IVA disease.[20] Other important factors include nodal status, tumor size, and lymphovascular space invasion. Other prognosticators, such as biomarkers including HPV DNA, are currently under investigation. In 1 study of 19 women with HPV-positive invasive squamous cell carcinoma, the presence of detectable plasma HPV DNA at the completion of standard treatment was associated with inferior progression-free survival.[30] Posttreatment surveillance with physical examination is essential with the goal of early detection of recurrence and mitigation of treatment-related toxicity. Posttreatment PET/CT at 3 months postchemoradiotherapy is recommended.[24] Additional imaging is generally reserved for patients with symptoms of recurrence.

Vulvar Cancer

Vulvar cancer is the fourth most common gynecologic malignancy in US women, with approximately 6000 new cases per year.[2] Incidence is increasing in younger women because of the increase in HPV-mediated disease. Vulvar cancer staging comprises tumor size and depth of invasion, determined by (1) physical examination; (2) biopsy/surgical pathology; and (3) lymph node status evaluated by physical examination, imaging, or surgical removal via lymphadenectomy or sentinel lymph node biopsy.[31] Recently published NCCN guidelines highlight modern management approaches.[32]

For early-stage disease, surgical approaches have evolved in favor of vulvar conservation. Radical local excision is preferred for removal of the primary lesion.[32] For large or multifocal lesions, modified radical vulvectomy may be required. Nodal evaluation can be omitted if nodes are clinically negative on examination and stromal invasion is less than or equal to 1 mm (stage IA). For select women with stage IB or II disease, sentinel lymph node biopsy may be performed.[33] All others with clinically negative nodes undergo inguinofemoral lymphadenectomy.

Indications for adjuvant radiotherapy to the vulva include (1) tumor larger than 4 cm, or (2) positive or close margins (defined as ≤8 mm).[34,35] Indications for adjuvant radiotherapy to the lymph nodes include (1) 2 or more lymph nodes, or (2) extracapsular extension.[36] In practice, many experts treat with adjuvant radiotherapy even when a single node is positive because of low salvage rates for women with nodal recurrence.[37] The Groningen International Study on Sentinel Nodes in Vulvar Cancer (GROINS-V-II)/GOG-270 study is investigating completion inguinofemoral lymphadenectomy versus adjuvant radiotherapy in women with early-stage vulvar cancer with a single positive sentinel lymph node.

For women with locally advanced or unresectable disease, concurrent chemoradiotherapy to the vulva and nodes is favored.[32] Some clinicians perform a biopsy at the completion of chemoradiotherapy and consider surgery in the absence of a complete response.[38,39] Others use chemoradiotherapy as definitive treatment, reserving surgery for progressive or recurrent disease.[40,41]

The most important prognostic indicator for survival in women with vulvar cancer is inguinofemoral nodal involvement.[42] Outcomes seem to be improving over time, possibly because of the high radiosensitivity of HPV-positive tumors or because of shifting demographics as women are diagnosed at younger ages and at earlier stages.[43,44] Women treated for vulvar cancer require long-term follow-up with regular physical examination and annual cervical/vaginal cytology.[45]

Modern Radiotherapy Planning

External beam

The use of radiotherapy for gynecologic cancers dates back to the early twentieth century. Major advances including use of photons, CT-based planning, and multileaf collimation allowed higher doses to the target and lower doses to normal tissues. More recent advances, including intensity modulated radiotherapy (IMRT) and volumetric modulated arc therapy (VMAT), have yielded even more adaptive treatment. However, patient positioning, contouring, and setup reproducibility must be addressed to avoid errors with these highly conformal approaches.[46]

Patient immobilization External beam planning begins with proper patient position at the time of simulation. Gynecologic patients are typically immobilized supine in a wing board or Vac-loc bag. For posthysterectomy patients, a vaginal marker can be placed to identify the vaginal apex on CT, although the marker should not displace vaginal tissue. For vulvar radiotherapy, any scars or gross disease should be clearly marked with radio-opaque wires or markers.

Imaging/image fusion Axial CT images are obtained with digital reconstruction in sagittal and coronal planes. Sagittal imaging is particularly useful to verify that appropriate targets have been contoured. Intravenous and/or bowel contrast can be helpful in differentiating nodes from adjacent bowel. For definitive cases, fusion of other diagnostic imaging, including MRI and PET/CT, can be extremely helpful to identify target volumes.[47] If IMRT or other conformal approaches are planned, the patient should be simulated twice, with bladder full and bladder empty. The differences in target position between the bladder full/empty scans are used to generate an internal target volume.

Target delineation/contouring In the two-dimensional (2D) radiotherapy era, radiation fields were designed using bony anatomic landmarks. With the advent of three-dimensional (3D) imaging, target structures should be contoured to ensure radiotherapy field design reflects individual variations in patient anatomy. Target structures for all gynecologic sites are presented in **Table 2**. Normal tissues, including small bowel, bladder, rectum, sigmoid, and femoral heads, are also contoured. Limiting dose to the duodenum is appropriate when para-aortic nodes are being treated.[48] Pelvic bones can be contoured for bone marrow–sparing radiotherapy. For vulvar cancer, recently published consensus guidelines provide contouring recommendations.[49]

Beam arrangement/technique For uterine and cervical cancers, 3D conformal radiotherapy using a 4-field beam arrangement (anteroposterior (AP)-posteroanterior (PA)

Table 2
Primary gynecologic sites and at risk nodal basins to be included in contours for uterine, cervical, and vulvar cancers

Nodal Groups	Uterine	Cervix	Vulvar
Para-aortic	If common iliac nodes involved or uterine fundus involved	If common iliac nodes involved	—
Common iliac	✔	✔	—
External iliac	✔	✔	✔
Internal iliac	✔	✔	✔
Obturator	✔	✔	✔
Sacral	If cervix involved	✔	—
Inguinal	If lower vaginal involved	If lower vaginal involved	✔

and opposed laterals) has been the standard for many years. More recent evidence suggests that IMRT may decrease toxicity while maintaining excellent oncologic outcomes in the postoperative setting. The Radiation Therapy Oncology Group (RTOG) 0418 is a phase II, multi-institutional study that showed IMRT is safe and feasible with appropriate attention to quality assurance.[50] In the randomized TIME-C study, IMRT reduced gastrointestinal and genitourinary toxicity compared with the 4-field approach.[51] However, caution must be applied when extrapolating these results to the definitive setting (eg, uterus, cervix, upper vagina intact), because large variations in target position with bladder and rectal filling may lead to dose alterations with conformal techniques such as IMRT. For vulvar cancer, traditional fields include wide AP and narrow PA fields with supplemental electron dose to the inguinal nodes to achieve target dose while protecting the femoral heads. IMRT is increasingly used for this site, in part because of the reduction in normal tissue toxicity reported in retrospective series and the excellent results seen with use of IMRT for anal cancer.[52]

Dose and schedule A typical EBRT dose/fractionation is 45 to 50.4 Gy delivered at 1.8 Gy per fraction. If gross nodal disease is present, an additional tumor bed boost is recommended, either sequentially or as a simultaneous integrated boost.[53] Similarly, parametrial boost can be prescribed sequentially, as a simultaneous integrated boost, or deferred until after the first brachytherapy fraction dose distribution is reviewed. Integrated boost techniques are newer, with dosimetric and clinical outcomes studies showing favorable efficacy and tolerability.[54-56]

Dose constraints The allowable dose to normal structures is evolving as conformal approaches are increasingly studied. External beam dose constraints used on the EMBRACE II and TIME-C studies are shown in **Table 3**.

On-board imaging Verification of target positioning is critical, particularly with conformal approaches. Kilovoltage imaging matched to bony anatomy is insufficient to capture target variation caused by changes in bladder/rectal filling. Therefore, cone beam CT should be used. Thermoluminescent dosimeters should be used to verify that the prescribed dose is delivered to the vulva and other superficial targets.

Brachytherapy
Brachytherapy planning and delivery have evolved considerably, from the earliest era when radium sources were inserted in the operating room to modern-day use of iridium-192 via remote afterloaders. Applicators can be placed intracavitary (eg, in the vaginal vault following hysterectomy or in the uterus and vaginal fornices for intact cervical or uterine cancer) or interstitial (eg, needles directly in the tissue). This article focuses on brachytherapy for definitive cervical cancer, because this is an active area of investigation.

Definitive brachytherapy For intact cervical cancer, brachytherapy is an essential component of therapy, because administration of brachytherapy significantly improves survival.[57] Direct application of high-dose-rate (HDR) radiation allows delivery of high doses to the gross disease while minimizing the dose to surrounding normal tissues, including the bladder, rectum, and small bowel.

Brachytherapy may be initiated at the completion of EBRT or during EBRT once gross tumor reduction is optimized. Low-dose-rate, pulse-dose-rate, and HDR approaches have been used and seem to have similar efficacy and toxicity. However,

Table 3
External beam targets and normal tissue constraints for postoperative uterine and cervical cancer

	EMBRACE		TIME-C	
Structure	Hard Dose Constraints	Soft Dose Constraints	Per Protocol	Acceptable Variation
Target				
PTV45	V95%>95% Dmax<107%[a]	NA	NA	NA
PTV-N(#)	D98%>90% of prescribed LN dose Dmax<107% of prescribed LN dose	NA	NA	NA
OARs				
Bowel	Dmax<105% (47.3 Gy)[a]	When no lymph node boost: • V40 Gy <100 cm^{3b} • V30 Gy <350 cm^{3b} When lymph node boost or para-aortic irradiation: • V40 Gy <250 cm^{3b} • V30 Gy <500 cm^{3b} Dmax <57.5 Gy	Up to 30% receives 40 Gy	No more than 70% receives 40 Gy
Sigmoid	Dmax<105% (47.3 Gy)[a]	Dmax<57.5 Gy	NA	NA
Bladder	Dmax<105% (47.3 Gy)[a]	V40 Gy <75%[b] V30 Gy <85%[b] Dmax<57.5 Gy	Up to 35% receives 45 Gy	No more than 70% receives 45 Gy
Rectum	Dmax<105% (47.3 Gy)[a]	V40 Gy <85%[b] V30 Gy <95%[b] Dmax<57.5 Gy	Up to 80% receives 40 Gy	<100% receives 40 Gy
Bone marrow	NA	NA	Up to 90% receives 10 Gy	90% does not receive >25 Gy
Bone marrow	NA	NA	Up to 37% receives 40 Gy	Not more than 60% receives 40 Gy
Spinal cord	Dmax<48 Gy	NA	NA	NA
Femoral heads	Dmax<50 Gy	NA	NA	NA
Kidney	Dmean<15 Gy	Dmean<10 Gy	NA	NA
Body	Dmax<107%[a]	—	NA	NA
Vagina PIBS: 2 cm	NA	When vagina not involved: D$_{PIBS-2cm}$<5 Gy	NA	NA
Optional	NA	NA	NA	NA
Ovaries	<5–8 Gy	NA	NA	NA
Duodenum[b]	V55<15 cm^3	NA	NA	NA

Abbreviations: D98%, Dose covering 98% of the volume; Dmax, Maximum dose; Dmean, Mean dose; PIBS, posterior-inferior border of the pubic symphysis; PTV45, planning target volume for 45 Gy; PTV-N, Planning target volume for node; V30 Gy, Volume of tissue receiving 30Gy; V40 Gy, Volume of tissue receiving 40Gy; V55 Gy, Volume of tissue receiving 55 Gy; V95%, Percent volume receiving at least 95% of prescription dose.
[a] In case lymph nodes are not boosted.
[b] Soft constraints are not based on clinical evidence.

HDR has notable advantages compared with low-dose-rate, including decreased dose to staff because of the use of remote afterloaders and the ability to perform procedures in the outpatient setting.

A variety of applicators are available, including intrauterine tandem with vaginal ovoids, cylinder, or ring, all yielding slightly different dose distributions.[58] Specific applicators are selected based on patient anatomy, extent of disease, and physician preference. A more recent advance is the use of interstitial needles in combination with intracavitary applications to further shape and individualize the dose distribution. Placement of needles either with freehand or template techniques can improve dose coverage to large or irregularly shaped targets without increasing dose to the normal structures (**Fig. 3**).[59] Use of advanced MRI technologies, such as real-time MRI tumor tracking, to assist with placement of brachytherapy catheters has shown promising early results.[60] Dose to the bladder and rectum can be reduced by using shielded ovoids or by introducing packing between the normal organs and the applicators, but care must be taken not to displace the applicator from the cervical os during packing.

Although treatments were historically planned using the 2D films and the point-based Manchester system, technical advances have led to increased use of CT and/or MRI for 3D volumetric planning.[57,61] MRI provides much better definition of tissues, thereby allowing adaptive planning as the tumor regresses with each delivered fraction. In 2012, the Groupe Europeen de Curietherapie and the European Society for Radiotherapy and Oncology (GEC-ESTRO) published guidelines for optimal MRI-guided brachytherapy planning target volumes.[62] GEC-ESTRO targets and EMBRACE II dose constraints are provided in **Table 4**.

The total prescription dose is the combined external beam and brachytherapy biologically effective dose, as if it were delivered in 2-Gy fractions (EQD2). EQD2 targets and dose constraints are shown in **Table 4**.

Image-guided brachytherapy improves local control and reduces normal tissue toxicity (**Fig. 4**). The international RetroEMBRACE showed improvements in local control and reduced late toxicity for women with large tumors treated with image-guided brachytherapy relative to historical controls.[63] Early results of the prospective, multi-institutional EMBRACE study have identified improved dose-volume thresholds for urinary and rectal toxicity in women with locally advanced cervical cancer receiving MRI-guided brachytherapy.[64] The currently open EMBRACE II study is further optimizing therapeutic ratio using the latest EBRT and brachytherapy techniques.

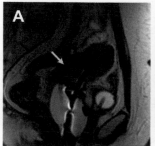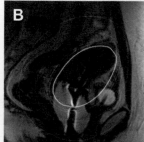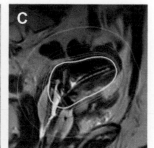

Fig. 3. Brachytherapy dose distribution with and without interstitial needles. (*A*) Gross cervical disease extending posteriorly toward rectum (*arrow*). (*B*) Dose distribution for tandem ovoid plan without interstitial needles. (*C*) Dose distribution with interstitial needles. (*Courtesy of* J. Chino, MD, Durham, NC.)

Table 4
Target definitions and dose constraints for intact cervical cancer brachytherapy

Target	Definition	Constraints
D90 CTV$_{HR}$ EQD2$_{10}$	Adaptive high-risk clinical target volume of the primary tumor	>90 Gy <95 Gy
D98 CTV$_{HR}$ EQD2$_{10}$	Adaptive high-risk clinical target volume of the primary tumor	>75
D98 GTV$_{res}$ EQD2$_{10}$	Residual (high signal) gross tumor volume of the primary tumor	>95 Gy
D98 CTV$_{IR}$ EQD2$_{10}$	Intermediate-risk clinical target volume of the primary tumor	>60 Gy
Point A EQD2$_{10}$	Point located 2 cm superior to the external cervical os and 2 cm lateral to the cervical canal	>65 Gy
OAR		
Bladder D2$_{cm^3}$ EQD2$_3$	Minimum dose in the most exposed 2 cm³ of bladder	<80 Gy
Rectum D2$_{cm^3}$ EQD2$_3$	Minimum dose in the most exposed 2 cm³ of rectum	<65 Gy
Rectovaginal point EQD2$_3$	—	<65 Gy
Sigmoid D2$_{cm^3}$ EQD2$_3$	Minimum dose in the most exposed 2 cm³ of sigmoid	<70 Gy
Bowel D2$_{cm^3}$ EQD2$_3$	Minimum dose in the most exposed 2 cm³ of bowel	<70 Gy

Target definitions are from GEC-ESTRO and dose constraints are from EMBRACE II.

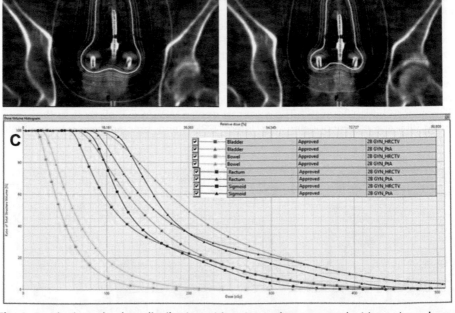

Fig. 4. Brachytheraphy dose distribution with point A plan compared with a volume-based plan. (*A*) Point A plan showing unnecessary dose to normal structures. (*B*) Volume-based plan conforming to high-risk clinical target volume (CTV) with minimal normal tissue exposure. (*C*) Dose/volume histogram comparing the 2 plans. High-risk CTV contoured in red. Planning was performed using CT and MRI, but only CT is shown here to highlight high-risk CTV contour. HRCTV, High risk clinical target volume.

Additional resources may be found at the American Brachytherapy Society Web site (www.americanbrachytherapy.org).

Despite these excellent results, use of brachytherapy is declining in the United States.[65,66] Stereotactic body radiotherapy (SBRT) boost is investigational, but the available data suggest worse outcomes with nonbrachytherapy approaches.[57] To date, no studies directly comparing SBRT with brachytherapy have been published.

SUMMARY

This article summarizes the role of radiotherapy in the management of uterine, cervical, and vulvar cancers with an emphasis on data from recent clinical trials. Modern technology, including IMRT and image-guided brachytherapy, offers greater precision to targeting tumor while reducing doses to organs at risk. Improvements in quality, safety, and efficacy of radiotherapy, in conjunction with advances in surgical approaches and systemic therapies, have the potential to translate into improved patient outcomes and more personalized gynecologic cancer care.

ACKNOWLEDGMENTS

The authors acknowledge Noelani Ho for her contributions toward preparation of the article, tables, and figures, and Oana Craciunescu, PhD, for her assistance with the images in this article.

REFERENCES

1. Bray F, Ferlay J, Soerjomataram I, et al. Global cancer statistics 2018: GLOBO-CAN estimates of incidence and mortality worldwide for 36 cancers in 185 countries. CA Cancer J Clin 2018;68(6):394–424.
2. Siegel RL, Miller KD, Jemal A. Cancer statistics, 2018. CA Cancer J Clin 2018; 68(1):7–30.
3. Morice P, Leary A, Creutzberg C, et al. Endometrial cancer. Lancet 2016; 387(10023):1094–108.
4. Lancaster JM, Powell CB, Chen LM, et al. Society of Gynecologic Oncology statement on risk assessment for inherited gynecologic cancer predispositions. Gynecol Oncol 2015;136(1):3–7.
5. ACOG committee opinion no. 557: management of acute abnormal uterine bleeding in nonpregnant reproductive-aged women. Obstet Gynecol 2013; 121(4):891–6.
6. Creasman W. Revised FIGO staging for carcinoma of the endometrium. Int J Gynaecol Obstet 2009;105(2):109.
7. McMeekin D, Benedet J, Broaddus R, et al. Corpus uteri. In: Stephen E, Byrd D, Compton C, et al, editors. AJCC cancer staging handbook. 7 edition. New York: Springer-Verlag; 2010. p. 718.
8. Rossi EC, Kowalski LD, Scalici J, et al. A comparison of sentinel lymph node biopsy to lymphadenectomy for endometrial cancer staging (FIRES trial): a multicentre, prospective, cohort study. Lancet Oncol 2017;18(3):384–92.
9. Holloway RW, Abu-Rustum NR, Backes FJ, et al. Sentinel lymph node mapping and staging in endometrial cancer: A Society of Gynecologic Oncology literature review with consensus recommendations. Gynecol Oncol 2017;146(2):405–15.
10. Mäenpää MM, Nieminen K, Tomás EI, et al. Robotic-assisted vs traditional laparoscopic surgery for endometrial cancer: a randomized controlled trial. Am J Obstet Gynecol 2016;215(5):588.e1-7.

11. Janda M, Gebski V, Davies LC, et al. Effect of total laparoscopic hysterectomy vs total abdominal hysterectomy on disease-free survival among women with stage I Endometrial Cancer: A Randomized Clinical Trial Laparoscopic vs Abdominal Hysterectomy for Stage I Endometrial Cancer Laparoscopic vs Abdominal Hysterectomy for Stage I Endometrial Cancer. JAMA 2017;317(12):1224–33.

12. Koh WJ, Abu-Rustum NR, Bean S, et al. Uterine neoplasms, version 1.2018, NCCN clinical practice guidelines in oncology. J Natl Compr Canc Netw 2018; 16(2):170–99.

13. McMeekin DS, Filiaci VL, Aghajanian C, et al. 1A randomized phase III trial of pelvic radiation therapy (PXRT) versus vaginal cuff brachytherapy followed by paclitaxel/carboplatin chemotherapy (VCB/C) in patients with high risk (HR), early stage endometrial cancer (EC): A Gynecologic Oncology Group trial. Gynecol Oncol 2014;134(2):438.

14. Randall ME, Filiaci V, McMeekin DS, et al. Phase III Trial: adjuvant pelvic radiation therapy versus vaginal brachytherapy plus paclitaxel/carboplatin in high-intermediate and high-risk early stage endometrial cancer. J Clin Oncol 2019; 37(21):1810–8.

15. de Boer SM, Powell ME, Mileshkin L, et al. Adjuvant chemoradiotherapy versus radiotherapy alone for women with high-risk endometrial cancer (PORTEC-3): final results of an international, open-label, multicentre, randomised, phase 3 trial. Lancet Oncol 2018;19(3):295–309.

16. de Boer SM, Powell ME, Mileshkin L, et al. Toxicity and quality of life after adjuvant chemoradiotherapy versus radiotherapy alone for women with high-risk endometrial cancer (PORTEC-3): an open-label, multicentre, randomised, phase 3 trial. Lancet Oncol 2016;17(8):1114–26.

17. Matei D, Filiaci VL, Randall M, et al. A randomized phase III trial of cisplatin and tumor volume directed irradiation followed by carboplatin and paclitaxel vs. carboplatin and paclitaxel for optimally debulked, advanced endometrial carcinoma. J Clin Oncol 2017;35(15_suppl):5505.

18. Matei D, Filiaci V, Randall ME, et al. Adjuvant Chemotherapy plus Radiation for Locally Advanced Endometrial Cancer. N Engl J Med 2019;380(24):2317–26.

19. Goodman CR, Hatoum S, Seagle B-LL, et al. Association of chemotherapy and radiotherapy sequence with overall survival in locoregionally advanced endometrial cancer. Gynecol Oncol 2019;153(1):41–8.

20. Cohen PA, Jhingran A, Oaknin A, et al. Cervical cancer. Lancet 2019;393(10167): 169–82.

21. Bhatla N, Aoki D, Sharma DN, et al. Cancer of the cervix uteri. Int J Gynaecol Obstet 2018;143(Suppl 2):22–36.

22. Woo S, Suh CH, Kim SY, et al. Magnetic resonance imaging for detection of parametrial invasion in cervical cancer: An updated systematic review and meta-analysis of the literature between 2012 and 2016. Eur Radiol 2018;28(2):530–41.

23. Gee MS, Atri M, Bandos AI, et al. Identification of distant metastatic disease in uterine cervical and endometrial cancers with FDG PET/CT: analysis from the ACRIN 6671/GOG 0233 multicenter trial. Radiology 2018;287(1):176–84.

24. Koh WJ, Abu-Rustum NR, Bean S, et al. Cervical cancer, version 3.2019, NCCN clinical practice guidelines in oncology. J Natl Compr Canc Netw 2019;17(1): 64–84.

25. Ramirez PT, Frumovitz M, Pareja R, et al. Minimally invasive versus abdominal radical hysterectomy for cervical cancer. N Engl J Med 2018;379(20):1895–904.

26. Melamed A, Margul DJ, Chen L, et al. Survival after minimally invasive radical hysterectomy for early-stage cervical cancer. N Engl J Med 2018;379(20): 1905–14.

27. U.S. Food & Drug Administration. FDA approves pembrolizumab for advanced cervical cancer with disease progression during or after chemotherapy. 2019. Available at: https://www.fda.gov/drugs/informationondrugs/approveddrugs/ucm610572.htm.

28. Chung HC, Ros W, Delord JP, et al. Efficacy and safety of pembrolizumab in previously treated advanced cervical cancer: results from the phase II KEYNOTE-158 study. J Clin Oncol 2019;37(17):1470–8.

29. Hollebecque A, Meyer T, Moore KN, et al. An open-label, multicohort, phase I/II study of nivolumab in patients with virus-associated tumors (CheckMate 358): Efficacy and safety in recurrent or metastatic (R/M) cervical, vaginal, and vulvar cancers. J Clin Oncol 2017;35(15_suppl):5504.

30. Han K, Leung E, Barbera L, et al. Circulating human papillomavirus DNA as a biomarker of response in patients with locally advanced cervical cancer treated with definitive chemoradiation. JCO Precis Oncol 2018;(2):1–8.

31. Pecorelli S. Revised FIGO staging for carcinoma of the vulva, cervix, and endometrium. Int J Gynaecol Obstet 2009;105(2):103–4.

32. Koh WJ, Greer BE, Abu-Rustum NR, et al. Vulvar cancer, version 1.2017, NCCN clinical practice guidelines in oncology. J Natl Compr Canc Netw 2017;15(1): 92–120.

33. Te Grootenhuis NC, van der Zee AGJ, van Doorn HC, et al. Sentinel nodes in vulvar cancer: Long-term follow-up of the GROningen INternational Study on Sentinel nodes in Vulvar cancer (GROINSS-V) I. Gynecol Oncol 2016; 140(1):8–14.

34. Chapman BV, Gill BS, Viswanathan AN, et al. Adjuvant radiation therapy for margin-positive vulvar squamous cell carcinoma: defining the ideal dose-response using the national cancer data base. Int J Radiat Oncol Biol Phys 2017;97(1):107–17.

35. Ignatov T, Eggemann H, Burger E, et al. Adjuvant radiotherapy for vulvar cancer with close or positive surgical margins. J Cancer Res Clin Oncol 2016;142(2): 489–95.

36. Kunos C, Simpkins F, Gibbons H, et al. Radiation therapy compared with pelvic node resection for node-positive vulvar cancer: a randomized controlled trial. Obstet Gynecol 2009;114(3):537–46.

37. Parthasarathy A, Cheung MK, Osann K, et al. The benefit of adjuvant radiation therapy in single-node-positive squamous cell vulvar carcinoma. Gynecol Oncol 2006;103(3):1095–9.

38. Montana GS, Thomas GM, Moore DH, et al. Preoperative chemo-radiation for carcinoma of the vulva with N2/N3 nodes: a gynecologic oncology group study. Int J Radiat Oncol Biol Phys 2000;48(4):1007–13.

39. Moore DH, Ali S, Koh WJ, et al. A phase II trial of radiation therapy and weekly cisplatin chemotherapy for the treatment of locally-advanced squamous cell carcinoma of the vulva: a gynecologic oncology group study. Gynecol Oncol 2012; 124(3):529–33.

40. Wahlen SA, Slater JD, Wagner RJ, et al. Concurrent radiation therapy and chemotherapy in the treatment of primary squamous cell carcinoma of the vulva. Cancer 1995;75(9):2289–94.

41. Russell AH, Mesic JB, Scudder SA, et al. Synchronous radiation and cytotoxic chemotherapy for locally advanced or recurrent squamous cancer of the vulva. Gynecol Oncol 1992;47(1):14–20.

42. PDQ Adult Treatment Editorial Board. Vulvar cancer treatment (PDQ(R)): health professional version. PDQ cancer information summaries. Bethesda (MD): National Cancer Institute (US); 2019.

43. Landrum LM, Lanneau GS, Skaggs VJ, et al. Gynecologic Oncology Group risk groups for vulvar carcinoma: improvement in survival in the modern era. Gynecol Oncol 2007;106(3):521–5.

44. Lee LJ, Howitt B, Catalano P, et al. Prognostic importance of human papillomavirus (HPV) and p16 positivity in squamous cell carcinoma of the vulva treated with radiotherapy. Gynecol Oncol 2016;142(2):293–8.

45. Salani R, Khanna N, Frimer M, et al. An update on post-treatment surveillance and diagnosis of recurrence in women with gynecologic malignancies: Society of Gynecologic Oncology (SGO) recommendations. Gynecol Oncol 2017; 146(1):3–10.

46. Viswanathan AN, Lee LJ, Eswara JR, et al. Complications of pelvic radiation in patients treated for gynecologic malignancies. Cancer 2014;120(24):3870–83.

47. Song Y, Erickson B, Chen X, et al. Appropriate magnetic resonance imaging techniques for gross tumor volume delineation in external beam radiation therapy of locally advanced cervical cancer. Oncotarget 2018;9(11):10100–9.

48. Verma J, Sulman EP, Jhingran A, et al. Dosimetric predictors of duodenal toxicity after intensity modulated radiation therapy for treatment of the para-aortic nodes in gynecologic cancer. Int J Radiat Oncol Biol Phys 2014;88(2):357–62.

49. Gaffney DK, King B, Viswanathan AN, et al. Consensus recommendations for radiation therapy contouring and treatment of vulvar carcinoma. Int J Radiat Oncol Biol Phys 2016;95(4):1191–200.

50. Klopp AH, Moughan J, Portelance L, et al. Hematologic toxicity in RTOG 0418: a phase 2 study of postoperative IMRT for gynecologic cancer. Int J Radiat Oncol Biol Phys 2013;86(1):83–90.

51. Klopp AH, Yeung AR, Deshmukh S, et al. Patient-reported toxicity during pelvic intensity-modulated radiation therapy: NRG oncology-RTOG 1203. J Clin Oncol 2018;36(24):2538–44.

52. Rao YJ, Chundury A, Schwarz JK, et al. Intensity modulated radiation therapy for squamous cell carcinoma of the vulva: Treatment technique and outcomes. Adv Radiat Oncol 2017;2(2):148–58.

53. Jurgenliemk-Schulz IM, Beriwal S, de Leeuw AAC, et al. Management of nodal disease in advanced cervical cancer. Semin Radiat Oncol 2019;29(2):158–65.

54. Cheng JY, Huang EY, Hsu SN, et al. Simultaneous integrated boost (SIB) of the parametrium and cervix in radiotherapy for uterine cervical carcinoma: a dosimetric study using a new alternative approach. Br J Radiol 2016;89(1068): 20160526.

55. Vergalasova I, Light K, Chino J, et al. Simultaneous integrated boost (SIB) for treatment of gynecologic carcinoma: Intensity-modulated radiation therapy (IMRT) vs volumetric-modulated arc therapy (VMAT) radiotherapy. Med Dosim 2017;42(3):230–7.

56. Boyle J, Craciunescu O, Steffey B, et al. Methods, safety, and early clinical outcomes of dose escalation using simultaneous integrated and sequential boosts in patients with locally advanced gynecologic malignancies. Gynecol Oncol 2014;135(2):239–43.

57. Holschneider CH, Petereit DG, Chu C, et al. Brachytherapy: A critical component of primary radiation therapy for cervical cancer: From the Society of Gynecologic Oncology (SGO) and the American Brachytherapy Society (ABS). Brachytherapy 2019;18(2):123–32.
58. Viswanathan AN, Thomadsen B. American Brachytherapy Society consensus guidelines for locally advanced carcinoma of the cervix. Part I: general principles. Brachytherapy 2012;11(1):33–46.
59. Fokdal L, Sturdza A, Mazeron R, et al. Image guided adaptive brachytherapy with combined intracavitary and interstitial technique improves the therapeutic ratio in locally advanced cervical cancer: Analysis from the retroEMBRACE study. Radiother Oncol 2016;120(3):434–40.
60. de Arcos J, Schmidt EJ, Wang W, et al. Prospective clinical implementation of a novel magnetic resonance tracking device for real-time brachytherapy catheter positioning. Int J Radiat Oncol Biol Phys 2017;99(3):618–26.
61. Tod MC, Meredith WJ. A dosage system for use in the treatment of cancer of the uterine cervix. Br J Radiol 1938;11(132):809–24.
62. Dimopoulos JC, Petrow P, Tanderup K, et al. Recommendations from Gynaecological (GYN) GEC-ESTRO Working Group (IV): Basic principles and parameters for MR imaging within the frame of image based adaptive cervix cancer brachytherapy. Radiother Oncol 2012;103(1):113–22.
63. Sturdza A, Potter R, Fokdal LU, et al. Image guided brachytherapy in locally advanced cervical cancer: Improved pelvic control and survival in RetroEMBRACE, a multicenter cohort study. Radiother Oncol 2016;120(3):428–33.
64. Mazeron R, Fokdal LU, Kirchheiner K, et al. Dose-volume effect relationships for late rectal morbidity in patients treated with chemoradiation and MRI-guided adaptive brachytherapy for locally advanced cervical cancer: Results from the prospective multicenter EMBRACE study. Radiother Oncol 2016;120(3):412–9.
65. Gill BS, Lin JF, Krivak TC, et al. National Cancer Data Base analysis of radiation therapy consolidation modality for cervical cancer: the impact of new technological advancements. Int J Radiat Oncol Biol Phys 2014;90(5):1083–90.
66. Robin TP, Amini A, Schefter TE, et al. Disparities in standard of care treatment and associated survival decrement in patients with locally advanced cervical cancer. Gynecol Oncol 2016;143(2):319–25.

The Evolving Role of Radiotherapy for Head and Neck Cancer

David L. Schwartz, MD[a,b],*, D. Neil Hayes, MD, MS, MPH[c,d,e,f,g]

KEYWORDS

- Head and neck cancer • Radiotherapy • Advances • Review

KEY POINTS

- Head and neck cancer is a nuanced disease site that benefits from specialized radiotherapy expertise and multidisciplinary care.
- Radiotherapy alone or in combination with systemic treatment is a cornerstone of locoregional head and neck cancer management.
- Advances in radiotherapy techniques, in combination with cytotoxic and newer biologic/immunologic agents, promise to make personalized therapy possible, particularly for favorable human papilloma virus–associated oropharyngeal cancers.
- Targeted biologic therapy and immune-oncology agents hold particular promise for individualized radiosensitization of head and neck cancer.

INTRODUCTION

Head and neck cancer is the sixth most common cancer diagnosis worldwide.[1] Oral cavity cancer is the most frequent cancer killer in southern Asia and the second most frequent in France, owing to the continued prevalence of cigarettes, smokeless tobacco products, and alcohol. Beyond statistics, the disease extracts a heavy toll on

Disclosure: D.L. Schwartz has received royalties from UptoDate and research funding from Elekta (Sweden). D.N. Hayes is on the Merck advisory board and is a founder, stockholder, and consultant for GeneCentric.
[a] Department of Radiation Oncology, UTHSC College of Medicine, 1265 Union Avenue, Memphis, TN 38104, USA; [b] Department of Preventive Medicine, UTHSC College of Medicine, 1265 Union Avenue, Memphis, TN 38104, USA; [c] Hematology/Oncology, Department of Medicine, UTHSC College of Medicine, 19 South Manassas Street, Cancer Research Building, 324, Memphis, TN 38103, USA; [d] Department of Genetics/Genomics/Informatics, UTHSC College of Medicine, Memphis, TN, USA; [e] Department of Preventive Medicine, UTHSC College of Medicine, Memphis, TN, USA; [f] Department of Pathology, UTHSC College of Medicine, Memphis, TN, USA; [g] Department of Computational Biology, St. Jude Children's Research Hospital, Memphis, TN, USA
* Corresponding author. UTHSC College of Medicine, 1265 Union Avenue, Memphis, TN 38104.
E-mail address: dschwar4@uthsc.edu

Hematol Oncol Clin N Am 34 (2020) 91–108
https://doi.org/10.1016/j.hoc.2019.08.019
0889-8588/20/© 2019 Elsevier Inc. All rights reserved.

the most elemental of human functions, including speech, eating, sight, hearing, and appearance.

Head and neck cancer defies broad description. The term encompasses a diverse spectrum of diseases that behave in varied ways based on subtle differences in anatomic location and host characteristics. Growing understanding of the role of human papillomavirus (HPV) infection and host immune surveillance across specific types of head and neck cancer have positioned the field in the thick of new oncologic treatment trends. The disease most commonly presents as squamous cell carcinoma emanating from the mucosal lining of the upper aerodigestive tract, typically in the oral cavity, larynx, or pharynx. Such cancers are the focus of this review. However, the term also includes cancers of regional skin (the most common of head and neck cancer sites by raw incidence), salivary glands, thyroid gland, paranasal sinuses, periorbital structures, peripheral nerves, and connective tissues.

Radiotherapy and surgery, either alone or in combination, can eliminate locoregional disease, especially in its early stages. Systemic cytotoxic, biologic, and immunologic agents are now used at all phases of treatment. Understanding of how best to deliver radiation, either alone or in combination with other modalities, has matured. The sum of these trends has been a steady improvement in the curative and functional patient outcomes for a disease long fraught with failure.

DEFINITIVE RADIOTHERAPY
Radiotherapy Alone

Conventional daily radiation alone historically provides 70% to 95% long-term local control and 50% overall survival (OS) for patients with early stage I to II head and neck disease. Local control is limited to 20% to 50% and OS to less than 10% to 25% for advanced stage III to IV disease. At present, radiation alone is reserved for early or favorable intermediate-stage laryngeal or oropharyngeal primary disease, or for poor-performance patients with locally advanced disease not considered to be candidates for surgery or concurrent chemoradiotherapy.

Limited-field radiation can control more than 90% of stage T1 glottic laryngeal cancers[2] and up to 80% of T2 lesions.[3] Radiation by itself can also provide excellent results for oropharyngeal cancers. Selek and colleagues[4] showed 85% local control and 77% disease-specific survival at 5 years in 175 stage I/II oropharyngeal cases treated at M.D. Anderson Cancer Center. Garden and colleagues[5] reviewed 857 patients with oropharyngeal cancer, including 324 patients who were treated with radiation alone for T1/2N1-2b, T3N0 disease. Following radiation alone, progression-free survival (PFS) was 90% for T1, 83% for T2, and 70% for patients with T3 disease. O'Sullivan and colleagues[6] also confirmed excellent local control (95%) and OS (86%) in minimal smokers treated with radiation alone for HPV-associated stage IV oropharyngeal disease.

Intensifying the frequency of radiation delivery improves control of advanced disease when not given with chemotherapy. The Radiation Therapy Oncology Group (RTOG) completed its landmark 90-03 phase III trial comparing once-daily radiation with altered fractionation approaches in 1073 patients with stage II to IV disease of the oropharynx, supraglottic larynx, oral cavity, and hypopharynx.[7] Altered fractionation provided improved locoregional control (54% vs 46%, $P \leq .05$) with a trend toward improved disease-free survival (38% vs 32%, $P \geq .054$) at 2 years. OS was equivalent in all treatment arms. Based on this local control benefit, once-daily radiation is no longer considered standard of care for patients receiving radiation alone for stage II to IV disease of these sites. However, 90-03 did show more intense acute toxicity with altered fractionation, so daily radiation may still be considered for managing locoregional disease in medically infirm patients.

Successive meta-analyses[8,9] have gone on to show improved local control and survival with hyperfractionation compared with daily radiation alone, although survival outcomes remain inferior to chemoradiotherapy. Combined modality treatment, therefore, remains standard of care for locally advanced head and neck cancer. The addition of chemotherapy obviates aggressive fractionation (discussed further later).

Radiotherapy Combined with Chemotherapy

No matter how radiotherapy is clinically delivered, the rationale for combining it with sensitizing chemotherapy is compelling. Historical clinical experience before the late 1990s used induction chemotherapy before radiation, or single-agent therapy concurrently with once-daily radiation. This chemoradiotherapy (CRT) experience was haphazard, with institutions using varying agents, doses, and schedules, resulting in no substantive consensus. Systematic reviews were ultimately required to show a survival benefit to the use of chemotherapy during this era, but only when given concurrently with radiation.[10–12] An updated meta-analysis by Pignon and colleagues[13] encompassing 16,485 cases enrolled onto 87 trials solidified this conclusion, showing a 4.5% absolute survival benefit at 5 years with the addition of chemotherapy. Timing of chemotherapy was predictive for survival ($P<.0001$), with most the benefit seen following concurrent treatment (6.5% absolute survival benefit at 5 years).

Historically, intermediate-stage to advanced-stage laryngeal or hypopharyngeal cancer was managed with total laryngectomy or laryngopharyngectomy. Radiotherapy served as the only means by which to treat without certain loss of voice. In the 1980s, the term organ sparing (or voice/larynx sparing) was coined for a strategy designed to triage patients according to chemosensitivity away from laryngectomy toward definitive radiation.

The landmark phase III Department of Veterans Affairs (VA) Larynx Study Group Trial[14] set out to show survival equivalency in 332 patients with stage III to IV disease randomized either to laryngectomy or to 3 cycles of cisplatin/5-fluorouracil (5-FU) before 70 Gy once-daily radiation alone. More than 80% of patients had a partial or total response to 2 cycles of induction and went on to radiation. Survival was equal in both study groups, and two-thirds of these patients randomized to organ sparing enjoyed larynx preservation 2 years following treatment. The European Organization for Research and Treatment of Cancer (EORTC) conducted a similar trial for patients with advanced pyriform sinus cancer.[15] Organ preservation therapy with induction chemotherapy again provided survival equivalent to laryngectomy. This approach became standard of care in North America for stage III to IV laryngeal and selected hypopharyngeal disease without T4 features, and remains an accepted (albeit less preferred) alternative to concurrent CRT.

Concurrent CRT is also the current standard for advanced nasopharyngeal and oropharyngeal disease. Randomized trials from North American and Europe have shown the largest and most consistent improvement in local control and OS with concurrent treatment.[13] Platinum agents have served longest as the chemotherapy workhorse in this disease site.[16] The Intergroup 0099 trial reported by Al-Sarraf and colleagues[17] was among the earliest successful trials, showing a 78% versus 47% survival benefit at 3 years with concurrent and adjuvant cisplatin-based treatment of advanced nasopharyngeal disease. RTOG 91-11, a 3-arm phase III trial for low-bulk stage III to IV laryngeal disease, was later reported by Forastiere and colleagues.[18,19] This study compared the VA Larynx trial induction chemotherapy regimen with either radiation alone or with combined 70 Gy and cisplatin 100 mg/m^2 for 3 cycles (the current gold standard chemotherapy regimen for concurrent head and neck treatment). Combined chemoradiation provided significantly improved larynx preservation (84% vs 72%) and local disease control (80% vs 64%) versus the VA induction regimen at 2 years. No OS differences were detected, potentially because of effective salvage of failures after radiation alone with laryngectomy.[20]

These trials used standard once-daily radiation given apprehension over the potential overlapping mucosal toxicity of accelerated fractionation and cisplatin/5-FU chemotherapy. The lure of further local control benefit led Brizel and colleagues[21] to conduct a randomized trial testing hyperfractionated (twice daily) radiation with concurrent and adjuvant cisplatin/5-FU compared with hyperfractionated radiation alone. Acute and chronic morbidity was manageable. Despite a slightly lower total radiation dose (70 vs 75 Gy), combined treatment yielded improved locoregional control and relapse-free survival at 3 years compared with radiation alone. European groups subsequently reported prospective outcomes for concurrent chemotherapy and accelerated radiotherapy[22–25]; however, these series used nonstandard regimens that narrowed applicability to North American practice and/or did not conclusively suggest improvement compared with daily fractionation. RTOG 99-14 meanwhile showed feasibility of 72 Gy concomitant boost delivered with cisplatin 100 mg/m^2 for 2 cycles.[26] This regimen was then definitively tested by RTOG against standard once-daily radiation and cisplatin 100 mg/m^2 for 3 cycles in 743 patients via a randomized phase III trial (RTOG 0129).[27,28] However, no improvements in OS, PFS, locoregional control, or distant disease control were observed. Accordingly, daily radiation fractionation remains standard of care with concurrent chemotherapy.

An important research focus emerged in the early 2000s as a result of promising early-phase trial results with the use of taxane-based induction chemotherapy followed by radiation or concurrent chemoradiotherapy. Haddad and colleagues[29] summarized experience with various induction combinations of intermediate-dose and high-dose docetaxel, cisplatin, and 5-FU before radiation-based locoregional management. After initial phase II reports showed encouraging activity with taxane-based induction,[30] a pair of multi-institutional phase III trials confirmed improved PFS and OS with the addition of docetaxel to platinum/5-FU (TPF) induction before radiation alone[31] or concurrent carboplatin and radiation.[32] Several randomized phase III trials have more recently tested concurrent chemoradiotherapy with or without taxane-based induction. The North American DeCIDE[33] and PARADIGM[34] trials both tested the addition of TPF to alternative aggressive taxane-based chemoradiotherapy regimens, whereas Spanish investigators tested the addition of TPF to concurrent cisplatin/radiation.[35] All 3 trials failed to conclusively show improvement in any survival outcomes with the addition of induction chemotherapy. In light of these results, as well as the steep morbidity and financial cost of aggressive induction, this approach has largely lost favor to concurrent chemoradiotherapy. Nonetheless, induction chemotherapy may yet have a role to play in helping to triage selected patients with favorable HPV-associated oropharyngeal cancer toward deintensified treatment (discussed further later). It also remains controversial as to whether aggressive TPF induction remains a viable organ preservation strategy for locally advanced (selected T2N+ and T3/T4) laryngeal and hypopharyngeal cancer. European data from the randomized GORTEC 2000-01[36] confirmed more than 70% larynx preservation at 10 years following TPF induction and radiotherapy alone for stage III/IV disease. These results could not be improved on by the addition of sensitizing systemic therapy to radiation in the subsequent TREMPLIN randomized phase II trial,[37] and it remains unsettled as to what strategies should now be tested to improve organ preservation in this disease site.

Organ Preservation for Human Papilloma Virus–Associated Cancers

As transoral and reconstructive surgical techniques continue to evolve, the association between radiotherapy and organ preservation therapy may loosen. Careful patient selection is, and will remain, critical for optimal management within the context of a broader spectrum of treatment pathways. Selection is particularly relevant to patients with HPV-associated oropharyngeal cancer, in whom excellent disease prognosis and young patient age add urgency to reducing acute treatment toxicity and long-term functional disability without sacrificing current high standards in disease control.

Host-related and disease-related factors weigh heavily on treatment selection. Younger, healthier, motivated patients with exophytic, minimally infiltrative disease (especially of the tonsil, tongue base, and larynx) are suitable candidates for transoral surgery and/or radiotherapy. Presence of low-volume primary disease potentially argues for radiation alone.[38] In contrast, advanced primary or nodal disease requires concurrent chemoradiation. Patients with infiltrative oral cavity involvement and/or very poor swallowing or laryngeal function are best managed surgically.

Treatment deintensification for favorable HPV-associated oropharyngeal cancer is under intense scrutiny. The multi-institutional phase II E1308 trial[39] tested whether patients with T1-3N0-2b HPV-positive oropharyngeal disease with complete primary tumor response to paclitaxel/cisplatin and cetuximab (a humanized monoclonal antibody to epidermal growth factor receptor [EGFR], discussed further later) induction could be safely treated to tiered doses of 54 to 70 Gy. Fifty-one of 80 evaluable cases showed complete response and received 54 Gy to the primary tumor. These patients had 80% PFS and 94% OS rates at 2 years, and had improved swallowing and nutritional status. Chera and colleagues[40] reported a multi-institutional phase II trial that treated 43 patients with T0-3N0-2c HPV-positive oropharyngeal cancer to 60 Gy and concurrent cisplatin. The primary study end point was pathologic complete response rate based on biopsy of primary site and lymph node dissection of involved nodes; this was achieved in 37 out of 43 (86%) patients with a favorable toxicity profile.

Villaflor and colleagues[41] took a different tack to treatment deintensification, focusing on reducing the volume of treatment rather than dose de-escalation. This institutional phase I/II trial enrolled 94 patients to receive cisplatin/paclitaxel/cetuximab induction chemotherapy (the first 50 patients were randomized to plus or minus everolimus, an oral mammalian target of rapamycin inhibitor). Patients with greater than or equal to 50% response received TFHX (paclitaxel, 5-FU, hydroxyurea, and 1.5 Gy twice daily radiotherapy every other week) to 75 Gy with the single planning target volume (PTV1) covering only gross disease. Patients with less than 50% response were treated with TFHX encompassing PTV1 and the next nodal station at risk (PTV2) to a dose of 45 Gy followed by a sequential boost of 75 Gy to PTV1. Thirty-seven of 89 (41.6%) patients were responders. PFS and OS at 2 years were 86.0% and 83.5% for responders, and 68.7% and 85.4% for nonresponders. Responders showed particularly good late swallowing function preservation.

Many ongoing phase II/III trials are testing a variety of approaches to treatment de-escalation for HPV-associated oropharyngeal cancers. These strategies include induction chemotherapy to select responsive patients for dose-reduced radiation (Quarterback, NCT01706939 and Quarterback 2, NCT02945631), upfront reduced-dose intensity-modulated radiation therapy (IMRT) with or without cisplatin (NRG HN002, NCT02254278), and primary transoral robotic surgery with or without radiation as a reduced-dose adjuvant (ECOG 3311, NCT01898494; PATHOS, NCT02215265;

ORATOR, NCT01590355; EORTC 1420, NCT02984410). One other popular approach has been the substitution of targeted biologic therapy (such as EGFR inhibition) for cytotoxic chemotherapy concurrent with radiation, under the assumption that this combination remains potent, but less toxic (discussed further later).

POSTOPERATIVE RADIOTHERAPY

Adjuvant radiation improves local control and survival following resection of advanced disease.[42-45] Radiation is typically indicated for positive/close margins, extracapsular nodal disease spread, 2 or more positive nodes, T3/T4 features (particularly bone/cartilage invasion), vascular/perineural invasion, infiltrative oral cavity disease (>3–7 mm invasion depth), and/or young age. These indications apply only to patients undergoing modified radical neck dissections. If a patient has had a selective neck dissection (far more common these days), radiation should be considered for any positive nodal disease. Limited evidence suggests that some cases of N1 disease may be successfully treated with selective dissection alone.[46,47]

Locoregional disease relapse following surgery is particularly common in patients with positive surgical margins, extracapsular nodal disease, or multiple positive nodes. Based on retrospective analyses,[48,49] adjuvant radiation reduces the relative risk of relapse by approximately 50%. However, locoregional recurrence rates remain as high as 35% to 60% in this population,[50] prompting the addition of chemotherapy to postoperative radiation. Two landmark multi-institutional phase III trials recently showed improved outcomes with this approach. In the first trial,[51] the EORTC randomized 334 subjects to 66 Gy with or without cisplatin 100 mg/m^2 for 3 cycles. Estimated 3-year local control (85% vs 70%), disease-free survival (60% vs 40%), and OS (65% vs 50%) were improved by the addition of cisplatin. Acute toxicity was exacerbated by chemotherapy, but severity of late effects purportedly remained equivalent. The RTOG conducted a complementary trial,[52] randomizing 459 patients to nearly identical treatment arms to the EORTC trial: 60 to 66 Gy with or without cisplatin 100 mg/m^2 to 3 cycles. Chemotherapy improved estimated 2-year local control (82% vs 72%, $P = .01$) and disease-free survival (70% vs 60%, $P = .05$). As with the EORTC trial, this was at the cost of higher acute grade 3 or greater toxicity. Joint reanalysis of both trials suggested significant clinical benefit to combined adjuvant therapy for patients with either positive surgical margins or extracapsular nodal disease.[53]

Adjuvant chemoradiotherapy continues to be studied by NRG Oncology with the ongoing RTOG 1216 phase II/III trial (NCT01810913, testing the substitution of docetaxel for cisplatin, with or without cetuximab, for high-risk disease including positive margins and/or extracapsular nodal disease) and RTOG 0920 phase III trial (NCT00956007, testing the addition of cetuximab for intermediate-risk disease without positive margins or extracapsular nodal disease). Recent institutional data[54] have suggested that HPV-associated oropharyngeal cancer with extracapsular nodal disease and negative surgical margins removed via transoral resection may not require the addition of chemotherapy to adjuvant radiation. The ongoing ADEPT phase III trial (NCT01687413) is randomizing such patients with T1/T2 primary disease to cisplatin/radiotherapy or radiotherapy alone.

REIRRADIATION

When head and neck disease relapses following irradiation, it typically recurs locoregionally. Even if disease is cured, secondary head and neck malignancies occur in up to 40% of patients.[55,56] Surgery has served as the only proven form of salvage for either situation, particularly for laryngeal disease.[57]

Multiple institutions have shown the feasibility of aggressive head and neck reirradiation.[58–61] Disease response seems to be more frequent and durable with reirradiation than with chemotherapy alone, but requires concurrent chemotherapy for optimal results.[62–66] Survival longer than 2 years has been observed in a finite minority (15%–20%) of patients. The RTOG 96-10 phase II study[67] was the first to use reirradiation in the cooperative group setting, using a split-course hyperfractionated radiation regimen with concurrent hydroxyurea and 5-FU in 81 patients with recurrent disease or second primaries. Median survival was approximately 8 months, but 16% of patients survived past 2 years. Six patients (7%) died of treatment-related sepsis or tumor site hemorrhage, but acute toxicity was typically no greater than grade 3. The RTOG concluded reirradiation to be feasible across institutions, and subsequently completed a follow-up phase II trial, RTOG 99-11. This trial examined uninterrupted hyperfractionated radiation with concurrent paclitaxel/cisplatin. Durable 2-year survival was reported as 25%.[68]

More recent results from experienced centers with the use of extremely localized hypofractionated (1–5 fractions) stereotactic treatment, with or without sensitizing therapy, suggest good tolerance and encouraging local disease control in highly selected patients.[69,70] This treatment is currently being studied in the cooperative group setting by the NRG-sponsored KEYSTROKE phase II trial (NCT03546582).

NEW DIRECTIONS
Targeted Biologic Therapy

EGFR is overexpressed or activated in 80% to 100% of head and neck cancers.[71] Interventions targeting EGFR, including monoclonal antibodies (cetuximab and panitumumab) and small molecule kinase inhibitors (gefitinib and erlotinib), have undergone intensive clinical testing. These agents show single-agent activity ranging from 4% to 11% in patients with metastatic disease.[72–74] Addition of cisplatin-based chemotherapy increases response rates to 10% to 26%[75–78] and improves survival compared with chemotherapy alone.[79] The addition of cetuximab also potentially improves disease response to taxane-based induction.[80,81] An important lesson from early trials was that EGFR targeting seems to work best when combined with cytotoxic treatment.

Data specific to combined EGFR blockade/radiotherapy in the curative setting have rapidly matured. A seminal phase III trial from Bonner and colleagues[82,83] randomizing 424 advanced-stage patients to radiation with or without cetuximab confirmed a significant OS benefit (46% vs 36% at 5 years) following combined therapy relative to radiation alone. This increased efficacy came with no additional reported mucosal toxicity burden. Concurrent cetuximab/radiation is now a standard-of-care treatment option, particularly for frail patients judged to be poor candidates for platinum chemotherapy. However, single-agent EGFR inhibition seems from recent randomized data to remain incrementally inferior to standard platinum-based CRT,[84] even with the addition of aggressive TPF induction chemotherapy,[85] in unselected patients with locally advanced disease.

Recent phase III data from the GORTEC 2007-1 trial[86] suggested that the addition of concurrent platinum chemotherapy can improve on the results of cetuximab/radiation for advanced-stage disease. Thus, an important step has been to test the addition of EGFR blockade to CRT. The ECOG 3303 phase II trial[87] confirmed the safety and activity of including cetuximab with concurrent cisplatin/radiation, whereas a phase II trial reported by Martins and colleagues[88] confirmed the safety of adding erlotinib to concurrent cisplatin/radiation. This finding prompted several randomized trials to directly test the addition of cetuximab to concurrent cisplatin/radiotherapy. The RTOG 0522 phase III trial enrolled 940 patients with stage III or IV (T2N2-3M0 or T3–T4, any N, M0) disease to modestly accelerated radiation (70–72 Gy over 6 weeks)/cisplatin 100 mg/m^2 every 3 weeks, with or without a 400 mg/m^2 loading dose of cetuximab followed by 250 mg/m^2/wk during radiotherapy.[89] The addition of cetuximab resulted in more frequent interruptions in chemoradiation (26.9% vs 15.1% for CRT alone) and more grade 3 to 4 radiation mucositis (43.2% vs 33.3% for CRT alone). No differences were found in 3-year PFS (61.2% vs 58.9% for CRT alone, $P = .76$), 3-year OS (72.9% vs 75.8% for CRT alone, $P = .32$), and locoregional failure (19.9% vs 25.9% for CRT alone, $P = .97$). Negative results were also reported for the similarly designed CONCERT-1 randomized phase II trial, which added panitumumab to cisplatin/radiation.[90] As such, the addition of EGFR inhibition to concurrent CRT cannot currently be considered standard of care, although the addition of newer targeted agents to CRT remains an area of active investigation for advanced-stage, high-risk HPV-unassociated disease.

As noted earlier, single-agent EGFR inhibitor/radiation seems modestly inferior to platinum-based CRT for unselected advanced-stage disease. However, patients with favorable HPV-associated oropharyngeal disease have consistently been shown to do well across EGFR radiosensitization trials[91]; accordingly, single-agent EGFR inhibitor/radiation has been hypothesized to represent a potential strategy for treatment deintensification, delivering the efficacy of platinum chemotherapy with less mucosal and functional toxicity for this selected subgroup. The maturing Trans-Tasman TROG 12.01 phase III (NCT01855451) trial is directly testing 70 Gy combined with single-agent cisplatin (every 3 week or weekly scheduling, respectively) or standard-dose weekly cetuximab. However, the much larger RTOG 1016 phase III trial has recently reported inferior survival outcomes with cetuximab/radiation.[92] This trial randomized 849 patients with T1-2N2a-3M0 or T3 to T4, any N, M0 HPV-positive disease to 70 Gy/cisplatin every 3 weeks or 70 Gy weekly cetuximab. Estimated 5-year OS was 77.9% (95% confidence interval [CI], 73.4–82.5) in the cetuximab group versus 84.6% (95% CI, 80.6–88.6) in the cisplatin group. Five-year PFS was significantly lower (67.3%; 95% CI, 62.4–72.2; vs 78.4%; 95% CI, 73.8–83.0) and locoregional failure was significantly higher (17.3%; 95% CI, 13.7–21.4; vs 9.9%; 95% CI, 6.9–13.6) in the cetuximab group. Furthermore, acute and late moderate to severe toxicity rates seemed similar across both treatment arms. These results were corroborated by the similarly designed UK De-ESCALaTE HPV phase III trial.[93] Thus, 2 cycles of 100 mg/m^2 cisplatin administered every 3 weeks currently remains standard of care for concurrent CRT for either HPV-associated or HPV-unassociated locally advanced head and neck cancer.

A looming challenge will be to elucidate optimal agent selection, dosing, sequencing, and response assessment for this new generation of treatment. Toward this end, key pilot publications in the early 2000s[94,95] showed that large-scale tumor gene expression profiling can predict for nodal metastasis and clinical disease behavior. Expression arrays and other profiling technologies are now providing high-order biomarker information for disease detection and treatment selection for individual patients and clinical trial design.[96,97]

Immuno-Oncology

Host immune dysfunction has been directly associated with the development and progression of head and neck cancer.[98] Programmed death receptor-1 (PD-1) binding with its ligands PD-L1 and PD-L2 deactivates T cells and has been directly

Table 1
Key head and neck phase III trials and meta-analyses

Trial/Reference	Year	Analyzable Patients (N)	Disease Stage/Site	Treatment Arms	Locoregional Control	OS
VA Larynx Study Group[14]	1991	332	Stage III-IV larynx	CDDP/5-FU × 3 → 70 Gy vs laryngectomy	66% larynx preservation at 2 y (P = NS)	68% at 2 y for both arms (P = NS)
Al-Sarraf et al[17]	1998	147	Stage III-IV nasopharynx	70 Gy + CDDP × 3 → CDDP/5-FU × 2 vs 70 Gy alone	NA	78% vs 47% at 3 y (P = .005)
RTOG 91-11[18,19]	2003	520	Stage III-IV larynx	70 Gy/CDDP × 3 vs CDDP/5-FU × 3 → 70 Gy vs 70 Gy alone	68% vs 55% vs 51% at 5 y (P = .002)	55% vs 58% vs 54% at 5 y (P = NS)
Pignon et al,[13]	2009	16,485	Any site (meta-analysis of 87 trials)	Concurrent, induction, and adjuvant CRT vs RT alone	0.74 (concurrent) vs 1.03 (induction) HR (P = .0001)	0.81 vs 0.96 vs 1.06 HR (P<.0001)
RTOG 0129[27,28]	2010	721	Stage III-IV oral cavity, oropharynx, larynx, hypopharynx	72 Gy in 42 fxs/CDDP × 2 vs 70 Gy in 35 fxs/CDDP × 3	39% vs 37% at 8 y (P = NS)	48% vs 48% at 8 y (P = NS)
RTOG 9501[52]	2004	416	Any site (high-risk postoperative)	60-66 Gy/CDDP × 3 vs 60-66 Gy alone	82% vs 72% at 2 y (P = .01)	65% vs 57% at 2 y (P = NS)
EORTC 22931[51]	2004	334	Any site (high-risk postoperative)	66 Gy/CDDP × 3 vs 66 Gy alone	82% vs 69% at 5 y (P = .007)	53% vs 40% at 5 y (P = .02)
Bonner et al,[82,83]	2006	424	Stage III-IV oropharynx, larynx, hypopharynx	70-72 Gy/cetuximab vs 70-72 Gy alone	47% vs 34% at 3 y (P<.01)	46% vs 36% at 5 y (P = .02)
GORTEC 2007-1[86]	2018	406	Stage III-IV oral cavity, oropharynx, larynx, hypopharynx	70 Gy/cetuximab + carboplatin/5-FU × 3 vs 70 Gy/cetuximab	78% vs 61% at 3 y (P<.001)	61% vs 55% at 3 y (P = NS)

(continued on next page)

Table 1
(continued)

Trial/Reference	Year	Analyzable Patients (N)	Disease Stage/Site	Treatment Arms	Locoregional Control	OS
RTOG 0522[89]	2014	891	Stage III–IV oropharynx, larynx, hypopharynx	70–72 Gy/CDDP × 2 + cetuximab vs 70–72/ CDDP × 2	80% vs 76% at 3 y (P = NS)	73% vs 76% at 3 y (P = NS)
RTOG 1016[92]	2019	805	T1–T2, N2a–N3 or T3–T4, N0–N3 HPV-associated oropharynx	70 Gy/cetuximab vs 70 Gy/ CDDP × 2	83% vs 90% at 5 y (P = .0005)	78% vs 85% at 5 y (P = .02)
De-ESCALaTE[93]	2019	321	T3–T4, N0 or T1–T4, N1–N3 HPV-associated oropharynx	70 Gy/cetuximab vs 70 Gy/ CDDP × 3	84% vs 94% at 2 y (P = .0007)	89% vs 98% at 2 y (P = .001)
CheckMate 141[106]	2016	361	Platinum-refractory recurrent head and neck disease	Nivolumab vs standard-of-care chemotherapy (MTX, docetaxel, or cetuximab)	13.3% vs 5.8% response rate	36% vs 17% at 12 mo (P = .01)
KEYNOTE-040[105]	2019	495	Platinum-refractory metastatic or recurrent head and neck disease	Pembrolizumab vs standard-of-care chemotherapy (MTX, docetaxel, or cetuximab)	14.6% vs 10.1% response rate	37% vs 26% at 12 mo (P = .02)

Abbreviations: CDDP, cisplatin; fxs, fractions; MTX, methotrexate; NA, not available; NS, nonsignificant; RT, radiotherapy.

implicated in head and neck tumor immune evasion.[99] Overexpression of PD-L1 occurs in many head and neck cancers.[100] Increased expression of immune checkpoint ligands cytotoxic T lymphocyte–associated protein 4 (CTLA-4) and PD-1 in tumor infiltrating T cells has been reported in patients with head and neck cancer,[101] and may serve as a favorable prognostic feature in HPV-associated head and neck cancers.[102]

Anti–PD-1 monoclonal antibodies nivolumab and pembrolizumab have been investigated in recurrent/metastatic disease. The KEYNOTE-012 phase Ib trial showed efficacy and safety of pembrolizumab in recurrent/metastatic head and neck cancers.[103,104] Overall response was 22% for PD-L1–positive tumors ($\geq$1%), compared with 4% for PD-L1–negative cancers (<1%) ($P = .021$). Interestingly, HPV-associated tumors were also more likely to respond than HPV-negative cancers (32% vs 14%). The follow-up phase III KEYNOTE-040 trial directly compared pembrolizumab with standard single-agent therapy (methotrexate, docetaxel, or cetuximab).[105] Median OS was 8.4 months with pembrolizumab versus 6.9 months with standard of care ($P = .0161$). The CheckMate 141 phase III trial assigned 361 patients with recurrent, platinum-refractory disease to receive nivolumab or standard single-agent methotrexate, docetaxel, or cetuximab.[106] Median OS was 7.5 months for nivolumab versus 5.1 months for standard therapy (hazard ratio [HR] = 0.70; $P = .01$). Treatment-related grade 3 to 4 toxicity occurred in 13% patients in the nivolumab group versus 35.1% in the standard-therapy group.

Table 1. summarizes important phase III/meta-analysis data in head and neck cancer, including the recent addition of seminal randomized immuno-oncology trial results to this progress. There are currently many prioritized multi-institutional trials testing potential roles for checkpoint inhibitors in the curative setting. Some highlights include NRG-HN003 (NCT02775812), a phase I trial determining optimal dosing of pembrolizumab given in combination with concurrent cisplatin and IMRT in the adjuvant setting for high-risk, stage III to IV disease; NRG-HN004 (NCT03258554), a phase II/III trial comparing concurrent radiation/cetuximab with radiation/durvalumab (an inhibitory monoclonal antibody to PD-L1) in the definitive setting for stage III to IVB patients judged not to be candidates for cisplatin; RTOG 3504 (NCT02764593), a dose-finding phase I trial confirming safety of concurrent radiation/nivolumab in combination with either weekly cisplatin, high-dose cisplatin every 3 weeks, or cetuximab in the definitive setting for intermediate-risk/high-risk patients; and JAVELIN (NCT02952586), a phase III placebo-controlled trial comparing concurrent radiation/cisplatin with or without avelumab (an inhibitory monoclonal antibody to PD-L1) in the definitive setting for high-risk patients.

SUMMARY

The length and quality of head and neck cancer survivorship continue to meaningfully improve. Radiotherapy has proved pivotal to these improved outcomes because of advances in treatment delivery, fractionation schemas, radiosensitizing systemic therapy, and thoughtful interplay with technical surgical improvements. The future looks brighter still, with rapid ongoing progress in targeted biologic therapy, immuno-oncology, molecular-genetic tumor characterization for personalized treatment, and holistic social support strategies to improve patient access to advances regardless of financial need. Head and neck cancer, a disease once fraught with nihilism and failure, is evolving into a major success story of modern multidisciplinary cancer care.

Continued dedication on the part of providers, patients, and society as a whole will be required to leverage this progress to its fullest.

REFERENCES

1. Gupta B, Johnson NW, Kumar N. Global epidemiology of head and neck cancers: a continuing challenge. Oncology 2016;91:13–23.
2. Mendenhall WM, Werning JW, Hinerman RW, et al. Management of T1-T2 glottic carcinomas. Cancer 2004;100:1786–92.
3. Garden AS, Forster K, Wong PF, et al. Results of radiotherapy for T2N0 glottic carcinoma: does the "2" stand for twice-daily treatment? Int J Radiat Oncol Biol Phys 2003;55:322–8.
4. Selek U, Garden AS, Morrison WH, et al. Radiation therapy for early-stage carcinoma of the oropharynx. Int J Radiat Oncol Biol Phys 2004;59:743–51.
5. Garden AS, Fuller CD, Rosenthal DI, et al. Radiation therapy (with or without neck surgery) for phenotypic human papillomavirus-associated oropharyngeal cancer. Cancer 2016;122:1702–7.
6. O'Sullivan B, Huang SH, Perez-Ordonez B, et al. Outcomes of HPV-related oropharyngeal cancer patients treated by radiotherapy alone using altered fractionation. Radiother Oncol 2012;103:49–56.
7. Fu KK, Pajak TF, Trotti A, et al. A Radiation Therapy Oncology Group (RTOG) phase III randomized study to compare hyperfractionation and two variants of accelerated fractionation to standard fractionation radiotherapy for head and neck squamous cell carcinomas: first report of RTOG 9003. Int J Radiat Oncol Biol Phys 2000;48:7–16.
8. Baujat B, Bourhis J, Blanchard P, et al. Hyperfractionated or accelerated radiotherapy for head and neck cancer. Cochrane Database Syst Rev 2010;(12):CD002026.
9. Lacas B, Bourhis J, Overgaard J, et al. Role of radiotherapy fractionation in head and neck cancers (MARCH): an updated meta-analysis. Lancet Oncol 2017;18: 1221–37.
10. Pignon JP, Bourhis J, Domenge C, et al. Chemotherapy added to locoregional treatment for head and neck squamous-cell carcinoma: three meta-analyses of updated individual data. MACH-NC Collaborative Group. Meta-analysis of chemotherapy on head and neck cancer. Lancet 2000;355:949–55.
11. Munro AJ. An overview of randomised controlled trials of adjuvant chemotherapy in head and neck cancer. Br J Cancer 1995;71:83–91.
12. El-Sayed S, Nelson N. Adjuvant and adjunctive chemotherapy in the management of squamous cell carcinoma of the head and neck region. A meta-analysis of prospective and randomized trials. J Clin Oncol 1996;14:838–47.
13. Pignon JP, le Maitre A, Maillard E, et al. Meta-analysis of chemotherapy in head and neck cancer (MACH-NC): an update on 93 randomised trials and 17,346 patients. Radiother Oncol 2009;92:4–14.
14. Veterans Affairs Laryngeal Cancer Study Group. Induction chemotherapy plus radiation compared with surgery plus radiation in patients with advanced laryngeal cancer. N Engl J Med 1991;324:1685–90.
15. Lefebvre JL, Andry G, Chevalier D, et al. Laryngeal preservation with induction chemotherapy for hypopharyngeal squamous cell carcinoma: 10-year results of EORTC trial 24891. Ann Oncol 2012;23:2708–14.
16. Forastiere AA. Overview of platinum chemotherapy in head and neck cancer. Semin Oncol 1994;21:20–7.

17. Al-Sarraf M, LeBlanc M, Giri PG, et al. Chemoradiotherapy versus radiotherapy in patients with advanced nasopharyngeal cancer: phase III randomized Intergroup study 0099. J Clin Oncol 1998;16:1310–7.

18. Forastiere AA, Goepfert H, Maor M, et al. Concurrent chemotherapy and radiotherapy for organ preservation in advanced laryngeal cancer. N Engl J Med 2003;349:2091–8.

19. Forastiere AA, Zhang Q, Weber RS, et al. Long-term results of RTOG 91-11: a comparison of three nonsurgical treatment strategies to preserve the larynx in patients with locally advanced larynx cancer. J Clin Oncol 2013;31:845–52.

20. Weber RS, Berkey BA, Forastiere A, et al. Outcome of salvage total laryngectomy following organ preservation therapy: the Radiation Therapy Oncology Group trial 91-11. Arch Otolaryngol Head Neck Surg 2003;129:44–9.

21. Brizel DM, Albers ME, Fisher SR, et al. Hyperfractionated irradiation with or without concurrent chemotherapy for locally advanced head and neck cancer. N Engl J Med 1998;338:1798–804.

22. Jeremic B, Milicic B, Dagovic A, et al. Radiation therapy with or without concurrent low-dose daily chemotherapy in locally advanced, nonmetastatic squamous cell carcinoma of the head and neck. J Clin Oncol 2004;22:3540–8.

23. Huguenin P, Beer KT, Allal A, et al. Concomitant cisplatin significantly improves locoregional control in advanced head and neck cancers treated with hyperfractionated radiotherapy. J Clin Oncol 2004;22:4665–73.

24. Budach V, Stuschke M, Budach W, et al. Hyperfractionated accelerated chemoradiation with concurrent fluorouracil-mitomycin is more effective than dose-escalated hyperfractionated accelerated radiation therapy alone in locally advanced head and neck cancer: final results of the radiotherapy cooperative clinical trials group of the German Cancer Society 95-06 Prospective Randomized Trial. J Clin Oncol 2005;23:1125–35.

25. Bourhis J, Sire C, Graff P, et al. Concomitant chemoradiotherapy versus acceleration of radiotherapy with or without concomitant chemotherapy in locally advanced head and neck carcinoma (GORTEC 99-02): an open-label phase 3 randomised trial. Lancet Oncol 2012;13:145–53.

26. Ang KK, Harris J, Garden AS, et al. Concomitant boost radiation plus concurrent cisplatin for advanced head and neck carcinomas: radiation therapy oncology group phase II trial 99-14. J Clin Oncol 2005;23:3008–15.

27. Ang KK, Harris J, Wheeler R, et al. Human papillomavirus and survival of patients with oropharyngeal cancer. N Engl J Med 2010;363:24–35.

28. Nguyen-Tan PF, Zhang Q, Ang KK, et al. Randomized phase III trial to test accelerated versus standard fractionation in combination with concurrent cisplatin for head and neck carcinomas in the Radiation Therapy Oncology Group 0129 trial: long-term report of efficacy and toxicity. J Clin Oncol 2014;32:3858–66.

29. Haddad RI, Posner M, Hitt R, et al. Induction chemotherapy in locally advanced squamous cell carcinoma of the head and neck: role, controversy, and future directions. Ann Oncol 2018;29:1130–40.

30. Argiris A, Jayaram P, Pichardo D. Revisiting induction chemotherapy for head and neck cancer. Oncology (Williston Park) 2005;19:759–70.

31. Vermorken JB, Remenar E, van Herpen C, et al. Cisplatin, fluorouracil, and docetaxel in unresectable head and neck cancer. N Engl J Med 2007;357:1695–704.

32. Posner MR, Hershock DM, Blajman CR, et al. Cisplatin and fluorouracil alone or with docetaxel in head and neck cancer. N Engl J Med 2007;357:1705–15.

33. Cohen EE, Karrison TG, Kocherginsky M, et al. Phase III randomized trial of induction chemotherapy in patients with N2 or N3 locally advanced head and neck cancer. J Clin Oncol 2014;32:2735–43.

34. Haddad R, O'Neill A, Rabinowits G, et al. Induction chemotherapy followed by concurrent chemoradiotherapy (sequential chemoradiotherapy) versus concurrent chemoradiotherapy alone in locally advanced head and neck cancer (PARADIGM): a randomised phase 3 trial. Lancet Oncol 2013;14:257–64.

35. Hitt R, Grau JJ, Lopez-Pousa A, et al. A randomized phase III trial comparing induction chemotherapy followed by chemoradiotherapy versus chemoradiotherapy alone as treatment of unresectable head and neck cancer. Ann Oncol 2014;25:216–25.

36. Janoray G, Pointreau Y, Garaud P, et al. Long-term results of a multicenter randomized phase III trial of induction chemotherapy with cisplatin, 5-fluorouracil, +/- docetaxel for larynx preservation. J Natl Cancer Inst 2016;108.

37. Lefebvre JL, Pointreau Y, Rolland F, et al. Induction chemotherapy followed by either chemoradiotherapy or bioradiotherapy for larynx preservation: the TREMPLIN randomized phase II study. J Clin Oncol 2013;31:853–9.

38. Garden AS, Asper JA, Morrison WH, et al. Is concurrent chemoradiation the treatment of choice for all patients with Stage III or IV head and neck carcinoma? Cancer 2004;100:1171–8.

39. Marur S, Li S, Cmelak AJ, et al. E1308: phase II trial of induction chemotherapy followed by reduced-dose radiation and weekly cetuximab in patients with hpv-associated resectable squamous cell carcinoma of the oropharynx- ECOG-ACRIN Cancer Research Group. J Clin Oncol 2017;35:490–7.

40. Chera BS, Amdur RJ, Tepper J, et al. Phase 2 trial of de-intensified chemoradiation therapy for favorable-risk human papillomavirus-associated oropharyngeal squamous cell carcinoma. Int J Radiat Oncol Biol Phys 2015;93:976–85.

41. Villaflor VM, Melotek JM, Karrison TG, et al. Response-adapted volume de-escalation (RAVD) in locally advanced head and neck cancer. Ann Oncol 2016;27:908–13.

42. Barkley HT Jr, Fletcher GH, Jesse RH, et al. Management of cervical lymph node metastases in squamous cell carcinoma of the tonsillar fossa, base of tongue, supraglottic larynx, and hypopharynx. Am J Surg 1972;124:462–7.

43. Huang D, Johnson CR, Schmidt-Ullrich RK, et al. Incompletely resected advanced squamous cell carcinoma of the head and neck: the effectiveness of adjuvant vs. salvage radiotherapy. Radiother Oncol 1992;24:87–93.

44. Zelefsky MJ, Harrison LB, Fass DE, et al. Postoperative radiation therapy for squamous cell carcinomas of the oral cavity and oropharynx: impact of therapy on patients with positive surgical margins. Int J Radiat Oncol Biol Phys 1993;25:17–21.

45. Parsons JT, Mendenhall WM, Stringer SP, et al. An analysis of factors influencing the outcome of postoperative irradiation for squamous cell carcinoma of the oral cavity. Int J Radiat Oncol Biol Phys 1997;39:137–48.

46. Chepeha DB, Hoff PT, Taylor RJ, et al. Selective neck dissection for the treatment of neck metastasis from squamous cell carcinoma of the head and neck. Laryngoscope 2002;112:434–8.

47. Pellitteri PK, Robbins KT, Neuman T. Expanded application of selective neck dissection with regard to nodal status. Head Neck 1997;19:260–5.

48. Huang DT, Johnson CR, Schmidt-Ullrich R, et al. Postoperative radiotherapy in head and neck carcinoma with extracapsular lymph node extension and/or

positive resection margins: a comparative study. Int J Radiat Oncol Biol Phys 1992;23:737–42.

49. Lundahl RE, Foote RL, Bonner JA, et al. Combined neck dissection and postoperative radiation therapy in the management of the high-risk neck: a matched-pair analysis. Int J Radiat Oncol Biol Phys 1998;40:529–34.

50. Cooper JS, Pajak TF, Forastiere A, et al. Precisely defining high-risk operable head and neck tumors based on RTOG #85-03 and #88-24: targets for postoperative radiochemotherapy? Head Neck 1998;20:588–94.

51. Bernier J, Domenge C, Ozsahin M, et al. Postoperative irradiation with or without concomitant chemotherapy for locally advanced head and neck cancer. N Engl J Med 2004;350:1945–52.

52. Cooper JS, Pajak TF, Forastiere AA, et al. Postoperative concurrent radiotherapy and chemotherapy for high-risk squamous-cell carcinoma of the head and neck. N Engl J Med 2004;350:1937–44.

53. Bernier J, Cooper JS, Pajak TF, et al. Defining risk levels in locally advanced head and neck cancers: a comparative analysis of concurrent postoperative radiation plus chemotherapy trials of the EORTC (#22931) and RTOG (# 9501). Head Neck 2005;27:843–50.

54. Sinha P, Kallogjeri D, Gay H, et al. High metastatic node number, not extracapsular spread or N-classification is a node-related prognosticator in transorally-resected, neck-dissected p16-positive oropharynx cancer. Oral Oncol 2015;51:514–20.

55. Mellott A, Vokes E. Chemoprevention in head and neck cancer. Cancer Treat Res 2001;106:221–35.

56. Anderson WF, Hawk E, Berg CD. Secondary chemoprevention of upper aerodigestive tract tumors. Semin Oncol 2001;28:106–20.

57. Goodwin WJ Jr. Salvage surgery for patients with recurrent squamous cell carcinoma of the upper aerodigestive tract: when do the ends justify the means? Laryngoscope 2000;110:1–18.

58. Skolyszewski J, Korzeniowski S, Reinfuss M. The reirradiation of recurrences of head and neck cancer. Br J Radiol 1980;53:462–5.

59. Langlois D, Eschwege F, Kramar A, et al. Reirradiation of head and neck cancers. Presentation of 35 cases treated at the Gustave Roussy Institute. Radiother Oncol 1985;3:27–33.

60. Emami B, Bignardi M, Spector GJ, et al. Reirradiation of recurrent head and neck cancers. Laryngoscope 1987;97:85–8.

61. Stevens KR Jr, Britsch A, Moss WT. High-dose reirradiation of head and neck cancer with curative intent. Int J Radiat Oncol Biol Phys 1994;29:687–98.

62. De Crevoisier R, Bourhis J, Domenge C, et al. Full-dose reirradiation for unresectable head and neck carcinoma: experience at the Gustave-Roussy Institute in a series of 169 patients. J Clin Oncol 1998;16:3556–62.

63. De Crevoisier R, Domenge C, Wibault P, et al. Full dose reirradiation combined with chemotherapy after salvage surgery in head and neck carcinoma. Cancer 2001;91:2071–6.

64. Spencer S, Wheeler R, Peters G, et al. Phase 1 trial of combined chemotherapy and reirradiation for recurrent unresectable head and neck cancer. Head Neck 2003;25:118–22.

65. Milano MT, Vokes EE, Salama JK, et al. Twice-daily reirradiation for recurrent and second primary head-and-neck cancer with gemcitabine, paclitaxel, and 5-fluorouracil chemotherapy. Int J Radiat Oncol Biol Phys 2005;61:1096–106.

66. Kramer NM, Horwitz EM, Cheng J, et al. Toxicity and outcome analysis of patients with recurrent head and neck cancer treated with hyperfractionated split-course reirradiation and concurrent cisplatin and paclitaxel chemotherapy from two prospective phase I and II studies. Head Neck 2005;27:406–14.

67. Spencer SA, Harris J, Wheeler RH, et al. RTOG 96-10: reirradiation with concurrent hydroxyurea and 5- fluorouracil in patients with squamous cell cancer of the head and neck. Int J Radiat Oncol Biol Phys 2001;51:1299–304.

68. Langer CJ, Harris J, Horwitz EM, et al. Phase II trial of concurrent split course hyperfractionated radiotherapy, cisplatin, and paclitaxel in patients with recurrent, previously irradiated squamous cell carcinoma of the head and neck: results of RTOG 99-11. Proc Am Soc Clin Oncol 2004;23:488.

69. Baliga S, Kabarriti R, Ohri N, et al. Stereotactic body radiotherapy for recurrent head and neck cancer: a critical review. Head Neck 2017;39:595–601.

70. Roman AA, Jodar C, Perez-Rozos A, et al. The role of stereotactic body radiotherapy in reirradiation of head and neck cancer recurrence. Crit Rev Oncol Hematol 2018;122:194–201.

71. Rubin Grandis J, Melhem MF, Gooding WE, et al. Levels of TGF-alpha and EGFR protein in head and neck squamous cell carcinoma and patient survival. J Natl Cancer Inst 1998;90:824–32.

72. Baselga J, Pfister D, Cooper MR, et al. Phase I studies of anti-epidermal growth factor receptor chimeric antibody C225 alone and in combination with cisplatin. J Clin Oncol 2000;18:904–14.

73. Cohen EE, Rosen F, Stadler WM, et al. Phase II trial of ZD1839 in recurrent or metastatic squamous cell carcinoma of the head and neck. J Clin Oncol 2003;21:1980–7.

74. Soulieres D, Senzer NN, Vokes EE, et al. Multicenter phase II study of erlotinib, an oral epidermal growth factor receptor tyrosine kinase inhibitor, in patients with recurrent or metastatic squamous cell cancer of the head and neck. J Clin Oncol 2004;22:77–85.

75. Grunwald V, Hidalgo M. Developing inhibitors of the epidermal growth factor receptor for cancer treatment. J Natl Cancer Inst 2003;95:851–67.

76. Mendelsohn J, Baselga J. Status of epidermal growth factor receptor antagonists in the biology and treatment of cancer. J Clin Oncol 2003;21:2787–99.

77. Herbst RS, Arquette M, Shin DM, et al. Phase II multicenter study of the epidermal growth factor receptor antibody cetuximab and cisplatin for recurrent and refractory squamous cell carcinoma of the head and neck. J Clin Oncol 2005;23:5578–87.

78. Baselga J, Trigo JM, Bourhis J, et al. Phase II multicenter study of the antiepidermal growth factor receptor monoclonal antibody cetuximab in combination with platinum-based chemotherapy in patients with platinum-refractory metastatic and/or recurrent squamous cell carcinoma of the head and neck. J Clin Oncol 2005;23:5568–77.

79. Vermorken JB, Mesia R, Rivera F, et al. Platinum-based chemotherapy plus cetuximab in head and neck cancer. N Engl J Med 2008;359:1116–27.

80. Kies MS, Holsinger FC, Lee JJ, et al. Induction chemotherapy and cetuximab for locally advanced squamous cell carcinoma of the head and neck: results from a phase II prospective trial. J Clin Oncol 2010;28:8–14.

81. Haddad RI, Tishler RB, Norris C, et al. Phase I study of C-TPF in patients with locally advanced squamous cell carcinoma of the head and neck. J Clin Oncol 2009;27:4448–53.

82. Bonner JA, Harari PM, Giralt J, et al. Radiotherapy plus cetuximab for squamous-cell carcinoma of the head and neck. N Engl J Med 2006;354: 567–78.

83. Bonner JA, Harari PM, Giralt J, et al. Radiotherapy plus cetuximab for locoregionally advanced head and neck cancer: 5-year survival data from a phase 3 randomised trial, and relation between cetuximab-induced rash and survival. Lancet Oncol 2010;11:21–8.

84. Giralt J, Trigo J, Nuyts S, et al. Panitumumab plus radiotherapy versus chemoradiotherapy in patients with unresected, locally advanced squamous-cell carcinoma of the head and neck (CONCERT-2): a randomised, controlled, open-label phase 2 trial. Lancet Oncol 2015;16:221–32.

85. Geoffrois L, Martin L, De Raucourt D, et al. Induction chemotherapy followed by cetuximab radiotherapy is not superior to concurrent chemoradiotherapy for head and neck carcinomas: results of the GORTEC 2007-02 phase III randomized trial. J Clin Oncol 2018;36:3077–83.

86. Tao Y, Auperin A, Sire C, et al. Improved outcome by adding concurrent chemotherapy to cetuximab and radiotherapy for locally advanced head and neck carcinomas: results of the GORTEC 2007-01 phase III randomized trial. J Clin Oncol 2018;36:3084–90.

87. Egloff AM, Lee JW, Langer CJ, et al. Phase II study of cetuximab in combination with cisplatin and radiation in unresectable, locally advanced head and neck squamous cell carcinoma: Eastern Cooperative Oncology Group Trial E3303. Clin Cancer Res 2014;20:5041–51.

88. Martins RG, Parvathaneni U, Bauman JE, et al. Cisplatin and radiotherapy with or without erlotinib in locally advanced squamous cell carcinoma of the head and neck: a randomized phase II trial. J Clin Oncol 2013;31:1415–21.

89. Ang KK, Zhang Q, Rosenthal DI, et al. Randomized phase III trial of concurrent accelerated radiation plus cisplatin with or without cetuximab for stage III to IV head and neck carcinoma: RTOG 0522. J Clin Oncol 2014;32:2940–50.

90. Mesia R, Henke M, Fortin A, et al. Chemoradiotherapy with or without panitumumab in patients with unresected, locally advanced squamous-cell carcinoma of the head and neck (CONCERT-1): a randomised, controlled, open-label phase 2 trial. Lancet Oncol 2015;16:208–20.

91. Psyrri A, Rampias T, Vermorken JB. The current and future impact of human papillomavirus on treatment of squamous cell carcinoma of the head and neck. Ann Oncol 2014;25:2101–15.

92. Gillison ML, Trotti AM, Harris J, et al. Radiotherapy plus cetuximab or cisplatin in human papillomavirus-positive oropharyngeal cancer (NRG Oncology RTOG 1016): a randomised, multicentre, non-inferiority trial. Lancet 2019;393:40–50.

93. Mehanna H, Robinson M, Hartley A, et al. Radiotherapy plus cisplatin or cetuximab in low-risk human papillomavirus-positive oropharyngeal cancer (De-ESCALaTE HPV): an open-label randomised controlled phase 3 trial. Lancet 2019;393:51–60.

94. Chung CH, Parker JS, Karaca G, et al. Molecular classification of head and neck squamous cell carcinomas using patterns of gene expression. Cancer Cell 2004;5:489–500.

95. Roepman P, Wessels LF, Kettelarij N, et al. An expression profile for diagnosis of lymph node metastases from primary head and neck squamous cell carcinomas. Nat Genet 2005;37:182–6.

96. Hammerman PS, Hayes DN, Grandis JR. Therapeutic insights from genomic studies of head and neck squamous cell carcinomas. Cancer Discov 2015;5: 239–44.
97. Hayes DN, Van Waes C, Seiwert TY. Genetic landscape of human papillomavirus-associated head and neck cancer and comparison to tobacco-related tumors. J Clin Oncol 2015;33:3227–34.
98. Schoenfeld JD. Immunity in head and neck cancer. Cancer Immunol Res 2015; 3:12–7.
99. Lyford-Pike S, Peng S, Young GD, et al. Evidence for a role of the PD-1:PD-L1 pathway in immune resistance of HPV-associated head and neck squamous cell carcinoma. Cancer Res 2013;73:1733–41.
100. Strome SE, Dong H, Tamura H, et al. B7-H1 blockade augments adoptive T-cell immunotherapy for squamous cell carcinoma. Cancer Res 2003;63:6501–5.
101. Jie HB, Gildener-Leapman N, Li J, et al. Intratumoral regulatory T cells upregulate immunosuppressive molecules in head and neck cancer patients. Br J Cancer 2013;109:2629–35.
102. Badoual C, Hans S, Merillon N, et al. PD-1-expressing tumor-infiltrating T cells are a favorable prognostic biomarker in HPV-associated head and neck cancer. Cancer Res 2013;73:128–38.
103. Chow LQM, Haddad R, Gupta S, et al. Antitumor activity of pembrolizumab in biomarker-unselected patients with recurrent and/or metastatic head and neck squamous cell carcinoma: results from the phase Ib KEYNOTE-012 expansion cohort. J Clin Oncol 2016;34:3838–45.
104. Seiwert TY, Burtness B, Mehra R, et al. Safety and clinical activity of pembrolizumab for treatment of recurrent or metastatic squamous cell carcinoma of the head and neck (KEYNOTE-012): an open-label, multicentre, phase 1b trial. Lancet Oncol 2016;17:956–65.
105. Cohen EEW, Soulieres D, Le Tourneau C, et al. Pembrolizumab versus methotrexate, docetaxel, or cetuximab for recurrent or metastatic head-and-neck squamous cell carcinoma (KEYNOTE-040): a randomised, open-label, phase 3 study. Lancet 2019;393:156–67.
106. Ferris RL, Blumenschein G Jr, Fayette J, et al. Nivolumab for recurrent squamous-cell carcinoma of the head and neck. N Engl J Med 2016;375: 1856–67.

Radiation Therapy for Thoracic Malignancies

Victor Ho-Fun Lee, MD[a],*, Li Yang, MD[b], Yong Jiang, MD, PhD[b],
Feng-Ming (Spring) Kong, MD, PhD[a],*

KEYWORDS

- Non–small cell lung cancer • Radiation techniques • Chemotherapy
- Targeted therapy • Immune checkpoint inhibitors

KEY POINTS

- Radiation therapy is the most commonly used non-surgical modality in treatment of lung cancers.
- New techniques of radiation treatment have greatly improved therapeutic ratios leading to better treatment outcomes and more favourable toxicities.
- New techniques like stereotactic body radiation therapy and proton therapy are now increasingly adopted as the sole radical treatment for small solitary lung tumours.

INTRODUCTION

Lung cancer is the most common type of thoracic malignancy and the top cause of cancer mortality worldwide. Non–small cell lung cancer (NSCLC) comprises of about 80% of all lung cancer.[1] Radiotherapy has been commonly used in patients with NSCLC during the course of their disease. Traditionally radiotherapy was used as palliative treatment of those who developed severe symptoms due to dyspnea, hemoptysis, spinal cord compression, or superior vena cava obstruction. Unfortunately, classical radiation techniques irradiated large fields, which included critical structures in the chest, and thus limited doses that could be safely delivered. In other words, the therapeutic ratio brought by the conventional technique was very small and the therapeutic effect is also brief and transient.

With the advent of modern radiotherapy techniques such as 3-dimensional conformal radiotherapy (3DCRT) and intensity-modulated radiation therapy (IMRT) in which the radiation beams are directed from different angles that converge where the tumor is located, dose escalation can be more safely achieved with fewer side

[a] Department of Clinical Oncology, La Ka Shing Faculty of Medicine, The University of Hong Kong, Queen Mary Hospital, 1/F, Professorial Block, 102 Pokfulam Road, Hong Kong, China;
[b] Clinical Oncology Center, The University of Hong Kong-Shenzhen Hospital, Haiyuan 1st Road, Futien District, Shenzhen 518053, China
* Corresponding authors.
E-mail addresses: vhflee@hku.hk (V.H.-F.L.); kong0001@hku.hk (F.-M.K.)

Hematol Oncol Clin N Am 34 (2020) 109–125
https://doi.org/10.1016/j.hoc.2019.09.007
0889-8588/20/© 2019 Elsevier Inc. All rights reserved.

hemonc.theclinics.com

effects to normal organs. IMRT can efficiently deliver a high dose to tumors with a rapid falloff leading to effective sparing of unnecessary radiation to the normal organs nearby. In fact, use of IMRT for lung cancer has increased from 2% in 2002 to 25% in 2009 in the United States.[2] A retrospective study of 13,292 stage III patients treated between 2003 and 2005 based on the United States National Cancer Data Base revealed that conformal radiotherapy (including both 3DCRT and IMRT) produced better overall survival (OS) when compared with 2-dimensional techniques.[3] A more recent update from National Cancer Data Base that included 7492 patients treated between 2003 and 2011 confirmed the small but significant OS advantage and few side effects with IMRT (median 20.0 months vs 18.2 months, $P<.0001$).[4] Apart from that, use of IMRT, when compared with a non-IMRT technique, predicted for a decreased likelihood of radiation treatment interruption of more than or equal to 4 days. The ability to dose escalate while limiting dose to normal tissues is a critical and recurring theme in lung cancer radiotherapy.

The following review shows and summarizes how radiotherapy can be considered and applied for NSCLC in different clinical settings.

Definitive Radiotherapy

Definitive radiotherapy is now the standard-of-care treatment of patients with early stage (preferably stage I disease with tumor size ≤3 cm) NSCLC who are not physically fit or refuse radical surgery. A median survival of more than 30 months and a 5-year survival rate of about 30% can be achieved with definitive radiotherapy alone with conventional dose fractionation of 66 to 70 Gy in 33 to 35 fractions.[5,6] Local recurrence and distant metastases are the usual patterns of relapse.[7,8]

Stereotactic body radiation therapy (SBRT) delivered by a hypofractionated scheme in a small number of fractions (typically between 3 and 8 fractions over 1–2 weeks) allows radiation oncologists to perform even more precise and conformal radiotherapy to the tumor with a rapid dose falloff in the surrounding lung parenchyma and adjacent structures, leading to enhanced tumor cell killing because of a higher biological effective dose (aiming at BED_{10} of at least 100 Gy) directed to the tumors.[9–11] Multiple randomized-controlled trials have been conducted to compare SBRT versus surgery (lobar or sublobar resection) for stage I NSCLC either in an unselected or in a high-risk population.[12–14] Unfortunately, all the trials prematurely closed because of very low patient accrual despite efforts to adjust enrollment criteria to enable enhanced patient recruitment. Nevertheless, Chang and colleagues[15] performed a pooled survival analysis from two phase III trials (STARS and ROSEL), which showed similar 3-year recurrence-free survival with either SBRT or resection (86% and 80% respectively, $P = .54$). OS was in favor of SBRT (95% vs 79%, hazard ratio [HR], 0.14, 95% confidence interval [CI] 0.017–1.190, $P = .037$). Extra caution must be taken when interpreting these results due to small sample size, unbalanced cohorts in these 2 studies, risk of type I error of inference, and relatively short follow-up.

There are now 3 ongoing multicenter randomized trials (STABLE-MATES, VALOR, and POSTILV) to compare resection and SBRT and the results are still eagerly awaited.[16–18] Another British phase III randomized trial that compares SBRT and resection in high-risk patients with peripheral tumors (SABRToothv1, NCT02629458) has just completed patient accrual with a target population of 54 patients.[19] Hopefully, preliminary results will be released in a couple of years.

Proton beam therapy has gained increasing attention recently in North America, in virtue of better conformity and tumor coverage when compared with photon treatment.[20,21] A phase II randomized trial comparing SBRT and stereotactic body proton therapy (SBPT) was prematurely closed due to poor patient accrual and lack of insurance coverage.[22] The published result showed that the treatment outcomes including 3-year OS and local and regional control were at least comparable and even better with SBPT. However, SBPT should not be routinely recommended outside of a clinical trial setting.

The usual recommended dose for SBRT for early-stage NSCLC is between 54 and 60 Gy in 3 fractions as reported by the RTOG 0618 study,[23] whereas 50 to 60 Gy in 5 fractions is optimal for centrally located tumors (within 2 cm of the proximal bronchial tree) as disclosed by RTOG 0813 study.[24] For ultracentral tumors, conventionally defined as tumors abutting or invading the proximal bronchial tree/trachea, a wide range of choices from 35 Gy/5fractions to 60 Gy/15fractions can be considered based on data from phase II trials (**Table 1**).[25–30] **Table 2** shows the recommended dose constraints for the organs-at-risk concerned during SBRT planning for ultra-central tumors.

Radiotherapy in Combination with Chemotherapy for Unresectable Stage III Non–Small Cell Lung Cancer

Radical chemoradiation, especially concurrent chemoradiation, is the standard treatment of unresectable stage III NSCLC.[31,32] The well-known meta-analysis of 6 clinical trials demonstrated an absolute OS benefit of 4.5% at 5 years with concurrent when compared with sequential chemoradiation, confirming the additive antitumor effect of delivering chemotherapy and radiotherapy simultaneously.[31] **Table 3** shows the summary of clinical trials that investigated the efficacy of combined modality treatments in unresectable stage III NSCLC.[33–40] Of note, Asian representation- and oncogene-driven NSCLC (eg, epidermal growth factor receptor (EGFR)-mutant tumors) are underrepresented. Therefore, special caution has to be taken when it comes to generalizability and applicability of these data in different populations.

Two to four cycles of platinum-based doublet chemotherapy given concurrently or sequentially with radiotherapy are recommended, whereas a weekly schedule with low-dose paclitaxel and carboplatin for 7 weeks concurrent with radiotherapy is another option in less medically fit patients.[41] A recent phase III trial (PROCLAIM) showed similar efficacy but better toxicity profiles with pemetrexed compared with the older drug etoposide, for nonsquamous NSCLC.[39] In addition, pemetrexed produces better activity against specific oncogene-driven tumors, for example, those with anaplastic lymphoma kinase (ALK) rearrangements.[42]

Involved field nodal irradiation showed better overall survival when compared with elective nodal irradiation.[43] The recommended radiation dose as radical treatment is between 60 and 70 Gy in 1.8 to 2 Gy fractions. Further dose escalation to 74 Gy resulted in an inferior survival compared with the standard dose in RTOG 0617 and is not recommended.[38] The dose constraints to adjacent important normal organs/tissues are shown in **Table 4**. Of great importance, dose to the heart should be minimized as much as achievable because it correlates negatively with survival.[44] Multiple ongoing studies are underway. Besides, radiation pneumonitis is also a serious concern. Lung dosimetry alone may not be always reliable to predict greater than or equal to G3 toxicity.[38]

IMRT, wherever possible, is preferred to older radiation techniques due to its better lung and heart sparing. The exploratory analysis of RTOG 0617 trial showed that the heart dose (V40—the percentage volume of the heart that has received 40 Gy or more) was the only significant prognostic factor on OS in multivariable analysis, which can be better spared with IMRT.[45] IMRT may also produce improved planning target volume coverage to the tumors and better avoidance of the esophagus to radiation. Together with robust motion management techniques during RT, for example, gating

Table 1
Published trials on using stereotactic body radiotherapy for ultracentral non-small cell lung cancer

Study (Reference)	Number of Patients	Definition of Ultra-Central Tumors	Dose Fractionation	BED α/β = 10 (Gy)	Local Control Rate	Grade 3–5 SBRT-Related Adverse Events
Chaudhuri et al,[25] 2015	6	GTV abutting the PBT or trachea	50 Gy/4–5 fractions	100/112.5	100% at 2 y	None
Tekatli et al,[26] 2016	47	PTV overlapping the trachea or main bronchi	60 Gy/12 fractions	90	No local relapse	38% for ≥ grade 3 toxicities, including 21% possibly SBRT-related fatalities
Daly et al,[27] 2017	9	PTV overlapping the PBT or esophagus	50 Gy/5 fractions	100	Not available	22.2% for ≥ grade 3 toxicities
Raman et al,[28] 2018	26	PTV contacting or overlapping the PBT, trachea, esophagus, pulmonary artery, or vein	60 Gy/8 fractions 48 Gy/4 fractions	105 105.6	100% at 2 y	No ≥ grade 4 toxicity
Chang et al,[29] 2018	46	ITV abutting the PBT	30–49 Gy/5 fractions or ≥50 Gy/5 fractions	48–97 or 100	95.7% at 2 y	8.7% for ≥ grade 3 toxicity
Nguyen et al,[30] 2019	14	PTV overlapping the PBT or esophagus	50 Gy/5 fractions or 56 Gy/8 fractions	100 or 95.2	89%	14.3% for ≥ grade 3 toxicity and 7.1% for grade 5 toxicity

Abbreviations: GTV, gross tumor volume; ITV, internal target volume; PBT, proximal bronchial tree; PTV, planning target volume.

Table 2
Recommended dose constraints of organs at risk in SBRT planning for ultracentral non–small cell lung cancer

Organs at Risk	Volume	Maximum Volume (Gy)	Maximum Point Dose	Avoidance Endpoint
Spinal cord	<0.25 cc <0.5 cc	22.5 Gy (4.5 Gy/fraction)	30 Gy (6 Gy/ fraction)	Myelitis
Ipsilateral brachial plexus	<3 cc	30 Gy (6 Gy/fraction)	32 Gy (6.4 Gy/ fraction)	Neuropathy
Skin	<10 cc	30 Gy (6 Gy/fraction)	32 Gy (6.4 Gy/ fraction)	Ulceration
Esophagus, nonadjacent wall	<5 cc	27.5 Gy (5.5 Gy/fraction)	105% of PTV prescription	Stenosis/ fistula
Heart/pericardium	<15 cc	32 Gy (6.4 Gy/fraction)	105% of PTV prescription	Pericardium
Great vessels, nonadjacent wall	<10 cc	47 Gy (9.4 Gy/fraction)	105% of PTV prescription	Aneurysm
Trachea and ipsilateral bronchus, nonadjacent wall	<4 cc	18 Gy (3.6 Gy/fraction)	105% of PTV prescription	Stenosis/ fistula
Lung (right and left)	1500 cc	12.5 Gy (2.5 Gy/fraction)		Basic lung function
Lung (right and left)	1000 cc	13.5 Gy (2.7 Gy/fraction)		Pneumonitis

Abbreviation: PTV, planning target volume.
From Bezjak A, Paulus R, Gaspar LE, et al. Safety and efficacy of a five-fraction stereotactic body radiotherapy schedule for centrally located non-small-cell lung Cancer: NRG Oncology/RTOG 0813 Trial. J Clin Oncol 2019;37(15):1316-1325; with permission.

and 4-dimensional evaluation of the internal target volume and daily image guidance before treatment, modern RT techniques are highly recommended in this setting.[46] Furthermore, patients treated with IMRT reported less meaningful decline in quality of life outcomes up to 1 year after following radical treatment.[47]

Proton beam therapy has dosimetric advantages in reducing the doses to the heart and the lung, which may be much preferred for those with bulky tumors and other underlying lung diseases.[21] A recently published phase II trial of 64 patients treated with proton beam therapy and concurrent chemotherapy with paclitaxel and carboplatin showed promising results.[48] However, late toxicity of greater than or equal to grade 3 pneumonitis developed in 12% of patients. In addition, 2 (3%) patients developed bronchial stricture and another one (2%) suffered from grade 4 bronchial fistula. Nevertheless, radiation dose distribution by proton beam is more susceptible to motion changes, tissue density heterogeneity, and set-up uncertainties. Adaptive proton beam planning has to be considered for those radiosensitive tumors that respond readily during radiation therapy. Four-dimensional imaging tracking the patients' breathing cycles might have to be considered as well during adaptive planning.

Preoperative Radiotherapy

Preoperative radiotherapy alone has no role in stage I to II NSCLC. There is evidence for the use of preoperative concurrent chemoradiation before surgery in selected patients. The INT-0139 study comparing radical chemoradiation with preoperative

Table 3
Summary of clinical trials on chemoradiation for unresectable stage IIIA/IIIB non-small cell lung cancer

Start Year of Study	Study	Eligibility Criteria	N=	Asian (%)	IIIA (%)	IIIB (%)	Treatment Schedules	OS (mo)	PFS (mo)	TRM (%)	Other Study Details
							Unresectable Stage IIIA/IIIB				
1984	CALGB 8433[33]	• T3 or N2 (Stage III based on staging criteria defined at time of study)	155	NA	NA	NA	a. Chemotherapy followed by sequential radiotherapy	13.8[a]	8.2[a]	0	
							b. Radiotherapy	9.6	5.5	0	
1994	RTOG 9410[34]	• Medically or surgically inoperable • Included Stage II–IIIB	577	2.0	42	57.0	a. Chemoradiation (Cisplatin + Vinblastine + 60 Gy)	17.0[a]	Time to infield progression similar between concurrent and sequential treatment	3.6	• 2% study patients were stage II
							b. Chemoradiation (Cisplatin + Etoposide + 69.6 Gy BID radiotherapy)	15.6		3.2	
							c. Chemotherapy (Cisplatin + Vinblastine) followed by sequential radiotherapy 60 Gy	14.6		4.6	
1997	CALGB 39801[35]	• Unresectable stage III	366	0	49.0	47.0	a. Induction chemotherapy followed by chemoradiation	14.0	8.0	2.0	
							b. Chemoradiation	12.0	7.0	1.0	

Year	Study	Characteristics	N				Treatment					Notes
2001	SWOG S0023[36]	• Unresectable stage III • Unselected for EGFR mutation	243	0.8	48.1	51.9	a. Chemoradiation followed by chemotherapy + consolidation gefitinib	23.0	8.3	Chemoradiation: 2	2.0	• Squamous 29.6%, adenocarcinoma 31.3%
							b. Chemoradiation followed by chemotherapy	35.0[a]	11.7	Adjuvant Chemotherapy: 0	0	
2005	KCSG-LU05-04[37]	• Unresectable stage III	420	100	22.1	77.4	a. Chemoradiation followed by chemotherapy	21.8	9.1	Chemoradiation: 3.6	2.9	• Patients recruited from Korea, Taiwan, and mainland China
							b. Chemoradiation	20.6	8.1		0	
2007	RTOG 0617[38]	• Unresectable stage III • 53.5% 3DCRT, 46.5% IMRT	424	2.4	64.9	35.1	a. Chemoradiation (74 Gy) followed by chemotherapy	20.3	9.8	3.9		• 53.5% 3DCRT, 46.5% IMRT
							b. Chemoradiation (60 Gy) followed by chemotherapy	28.7[a]	11.8	1.4		
		• Unresectable stage III • Patients unselected for EGFR expression	465	2.8	65.4	34.6	c. Chemoradiation followed by chemotherapy + cetuximab	25.0	10.8	4.2		• 43.8% with available EGFR H-score (21.6% ≥ 200)
							d. Chemoradiation followed by chemotherapy	24.0	10.7	2.2		

(continued on next page)

Table 3
(continued)

Start Year of Study	Study	Eligibility Criteria	N=	Asian (%)	IIIA (%)	IIIB (%)	Treatment Schedules	OS (mo)	PFS (mo)	TRM (%)	Other Study Details
							Unresectable Stage IIIA/IIIB				
2008	PROCLAIM[39]	• Unresectable stage III • Nonsquamous only	598	20.4	47.2	52.3	a. Chemoradiation (cisplatin + pemetrexed) followed by chemotherapy	26.8	11.4	1.8	
							b. Chemoradiation (cisplatin + etoposide) followed by chemotherapy	25.0	9.8	1.1	
2014	PACIFIC[40]	• Unresectable stage III • Unselected for PD-L1 status	713	26.9	52.9	44.7	a. Chemoradiation followed by durvalumab	NR[a]	17.2[a]	4.4	• 36.7% patients had unknown PD-L1 status • 6% EGFR mutant
							b. Chemoradiation	28.7	5.6	6.4	

Abbreviations: BID, twice daily; EGFR, epidermal growth factor receptor; TRM, treatment-related mortality.
[a] Statistically significant difference.

Table 4
Recommended dose constraints to critical organs at risk in radical radiotherapy planning for stage III non–small cell lung cancer

Critical Organs At Risk	Dose Constraint
Spinal canal	≤48 Gy
Spinal canal PRV	≤50 Gy
Lungs	
V20	≤35%
V5	≤65%
Mean dose	≤18 Gy
Heart	
V60	≤33%
V45	≤66%
V40	≤100%
Brachial plexus	≤66 Gy

Abbreviation: PRV, planning organ at risk volume.

chemoradiation followed by surgery for N2 NSCLC produced a longer progression-free survival (PFS) without OS improvement.[49] However, subgroup analysis revealed that an OS advantage was observed in those who did not receive pneumonectomy.

On the other hand, researchers from South Korea also noted excellent survival outcomes in those who achieved successful N2 downstaging following neoadjuvant chemoradiation, regardless of the bulk and extent of N2 status.[50,51] However, other studies have suggested that adding radiotherapy to preoperative radiotherapy enhanced downstaging but not survival outcomes.[52–55]

Careful patient selection and dedicated management in a high-volume tertiary referral center with multidisciplinary discussion is highly desired to make the most appropriate treatment decision for stage III NSCLC and to minimize any breaks in radiotherapy especially when a preoperative strategy is considered.

Postoperative Radiotherapy

Adjuvant chemotherapy has been well established as standard treatment following surgery for node-positive stage II to III disease, supported by meta-analyses with a 5% improvement of OS with platinum-based doublet chemotherapy.[56] However, those with node-positive disease after resection still had a 20% to 40% risk of locoregional relapse, which in turn correlated with a worse OS.[56,57]

Therefore, it is intuitive and appealing to consider radiotherapy to sterilize the mediastinal nodal stations. Nevertheless, the evidence of postoperative radiotherapy for resected stage I to IIIA NSCLC is still controversial. Early meta-analysis of trials conducted in the 1960s to 1970s demonstrated a decrease in OS with postoperative radiotherapy, which was postulated to be related to the cardiopulmonary toxicities brought by the use of traditional radiation techniques considered out-fashioned nowadays.[58]

Two Surveillance, Epidemiology, and End Results (SEER) analyses and a secondary exploratory analysis of Adjuvant Navelbine International Trialist Association trial suggested a potential OS benefit in the modern cohort of stage IIIA (N2) disease.[59–61] Notwithstanding, the effect of postoperative RT in the era of postoperative chemotherapy on OS was not addressed by the SEER studies.

A review of 4483 patients with pathologic N2 NSCLC identified from National Cancer Data Base treated with complete resection followed by adjuvant chemotherapy with or without postoperative radiotherapy published in 2016 demonstrated that postoperative radiotherapy (HR 0.886, 95% CI 0.798–0.988, $P = .029$), in addition to other factors such as younger age, female sex, urban population, lower Charlson score, smaller tumor size, multiagent chemotherapy, and resection with at least a lobectomy, was prognostic of improved OS.[62]

The most recent systematic review and meta-analysis of 11 studies of 8928 patients with resectable stage III N2 NSCLC revealed a trend of improvement of OS with postoperative radiotherapy (HR 0.88, 95% CI 0.76–1.02, $P = .11$) and a significant improvement of disease-free survival (HR 0.78, 95% CI 0.66–0.92, $P = .003$). Subgroup analysis on Caucasian patients further confirmed the OS benefit with postoperative radiotherapy (HR 0.88, 95% CI 0.81–0.96, $P = .003$).[63]

The recommended radiation dose in postoperative radiotherapy or chemoradiation is between 50 and 54 Gy to the involved nodal stations, with or without an additional boost of 60 to the high-risk sites for those with positive resection margins. Adjuvant chemoradiation is often considered in cases of extracapsular extension or positive margins.

Combination of Radiation Therapy and Immunotherapy

Immunotherapy in the form of immune checkpoint inhibitors has established a novel treatment paradigm for advanced NSCLC. It has been discovered that radiotherapy stimulates the release of tumor-associated antigens and damage-associated molecular patterns, which can elicit an immunogenic response.[64,65] Besides, radiotherapy has been observed to enhance the antigen-presenting ability of the immune cells with a resultant increase in tumor recognition and antitumor activity.[66–70] Combination of radiotherapy and immune checkpoint inhibitor has exhibited synergistic antitumor responses in preclinical studies, probably arising from the enhanced activity and diversity of the antitumor T cells contributed by radiotherapy.[71,72] In fact, the exploratory analysis of the phase I dose-finding study of pembrolizumab in advanced or metastatic NSCLC in KEYNOTE-001 trial demonstrated that patients who received previous radiotherapy at any time point before their first cycle of pembrolizumab showed a significant improvement of OS and PFS.[73]

Immunotherapy as maintenance therapy after completion of concurrent chemoradiation is new standard for patients and oncologists in the United States. The pivotal phase III randomized controlled trial (PACIFIC) comparing durvalumab (a PD-L1 inhibitor) with observation after completion of concurrent chemoradiation for stage III inoperable NSCLC demonstrated an significant OS advantage (2-year rate 66.3% vs 55.6%).[40] However, the low Asian representation (27% of the whole study population) together with only 6% of EGFR-mutated NSCLC and the unknown proportion of ALK-rearranged tumors in this study has raised concerns about the applicability of these data to Asian patients. Intriguingly, the Japanese subset in this study enjoyed a significantly longer median PFS with durvalumab (HR 0.49, $P = .020$), consistent with that of the whole study population.[74] On the other hand, the incidence of radiation pneumonitis of any grade was higher in the Japanese population compared with the overall population (Placebo: 60% [Japanese] vs 24.8% [overall]; Durvalumab: 73.6% [Japanese] vs 33.9% [overall]), although the rates of pneumonitis/radiation pneumonitis leading to treatment discontinuation were similar. It may be that Japanese NSCLC represents a distinct and radiosensitive entity. Patients in this study were also unselected for the PD-L1 expression status in their tumors. A new PACIFIC2 trial adding durvalumab concurrently with cisplatin chemoradiation may help solve this query, as more Eastern participation into this international trial is highly expected (NCT03519971). Further questions remain undeciphered, including the optimal timing of initiating durvalumab maintenance treatment; there seemed to be an improvement in PFS in those who started durvalumab earlier ($\leq$2 weeks after completion of concurrent chemoradiation). Besides, the beneficial roles of durvalumab in patients treated with surgery after chemoradiation, sequential chemoradiation, and altered dose fractionation schemes are yet to be addressed. Future trials on these 3 issues (NCT03871153, NCT03693300, and NCT03801902, respectively) are now under way and the results are awaited.

Radiation Therapy for Stage IV Non–Small Cell Lung Cancer

Radiation therapy has been increasingly used for stage IV NSCLC, not just for palliative benefit but also in the context of more definitive approaches. For example, SBRT for tumor eradication of the resistant clones refractory to targeted therapy for mutation-driven NSCLC is one area of active interest.[75]

The first phase II randomized controlled trial used aggressive local consolidative therapy with either chemoradiation or surgical resection or maintenance systemic therapy/observation alone in those patients with less than or equal to 3 metastases who did not progress on standard first-line systemic therapy/observation.[76] First-line systemic therapy could be either greater than or equal to 4 cycles of platinum doublet therapy or greater than or equal to 3 months of EGFR/ALK inhibitor for patients with EGFR mutations/ALK rearrangements, respectively. The study was terminated early after recruitment of 49 patients because of efficacy with local consolidative therapy on the recommendation of the Data Safety Monitoring Board. The median PFS was 11.9 (90% CI 5.72–20.90) months with local consolidative therapy compared with only 3.9 (90% CI 0.18–0.66) for those without local consolidative therapy. OS data were yet to mature but the toxicity profiles were similar between the 2 arms.

These encouraging and promising results were further echoed in another phase II randomized study evaluating consolidative radiotherapy in the setting of oligometastases (primary tumor and up to 5 metastatic sites).[77] In this single-center study, patients received first-line systemic therapy and were subsequently randomized to consolidative radiotherapy with or without maintenance chemotherapy versus maintenance chemotherapy alone. Again the study was prematurely terminated, as an interim analysis detected a significant PFS improvement with SBRT plus maintenance chemotherapy compared with maintenance chemotherapy alone arm (9.7 months vs 3.5 months respectively, $P = .01$). The recently completed COMET study also compares the efficacy of standard of care versus SBRT in the setting of different combinations of oligometastases up to 5 lesions as defined.[78] The results of this Canadian study will be released in due course.

A cost-effectiveness analysis conducted in Switzerland suggested that local therapies including SBRT and surgery may be cost-effective in those responding to first-line systemic treatment.[79] Similar studies should be conducted in Asian countries where a much higher incidence of EGFR mutations is expected.[80,81]

SUMMARY

In summary, radiation techniques have advanced tremendously leading to substantial and significant improvement in therapeutic ratios, treatment outcomes, and quality of life in patients with NSCLC. Future research directions should focus on the combination of modern radiation techniques with other novel therapeutics, especially targeted therapy for oncogene-driven tumors and immune checkpoint inhibitors for those tumors with favorable predictive biomarkers. Studies on definitive treatment in oligometastatic patients are also warranted. International multicenter studies are warranted to prove the applicability, safety, and efficacy in patients across different ethnicities.

REFERENCES

1. Bray F, Ferlay J, Soerjomataram I, et al. Global cancer statistics 2018: GLOBOCAN estimates of incidence and mortality worldwide for 36 cancers in 185 countries. CA Cancer J Clin 2018;68(6):394–424.
2. Harris JP, Murphy JD, Hanion AL, et al. A population-based comparative effectiveness study of radiation therapy techniques in stage III non-small cell lung cancer. Int J Radiat Oncol Biol Phys 2014;88:872–4.
3. Sher DJ, Koshy M, Liptay MJ, et al. Influence of conformal radiotherapy technique on survial after chemoradiotherapy for patients with stage III non-small cell lung cancer in the National Cancer Data Base. Cancer 2014;120:2360–8.
4. Koshy M, Malik R, Spiotto M, et al. Association between intensity modulated radiation therapy and survival in patients with stage III non-small cell lung cancer treated with chemoradiotherapy. Lung Cancer 2017;108:222–7.
5. Maguire PD, Marks LB, Sibley GS, et al. 73.6Gy and beyond: hyperfrationated, accelerated radiotherapy for non-small-cell lung cancer. J Clin Oncol 2001;19: 705–11.
6. Bogart JA, Aronowitz JN. Localized non-small cell lung cancer: adjuvant radiotherapy in the era of effective systemic therapy. Clin Cancer Res 2005;11(13 Pt 2):5004s–10s.
7. Bradley JD, Wahab S, Lockett MA, et al. Elective nodal failures are uncommon in medically inoperable patients with Stage I non-small-cell lung carcinoma treated with limited radiotherapy fields. Int J Radiat Oncol Biol Phys 2003;56:342–7.
8. Kong FM, Ten Haken RK, Schipper MJ, et al. High-dose radiation improved local tumor control and overall survival in patients with inoperable/unresectable non-small-cell lung cancer: long-term results of a radiation dose escalation study. Int J Radiat Oncol Biol Phys 2005;63:324–33.
9. Videtic GM, Stephans KL. The role of stereotactic body radiotherapy in the management of non-small cell lung cancer: an emerging standard for the medically inoperable patient? Curr Oncol Rep 2010;12(4):235–41.
10. Chua KLM, Sin I, Fong KW, et al. Stereotactic body radiotherapy for early stage lung cancer-historical developments and future strategies. Chin Clin Oncol 2017; 6(Suppl 2):S20.
11. Nagata Y, Kimura T. Stereotactic body radiotherapy (SBRT) for Stage I lung cancer. Jpn J Clin Oncol 2018;48(5):405–9.
12. Fernando HC, Timmerman R. American College of Surgeons Oncology Group Z4099/Radiation Therapy Oncology Group 1021: a randomized study of sublobar resection compared with stereotactic body radiotherapy for high-risk stage I non-small cell lung cancer. J Thorac Cardiovasc Surg 2012;144:S35–8.
13. Trial of Either Surgery or Stereotactic Radiotherapy for Early Stage (IA) Lung Cancer (ROSEL). Available at: https://clinicaltrials.gov/ct2/show/NCT00687986. Accessed June 20, 2018.
14. Randomized Study to Compare CyperKnife to Surgical Resection in Stage I Non–Small Cell Lung Cancer (STARS). Available at: https://clinicaltrials.gov/. Accessed June 20, 2018.

15. Chang JY, Senan S, Paul MA, et al. Stereotactic ablative radiotherapy versus lo-bectomy for operable stage I non-small-cell lung cancer: a pooled analysis of two randomised trials. Lancet Oncol 2015;16:630–7.

16. Ca Sublobar Resection (SR) Versus Stereotactic Ablative Radiotherapy (SAbR) for Lung Cancer (STABLE-MATES). Available at: https://www.clinicaltrials.gov/ct2/show/NCT02468024. Accessed June 20, 2018.

17. Veteran Affairs Lung Cancer or Stereotactic Radiotherapy (VALOR). Available at: https://clinicaltrials.gov/ct2/show/NCT02984761. Accessed June 5, 2018.

18. Radical Resection vs. Ablative Stereotactic Radiotherapy in Patients with Oper-able Stage I NSCLC (POSTILV). Available at: https://clinicaltrials.gov/ct2/show/NCT01753414. Accessed June 20, 2018.

19. A Study to Determine the Feasibility and Acceptability of Conducting a Phase III Randomised Controlled Trial Comparing Stereotactic Ablative Radiotherapy with Surgery in paTients with Peripheral Stage I Non-Small Cell Lung Cancer cOnsid-ered Higher Risk of Complications from Surgical Resection (SABRTOOTHv1). Available at: https://clinicaltrials.gov/ct2/show/NCT02629458. Accessed July 31, 2019.

20. Liao Z, Lee JJ, Komaki R, et al. Bayesian adaptive randomization trial of passive scattering proton therapy and intensity-modulated photon radiotherapy for locally advanced non-small-cell lung cancer. J Clin Oncol 2018;36(18):1813–22.

21. Chang JY, Zhang X, Knopf A, et al. Consensus guidelines for implementing pencil-beam scanning proton therapy for thoracic malignancies on behalf of the PTCOG Thoracic and Lymphoma Subcommittee. Int J Radiat Oncol Biol Phys 2017;99:41–50.

22. Natavithya C, Gomez DR, Wei X, et al. Phase 2 study of stereotactic body radia-tion therapy and stereotactic body proton therapy for high-risk, medically inoper-able, early-stage non-small cell lung cancer. Int J Radiat Oncol Biol Phys 2018;101(3):558–63.

23. Timmerman RD, Paulus R, Pass HI, et al. Stereotactic body radiation therapy for operable early-stage lung cancer: findings from the NRG oncology RTOG 0618 trial. JAMA Oncol 2018;4(9):1263–6.

24. Bezjak A, Paulus R, Gaspar LE, et al. Safety and efficacy of a five-fraction stereo-tactic body radiotherapy schedule for centrally located non-small-cell lung Can-cer: NRG Oncology/RTOG 0813 trial. J Clin Oncol 2019;37:1316–25.

25. Chaudhuri AA, Tang C, Binkley MS, et al. Stereotactic ablative radiotherapy (SABR) for treatment of central and ultra-central lung tumors. Lung Cancer 2015;89(1):50–6.

26. Tekatli H, Haasbeek N, Dahele M, et al. Outcomes of hypofractionated high-dose radiotherapy in poor-risk patients with "ultracentral" non-small cell lung cancer. J Thorac Oncol 2016;11(7):1081–9.

27. Daly M, Novak J, Monjazeb A. P2.05-056 safety of stereotactic body radiotherapy for central, ultracentral, and paramediastinal lung tumors. J Thorac Oncol 2017;12(1):S1066.

28. Raman S, Yau V, Pineda S, et al. Ultracentral tumors treated with stereotactic body radiotherapy: Singleinstitution experience. Clin Lung Cancer 2018;19(5):e803–10.

29. Chang JH, Poon I, Erler D, et al. The safety and effectiveness of stereotactic body radiotherapy for central versus ultracentral lung tumors. Radiother Oncol 2018;129:277–83.

30. Nguyen KNB, Hause DJ, Novak J, et al. Tumor control and toxicity after SBRT for ultracentral, central, and paramediastinal lung tumors. Pract Radiat Oncol 2019; 9:e196–202.

31. Aupérin A, Le Péchoux C, Rolland E, et al. Meta-analysis of concomitant versus sequential radiochemotherapy in locally advanced non-small-cell lung cancer. J Clin Oncol 2010;28(13):2181–90.

32. Bezjak A, Temin S, Franklin G, et al. Definitive and adjuvant radiotherapy in locally advanced non-small-cell lung cancer: american society of clinical oncology clinical practice guideline endorsement of the american society for radiation oncology evidence-based clinical practice guideline. J Clin Oncol 2015;33(18): 2100–5.

33. Dillman RO, Herndon J, Seagren SL, et al. Improved survival in stage III non-small-cell lung cancer: seven-year follow-up of cancer and leukemia group B (CALGB) 8433 trial. J Natl Cancer Inst 1996;88(17):1210–5.

34. Curran WJ Jr, Paulus R, Langer CJ, et al. Sequential vs. concurrent chemoradiation for stage III non-small cell lung cancer: randomized phase III trial RTOG 9410. J Natl Cancer Inst 2011;103(19):1452–60.

35. Vokes EE, Herndon JE 2nd, Kelley MJ, et al. Induction chemotherapy followed by chemoradiotherapy compared with chemoradiotherapy alone for regionally advanced unresectable stage III Non-small-cell lung cancer: cancer and Leukemia Group B. J Clin Oncol 2007;25(13):1698–704.

36. Kelly K, Chansky K, Gaspar LE, et al. Phase III trial of maintenance gefitinib or placebo after concurrent chemoradiotherapy and docetaxel consolidation in inoperable stage III non-small-cell lung cancer: SWOG S0023. J Clin Oncol 2008;26(15):2450–6.

37. Ahn JS, Ahn YC, Kim JH, et al. Multinational randomized phase III trial with or without consolidation chemotherapy using docetaxel and cisplatin after concurrent chemoradiation in inoperable stage III non-small-cell lung cancer: KCSG-LU05-04. J Clin Oncol 2015;33:2660–6.

38. Bradley JD, Paulus R, Komaki R, et al. Standard-dose versus high-dose conformal radiotherapy with concurrent and consolidation carboplatin plus paclitaxel with or without cetuximab for patients with stage IIIA or IIIB non-small-cell lung cancer (RTOG 0617): a randomised, two-by-two factorial phase 3 study. Lancet Oncol 2015;16(2):187–99.

39. Senan S, Brade A, Wang LH, et al. PROCLAIM: randomized phase III trial of pemetrexed-cisplatin or etoposide-cisplatin plus thoracic radiation therapy followed by consolidation chemotherapy in locally advanced nonsquamous non-small-cell lung cancer. J Clin Oncol 2016;34(9):953–62.

40. Antonia SJ, Villegas A, Daniel D, et al. Overall survival with durvalumab after chemoradiotherapy in stage III NSCLC. N Engl J Med 2018;379:2342–50.

41. Belani CP, Choy H, Bonomi P, et al. Combined chemoradiotherapy regimens of paclitaxel and carboplatin for locally advanced non-small-cell lung cancer: a randomized phase II locally advanced multi-modality protocol. J Clin Oncol 2005; 23(25):5883–91.

42. Lee JO, Kim TM, Lee SH, et al. Anaplastic lymphoma kinase translocation: a predictive biomarker of pemetrexed in patients with non-small cell lung cancer. J Thorac Oncol 2011;6:1474–80.

43. Yuan S, Sun X, Li M, et al. A randomized study of involved-field irradiation versus elective nodal irradiation in combination with concurrent chemotherapy for inoperable stage III nonsmall cell lung cancer. Am J Clin Oncol 2007;30(3):239–44.

44. Speirs CK, DeWees TA, Rehman S, et al. Heart dose is an independent dosimetric predictor of overall survival in locally advanced non-small cell lung cancer. J Thorac Oncol 2017;12(2):293–301.

45. Chun SG, Hu C, Choy H, et al. Impact of intensity-modulated radiation therapy technique for locally advanced non-small-cell lung cancer: a secondary analysis of the NRG oncology RTOG 0617 randomized clinical trial. J Clin Oncol 2017;35: 56–62.

46. Johnson-Hart CN, Price GJ, Faivre-Finn C, et al. Residual setup errors towards the heart after image guidance linked with poorer survival in lung cancer patients: do we need stricter IGRT protocols? Int J Radiat Oncol Biol Phys 2018;102: 434–42.

47. Movsas B, Hu C, Sloan J, et al. Quality of life analysis of a radiation dose-escalation study of patients with non-small-cell lung cancer: a secondary analysis of the radiation therapy oncology group 0617 randomized clinical trial. JAMA Oncol 2016;2:359–67.

48. Chang JY, Verma V, Li M, et al. Proton beam radiotherapy and concurrent chemotherapy for unresectable stage III non-small cell lung cancer: final results of a phase 2 study. JAMA Oncol 2017;3:e172032.

49. Albain KS, Swann RS, Rusch VW, et al. Radiotherapy plus chemotherapy with or without surgical resection for stage III non-small-cell lung cancer: a phase III randomised controlled trial. Lancet 2009;374:379–86.

50. Kim HK, Cho JH, Choi YS, et al. Outcomes of neoadjuvant concurrent chemoradiotherapy followed by surgery for non-small-cell lung cancer with N2 disease. Lung Cancer 2016;96:56–62.

51. Lee H, Ahn YC, Pyo H, et al. Pretreatment clinical mediastinal nodal bulk and extent do not influence survival in N2-positive stage IIIA non-small cell lung cancer patients treated with trimodality therapy. Ann Surg Oncol 2014;21:2083–90.

52. Thomas M, Rube C, Hoffknecht P, et al. Effect of preoperative chemoradiation in addition to preoperative chemotherapy: a randomised trial in stage III non-small-cell lung cancer. Lancet Oncol 2008;9:636–48.

53. Pless M, Stupp R, Ris HB, et al. Induction chemoradiation in stage IIIA/N2 non small-cell lung cancer: a phase 3 randomised trial. Lancet 2015;386(9998): 1049–56.

54. Katakami N, Tada H, Mitsudomi T, et al. A phase 3 study of induction treatment with concurrent chemoradiotherapy versus chemotherapy before surgery in patients with pathologically confirmed N2 stage IIIA nonsmall cell lung cancer (WJTOG9903). Cancer 2012;118:6126–35.

55. Girard N, Mornex F, Douillard JY, et al. Is neoadjuvant chemoradiotherapy a feasible strategy for stage IIIA-N2 non-small cell lung cancer? Mature results of the randomized IFCT-0101 phase II trial. Lung Cancer 2010;69(1):86–93.

56. NSCLC Meta-analyses Collaborative Group, Arriagada R, Auperin A, Burdett S, et al. Adjuvant chemotherapy, with or without postoperative radiotherapy, in operable non-small-cell lung cancer: Two meta-analyses of individual patient data. Lancet 2015;375:1267–77.

57. Le Pechoux C. Role of postoperative radiotherapy in resected non-small cell lung cancer: a reassessment based on neew data. Oncologist 2011;16:672–81.

58. PORT Meta-analysis Trialists Group. Postoperative radiotherapy for non-small cell lung cancer. Cochrane Database Syst Rev 2015;(2):CD002142.

59. Lally BE, Zelterman D, Colasanto JM, et al. Postoperative radiotherapy for stage II or III non-small-cell lung caner using the surveillance, epidemiology, and end results database. J Clin Oncol 2006;24:2998–3006.

60. Lally BE, Detterbeck FC, Geiger AM, et al. The risk of death from heart diseae in patients with nonsmall cell lung cancer who receive postoperative radiotherapy: Analysis of the Surveillance , Epidemiology, and End Results database. Cancer 2007;110:911–7.
61. Douillard JY, Rosell R, De Lena M, et al. Impact of postoperative radiation therapy on survival in patietns with complete resection and stage I, II or IIIA non-small-cell lung cancer treated witih adjuvant chemotherapy: The Adjuvant Navelbine International Trialist Association (ANITA) randomized trial. Int J Radiat Oncol Biol Phys 2008;72:695–701.
62. Robinson CG, Patel AP, Bradley JD, et al. Postoperative radiotherapy for pathologic N2 non-small-cell lung cancer treated with adjuvant chemotherapy: a review of the National Cancer Data Base. J Clin Oncol 2015;33(8):870–6.
63. Zhang H, Zhang DX, Ju T, et al. The effect of postoperative radiotherapy on the survival of patients with resectable stage III-N2 non-small-cell lung cancer: a systematic review and meta-analysis. Neoplasma 2019;2019 [pii:18123N965].
64. Formenti SC, Demaria S. Radiation therapy to convert the tumor into an in situ vaccine. Int J Radiat Oncol Biol Phys 2012;84:879–80.
65. Demaria S, Golden EB, Formenti SC. Role of local radiation therapy in cancer immunotherapy. JAMA Oncol 2015;1:1325–32.
66. Reits EA, Hodge JW, Herberts CA, et al. Radiation modulates the peptide repertoire, enhances MHC class I expression, and induces successful antitumor immunotherapy. J Exp Med 2006;203:1259–71.
67. Sharabi AB, Lim M, DeWeese TL, et al. Radiation and checkpoint blockade immunotherapy: radiosensitisation and potential mechanisms of synergy. Lancet Oncol 2015;16:e498–509.
68. Sharabi AB, Nirschl CJ, Kochel CM, et al. Stereotactic radiation therapy augments antigen-specific pd-1-mediated antitumor immune responses via cross-presentation of tumor antigen. Cancer Immunol Res 2015;3:345–55.
69. Gupta A, Probst HC, Vuong V, et al. Radiotherapy promotes tumor-specific effector CD8+ T cells via dendritic cell activation. J Immunol 2012;189:558–66.
70. Liao YP, Wang CC, Butterfield LH, et al. Ionizing radiation affects human MART-1 melanoma antigen processing and presentation by dendritic cells. J Immunol 2004;173:2462–9.
71. Herter-Sprie GS, Koyama S, Korideck H, et al. Synergy of radiotherapy and PD-1 blockade in Kras-mutant lung cancer. JCI Insight 2016;16:e87415.
72. Twyman-Saint Victor C, Rech AJ, Maity A, et al. Radiation and dual checkpoint blockade activate non-redundant immune mechanisms in cancer. Nature 2015; 520:373–7.
73. Shaverdian N, Lisberg AE, Bornazyan K, et al. Previous radiotherapy and the clinical activity and toxicity of pembrolizumab in the treatment of non-small-cell lung cancer: a secondary analysis of the KEYNOTE-001 phase 1 trial. Lancet Oncol 2017;18:895–903.
74. Tokito T, MS, Kurata T, et al. Overall Survival with Durvalumab vs. Placebo after Chemoradiotherapy in Stage III NSCLC: PACIFIC. 58th annual meeting of Japanese Lung Cancer Society 2017: Yokohama, October 14–15, 2017. p. S1–4.
75. Ning MS, Gomez DR, Heymach JV, et al. Stereotactic ablative body radiation for oligometastatic and oligoprogressive disease. Transl Lung Cancer Res 2019;8:97–106.
76. Gomez DR, Blumenschein GR Jr, Lee JJ, et al. Local consolidative therapy versus maintenance therapy or observation for patients with oligometastatic non-smallcell lung cancer without progression after first-line systemic therapy:

a multicentre, randomised, controlled, phase 2 study. Lancet Oncol 2016;17: 1672–82.
77. Iyengar P, Wardak Z, Gerber DE, et al. Consolidative radiotherapy for limited metastatic non-small-cell lung cancer: a phase 2 randomized clinical trial. JAMA Oncol 2018;4:e173501.
78. Palma DA, Haasbeek CJ, Rodrigues GB, et al. Stereotactic ablative radiotherapy for comprehensive treatment of oligometastatic tumors (SABR-COMET): study protocol for a randomized phase II trial. BMC Cancer 2012;12:305.
79. Panje CM, Dedes KJ, Matter-Walstra K, et al. A cost-effectiveness analysis of consolidative local therapy in oligometastatic non-squamous non-small cell lung cancer (NSCLC). Radiother Oncol 2018;129:257–63.
80. Weickhardt AJ, Scheier B, Burke JM, et al. Local ablative therapy of oligoprogressive disease prolongs disease control by tyrosine kinase inhibitors in oncogene-addicted non-small-cell lung cancer. J Thorac Oncol 2012;7:1807–14.
81. Chan OSH, Lee VHF, Mok TSK, et al. The role of radiotherapy in epidermal growth factor receptor mutation-positive patients with oligoprogression: a matched-cohort analysis. Clin Oncol (R Coll Radiol) 2017;29:568–75.

Hematologic Malignancies

Yolanda D. Tseng, MPhil, MD[a], Andrea K. Ng, MD, MPH[b],*

KEYWORDS

- Hematologic malignancies • Hodgkin lymphoma • Non-Hodgkin lymphoma
- Leukemia • Multiple myeloma • Plasmacytoma

KEY POINTS

- Radiation therapy plays a key role in various settings of hematologic malignancies, including as primary, adjuvant, salvage, or palliative therapy.
- Optimal dose fractionation, target volume, and timing in relation to systemic therapy vary on a case-by-case basis.
- Advanced radiation therapy techniques allow more precise dose delivery to target sites while limiting doses to surrounding critical normal organs.

INTRODUCTION

Hematologic malignancies represent a wide range of disease entities, most of which are highly responsive to radiation therapy. Either alone or with systemic therapy, radiation therapy can play in a critical role in the primary treatment, salvage, or palliative setting. Whether radiation therapy should be included, and, if so, the optimal dose and volume, varies depending on the histologic subtypes, stage at presentation, patient performance status, response to systemic therapy if given, treatment intent, and patient preferences. This review focuses on the indications for radiotherapy among more commonly seen hematologic malignancies. Where appropriate, the recommended radiation dose and target volume according to available evidence and/or published guidelines are discussed. In addition, modern radiotherapy techniques for the more challenging treatments sites are examined, with goals of limiting doses to organs at risk while preserving target coverage.

ROLE OF RADIATION THERAPY IN HEMATOLOGIC MALIGNANCIES
Hodgkin Lymphoma

Limited stage
Patients with limited-stage Hodgkin lymphoma (HL) are generally divided into favorable and unfavorable prognostic groups. Summarized in **Table 1** are factors used in

Disclosure: The authors have nothing to disclose.
[a] Department of Radiation Oncology, Seattle Cancer Care Alliance Proton Therapy Center, University of Washington School of Medicine, 1570 North 115th Street, Seattle, WA 98133, USA; [b] Department of Radiation Oncology, Dana-Farber/Brigham and Women's Cancer Center, Harvard Medical School, 75 Francis Street, Boston, MA 02115, USA
* Corresponding author.
E-mail address: andrea_ng@dfci.harvard.edu

defining favorable prognosis, or low-risk disease, in patients with early-stage HL, according to the German Hodgkin Study Group (GHSG) and the European Organization for Research and Treatment of Cancer (EORTC), the two key cooperative groups on HL clinical trials.

The GHSG HD10, HD11, EORTC-French Groupe d'Étude des Lymphomes de l'Adulte (GELA) H9F trials addressed radiation dose de-escalation to 20 Gy after chemotherapy in early-stage HL.[1–4] In the GHSG HD10 trial,[2] there were no differences in 10-year progression-free survival (PFS) between 20 Gy versus 30 Gy after 2 or 4 cycles of adriamycin, bleomycin, vinblastine dacarbazine (ABVD) chemotherapy in patients with early-stage low-risk HL (10-year PFS, 87%).[3] In the EORTC-GELA H9F trial randomizing early-stage, favorable-prognosis patients to 36 Gy, 20 Gy, or no radiotherapy after 6 cycles of epirubicin, bleomycin, vinblastine, and prednisone (EBVP), the no-radiotherapy arm was closed early because of unacceptable relapse rates (5-year RFS, 68.9%), but there was no difference between the 36-Gy and 20-Gy arms (5-year RFS, 88.6% vs 84.2%).[4] However, nonstandard chemotherapy, EBVP, was used in this trial. In the GHSG HD11 trial,[1] which included early-stage patients with risk factors, 20 Gy was noninferior to 30 Gy after baseline bleomycin, etoposide, doxorubicin, cyclophosphamide, vincristine, procarbazine, and prednisone (BEACOPP)[3]; however, inferiority of 20 Gy cannot be excluded after ABVD (10-year PFS, 76% vs 84%). As such, a consolidative radiation dose of 20 Gy is adequate in patients with low-risk disease, but 30 Gy remains the standard dose after ABVD for early-stage HL with risk factors.

Recent trials have focused on adapting treatment based on PET response to chemotherapy. The United Kingdom Randomised Phase III Trial to Determine the Role of FDG–PET Imaging in Clinical Stages IA/IIA Hodgkin's Disease (RAPID), the EORTC/Lymphoma Study Association (LYSA)/Fondazione Italiana Linfomi (FIL) H10, and the GHSG HD16 trials tested omission of radiotherapy in early-stage patients with complete PET response to chemotherapy.[5–7] The RAPID trial compared 3 cycles of ABVD followed by radiotherapy versus 3 cycles of ABVD alone after a complete PET response.[5] By intent-to-treat analysis, the 3-year PFS rate was 94.6% in the radiotherapy group and 90.8% in the no-radiotherapy group ($P = .16$). However, the prespecified noninferiority margin of 7 percentage points was not met. The noninferiority of chemotherapy alone therefore could not be concluded. Moreover, by per-protocol analysis, after excluding patients who did not receive the assigned treatment, there was a significant difference favoring radiotherapy (3-year PFS 97.1% vs 90.8%, $P = .02$). In the EORTC/LYSA/FIL H10 trial,[6] for favorable patients with early complete PET response to ABVD, the 5-year PFS of the combined modality therapy arm was significantly higher than that of the

Table 1
Definition of favorable-prognosis early-stage Hodgkin lymphoma

	GHSG[2]	EORTC[6]
Age (y)	—	<50
ESR B Symptoms	<30 or <50 with no B symptoms	<30 or <50 with no B symptoms
Large Mediastinal Adenopathy	No	No
Extranodal sites	None	—
Number of sites	<3	<4

Abbreviations: EORTC, European Organization for Research and Treatment of Cancer; ESR, erythrocyte sedimentation rate; GHSG, German Hodgkin Study Group.

chemotherapy-alone arm (99% vs 87.1%). The corresponding 5-year PFSs were 92.1% and 89.6%, respectively, for unfavorable patients. Although this difference was not significant, the prespecified noninferiority margin was not met. Hence, non-inferiority of chemotherapy alone could not be concluded. In the GHSG HD16 trial,[7] patients with early-stage low-risk disease were randomized to ABVD times 2 followed by 20-Gy radiotherapy, versus ABVD times 2 alone if PET-negative disease was achieved. Among the 628 patients with PET-negative disease after ABVD times 2, the 5-year PFS was significantly higher in the radiotherapy arm (93.4% vs 86.1%; difference, 7.3%; 95% confidence interval, 1.6%–13.0%). Available data thus far indicate that, despite complete PET response to chemotherapy, radiotherapy cannot be safely omitted in early-stage patients.

Involved-field radiation therapy (IFRT) was used in both the RAPID and the GHSG HD16 trials, whereas involved-node radiation therapy (INRT) was used in the EORTC/LYSA/FIL H10 trial. The efficacy of INRT after ABVD has been shown in patients with early-stage HL, with a 4-year freedom from disease progression (FFP) of 96.4%.[8] Guidelines for INRT and involved-site radiation therapy (ISRT) are detailed in a report published by the International Radiation Oncology Lymphoma Group (ILROG).[9]

Advanced stage

Several prospective trials evaluated the role of radiation therapy for advanced-stage HL. The GHSG HD12 trial compared 2 BEACOPP variants with or without radiation therapy in advanced-stage patients.[10] Among the 950 patients with initial bulky disease (>5 cm) or residual disease after chemotherapy (>1.5 cm), the no-radiotherapy arm had a significantly inferior 10-year PFS (83.5% vs 88.6%). In the subgroup of patients with residual disease (>1.5 cm), the no-radiotherapy arm had a significantly inferior PFS (83.4% vs 89.7%) and overall survival (OS) (88.4% vs 94.4%).[11]

In the GHSG HD15 trial,[12] after dose-escalated BEACOPP and its variants, radiation therapy was limited to patients with residual disease of 2.5 cm and with residual PET avidity. A 4-year PFS rate of 92.1% was achieved with this approach, suggesting that radiotherapy is not needed after a complete metabolic response to BEACOPP. Among patients with PET-positive disease that received radiotherapy to the sites of residual disease, the 4-year PFS survival was 86.2%. This rate is favorable compared with the 3-year PFS of only 67.5% in patients with positive interim PET on the Response-adapted therapy for advanced Hodgkin lymphoma (RATHL) trial,[13] in whom only 11% received consolidative radiotherapy. In the GITIL/FIL HD 0607 trial,[14] patients with negative PET after 2 cycles of ABVD continued on a total of 6 cycles of ABVD, and those with a large nodal mass at diagnosis (≥5 cm) who remained PET negative were randomly assigned to radiotherapy or no further treatment. There was no difference in 3-year PFS between the 2 arms (97% v 93%; $P = .29$). Routine addition of radiation therapy after chemotherapy in patients with advanced-stage disease is therefore not indicated, but it should be considered in patients who lack complete metabolic response to chemotherapy.

Nodular lymphocyte-predominant Hodgkin lymphoma

Nodular lymphocyte-predominant HL (NLPHL) accounts for approximately 5% of all HL cases. More than half of the patients with NLPHL have early-stage disease at presentation. Compared with classic HL, NLPHL has a more indolent clinical course and a better overall prognosis.[15–18] For patients with stage I disease and those with stage II disease with contiguous sites of involvement, ISRT to doses of 30 to 36 Gy fractions of

1.8 to 2 Gy is the mainstay treatment. In the context of radiotherapy as the sole treatment modality, the clinical target volume (CTV) should encompass gross disease as well as suspected subclinical disease.[9]

Aggressive Non-Hodgkin Lymphoma

The most common subtype of aggressive non-Hodgkin lymphoma (NHL) is diffuse large B-cell lymphoma (DLBCL). The current standard chemotherapy regimen for DLBCL is rituximab, cyclophosphamide, doxorubicin, vincristine and prednisone (R-CHOP) chemotherapy. Several earlier randomized trials from the prerituximab era have addressed the role of radiotherapy in early-stage aggressive NHL.[19–22] The Southwest Oncology Group (SWOG) 8636 study compared 8 cycles of CHOP with 3 cycles of CHOP followed by radiation therapy,[22] with long-term follow-up showing continued events in both arms but no differences in PFS or OS rates.[23] However, a higher risk of cardiac-related mortality was observed in the 8 cycles of CHOP arm.[22] Two other studies compared the outcome of older patients with limited-stage DLBCL treated with prolonged chemotherapy versus abbreviated chemotherapy and radiotherapy.[24,25] Similar survival outcomes were achieved, but patients treated with abbreviated chemotherapy and radiotherapy were less likely to require second-line salvage therapy, and less likely to experience neuropathy, febrile neutropenia, or febrile neutropenia requiring hospitalization.

The German High-grade Non-Hodgkin Lymphoma Study Group (DSHNHL) reported on outcomes of patients with DLBCL with skeletal involvement. After a complete response to chemotherapy, those who received consolidative radiotherapy had a significantly improved 3-year event-free survival (EFS) (75% vs 36%; $P<.001$).[26] On multivariable analysis, the addition of radiotherapy reduced the risk of an event by 70% ($P<.001$). In a separate study, patients with bulky disease (≥7.5 cm) from the R-CHOP-14 times 6 arm of the RICOVER-60 trial formed the study population. Compared with patients who did not receive radiotherapy after a protocol amendment, those who received radiotherapy before the amendment had significantly higher rates of EFS (80% vs 54%; $P = .001$), PFS (88% vs 62%; $P<.001$), and OS (90% vs 65%; $P = .001$).[27] However, both of these studies were retrospective subgroup analyses and thus prone to selection bias. The UNFOLDER trial randomized patients with DLBCL to R-CHOP-14 versus R-CHOP-21.[28] Patients with initial bulky disease (≥7.5 cm) or extranodal involvement were further randomized to receive radiotherapy versus no radiotherapy. The final analysis, reported in abstract form, showed a significantly worse 3-year EFS in the chemotherapy-alone arm (68% vs 84%; $P = .001$), but there was no difference in 3-year PFS (89% vs 81%; $P = .221$). However, PET computed tomography (CT) assessment was not performed in the UNFOLDER trial. The LYSA Group randomized patients with nonbulky (<7 cm), early-stage DLBCL to radiotherapy versus no further treatment after a complete PET response to 4 to 6 cycles of R-CHOP-14.[29] This noninferiority trial was designed with an upper limit of 8% difference in EFS between the arms. The difference in 5-year EFS was not statistically significant between the 2 arms (92% vs 89%; $P = .18$). Whether the prespecified noninferiority criteria were met was not reported.

In summary, the key indications for adding consolidative radiotherapy after R-CHOP chemotherapy for DLBCL include initial bulky disease (≥7.5 cm), skeletal sites, and incomplete response to chemotherapy. In addition, radiotherapy is often considered in patients with low-risk (international prognostic index of 0–1), nonbulky, nodal limited-stage DLBCL, allowing patients to receive a more abbreviated course of chemotherapy.

The consolidative radiation doses used in earlier trials ranged from 30 Gy to as high as 55 Gy.[22] Lowry and colleagues[30] randomized 640 sites of aggressive NHL to 30 Gy in 15 fractions versus 40 to 45 Gy in 20 to 23 fractions. No significant differences in freedom from local progression and OS rates between the 2 arms were found, suggesting that 30 Gy is adequate after chemotherapy.

In the trials discussed earlier, IFRT was used, but more recent data support use of smaller fields. The British Columbia experience showed that the use of INRT less than or equal to 5 cm resulted in similar disease control compared with an earlier cohort of patients who received IFRT.[31] Verhappen and colleagues[32] found only 1 relapse outside of the INRT field but in the IFRT volume among 67 patients with stage I to II aggressive NHL treated with INRT. Guidelines for INRT/ISRT for nodal and extranodal NHL have been published by ILROG, with details on recommended dose, volumes, and techniques.[33,34]

Indolent Non-Hodgkin Lymphoma

Follicular lymphoma
About 20% to 25% of patients with follicular lymphoma present with stage I to II disease. Several retrospective series have shown that radiation therapy alone is curative in 35% to 40% of cases. A recent multi-institutional study on patients with stage I to II follicular lymphoma staged with PET-CT and treated with radiotherapy found 5-year FFP and OS to be 68.9% and 95.7%, respectively. For stage I patients, the 5-year FFP was 74.1%.[35] These findings reflect more favorable outcomes in modernly staged patients. A follow-up study from the same group found excellent results in patients who relapsed after primary radiotherapy and were salvaged with further radiotherapy, with a 3-year FFP of 73.9%.[36]

Earlier series have used larger radiation fields and higher doses of 35 to 40 Gy. Campbell and colleagues[37] reported on 95 patients with localized follicular lymphoma treated with INRT less than 5 cm alone, and found that only 1% of patients had regional-only recurrence. Lowry and colleagues[30] randomized 361 sites of indolent lymphoma to 24 Gy in 12 fractions versus 40 to 45 Gy in 20 to 30 fractions, showing no differences in rates of local progression, PFS, and OS, suggesting that 24 Gy is adequate for indolent lymphoma. The addition of rituximab to radiotherapy for early-stage follicular lymphoma seems to prolong PFS but not OS.[38] MacManus and colleagues[39] compared radiotherapy alone versus radiotherapy and Cyclophosphamide, vincristine, prednisone, rituximab [CVP (R)] in a randomized trial and showed a significantly improved PFS with the combined approach, but again without OS differences.

For patients with advanced-stage or recurrent follicular lymphoma, low-dose radiotherapy (2 Gy × 2) has overall response rates of 80% to more than 90%.[40–46] The advantages of this approach, in addition to a high response rate, include minimal treatment toxicity, patient convenience, and potential delay in need of starting systemic therapy. However, the FORT trial showed that 4 Gy was significantly inferior to 24 Gy for follicular or marginal zone lymphoma in terms of response rates (81% vs 74.1%; $P = .006$) and 2-year PFS rates (93.7% vs 80.4%; $P<.001$) in the 4-Gy arm.[47] These findings led to the conclusion that although 4 Gy remains a useful regimen in the palliative setting, 24 Gy is the standard dose for patients treated with curative intent.

Extranodal marginal zone lymphoma of mucosa-associated lymphoid tissue
Extranodal marginal zone lymphoma of mucosa-associated lymphoid tissue (MALT) accounts for about 8% to 10% of NHL. Doses of around 30 Gy to involved nodal

regions or extranodal sites yield local control rates of close to 100%, with a chance of long-term cure in about three-quarters of patients with limited-stage disease. However, the previously mentioned United Kingdom randomized trial, which included cases of MALT lymphoma, showed that 24 Gy is adequate.[30] Gastric MALT lymphoma, the most common disease site, has historically been treated to a dose of 30 Gy in 20 fractions,[48] although recent data suggest a lower dose of 24 Gy is acceptable.[49]

Relapses tend to occur at other extranodal sites in which MALT lymphomas tend to occur, or in a nonirradiated contralateral paired organ.[50] The likelihood of achieving a second remission in patients with limited relapses remains excellent with further local radiation therapy.

Leukemia

The most common scenario in which radiation therapy is used in the management of patients with leukemia include treatment of central nervous system (CNS) disease and other forms of extramedullary relapses.

Either whole-brain radiation therapy (WBRT) or cranial spinal irradiation (CSI) may be considered in patients with leukemia and history of CNS disease as part of treatment before allogeneic stem cell transplant (SCT), consolidation after salvage chemotherapy, or salvage treatment of relapsed/refractory disease. A retrospective study among pediatric patients with acute lymphoblastic leukemia and CNS involvement suggested a trend toward improved disease-free survival among patients receiving CSI compared with cranial boost alone before SCT.[51] In the pretransplant setting, the ILROG guidelines recommend WBRT of 23.4 Gy at 1.8 Gy per fraction, but a reduced dose of 18 Gy to the spine can be considered,[52] and total body irradiation dose, if given, should be factored into the CSI dose.

Myeloid sarcoma, also known as chloroma or granulocytic sarcoma, and leukemia cutis are extramedullary tumors comprising myeloid blasts, in most cases occurring concurrently with acute myeloid leukemia.[53] They are highly sensitive to radiation therapy and a dose of 24 Gy in 12 fractions, as recommended by ILROG, can produced durable local control.[54] In patients with limited life expectancy, a dose as low as 6 Gy can achieve effective short-term palliation.

Plasma Cell Neoplasm

Radiation therapy is often used for palliation of painful bony lesions and nerve root or cord compressions in patients with multiple myeloma. Guidelines on the optimal dose-fractionation scheme in the palliation of multiple myeloma have been proposed by ILROG.[55] In general, a dose of 20 Gy in 5 fractions can produce durable symptom control.

Solitary plasmacytoma accounts for 5% to 10% of all plasma cell dyscrasias. In patients with solitary plasmacytoma of the bone, local radiation therapy to doses of 45 to 50 Gy can provide effective local control of more than 80%. However, about half of these patients progress to multiple myeloma at 10 years, and, by 15 years, most develop multiple myeloma. Unlike solitary plasmacytoma of the bone, extraosseous solitary plasmacytoma is associated with a lower risk of progression to multiple myeloma, and has a more favorable disease-free survival.[56–60] Most series used doses of 40 to 50 Gy, which yielded local control rates of 85% to 90%. An ongoing randomized trial is exploring the impact of the addition of ixazomib, lenalidomide, and dexamethasone to zoledronic acid in patients with solitary plasmacytoma of the bone (Alliance A061402).

CONTEMPORARY RADIATION TECHNOLOGY FOR HEMATOLOGIC MALIGNANCIES

The concept of ISRT and INRT reflects use of three-dimensional (3D) treatment planning, integration of modern imaging, and advanced treatment delivery techniques.[9] The target volumes include the initially involved lymph nodes but excludes initially uninvolved, displaced organs after disease regression. The optimal radiation technique (discussed later) is case dependent. Comparative dosimetric studies between radiation techniques exist for certain anatomic sites such as the mediastinum,[61] which have helped elucidate the relative benefit of one radiation technique compared with another across a patient population. However, patient-specific plan comparisons will ultimately provide the most individualized and objective data.

Radiation Techniques for Treatment of Mediastinal Lymphoma

Given the risk of radiation-associated late effects, which are dose dependent, patient positioning, motion management, and radiation techniques are selected with the aim of reducing dose to the lung, heart, breast, and body. Positioning the arms down or akimbo (vs up) is associated with less breast tissue toward the patient's midline and may decrease breast doses in female patients, especially in the absence of axillary disease.[62] Respiratory and cardiac motion may affect the intrafractional position of the mediastinum. As such, motion management with either four-dimensional (4D) CT or deep-inspirational breath-hold (DIBH) is important to ensure adequate coverage of the moving target. In addition to minimizing respiratory motion, treatment with DIBH is associated with lower lung and heart doses compared with free breathing.[63–65]

The relative benefit of 3D conformal, intensity-modulated radiation therapy (IMRT)/ volumetric modulated arc therapy (VMAT), and proton therapy (PT) depends on the extent of mediastinal disease. Patients with mediastinal lymphoma may be categorized as having upper versus lower mediastinal disease (**Table 2**). Patients with exclusively upper mediastinal involvement may be adequately treated with 3D conformal techniques such as anterior and posterior fields with minimal dose to the breast. In contrast, patients with lower mediastinal involvement may require advanced radiation techniques to carve dose around the heart.

Proton therapy for mediastinal lymphoma

PT's unique physical dose distribution is characterized by rapid dose drop-off along the beam path at a certain depth in the patient (**Fig. 1**). PT delivery techniques include passive scattering, uniform scanning, and pencil-beam scanning (PBS) (**Table 3**). Although passive scattering is the most mature technique, many centers are moving toward PBS.

Table 2 Various definitions of lower mediastinal disease among patients with lymphoma	
	Lower/Whole Mediastinum
ILROG (Dabaja et al,[72] 2018)	Mediastinal disease spans below the origin of the left main stem coronary artery
Institut Gustav Roussy (Paumier et al,[64] 2012)	Mediastinal disease whose lower border extends beyond 3 cm below the carina
Authors' definition	Mediastinal disease that spans below the left pulmonary artery (ie, superior aspect of the heart as defined by the breast contouring atlas[74])

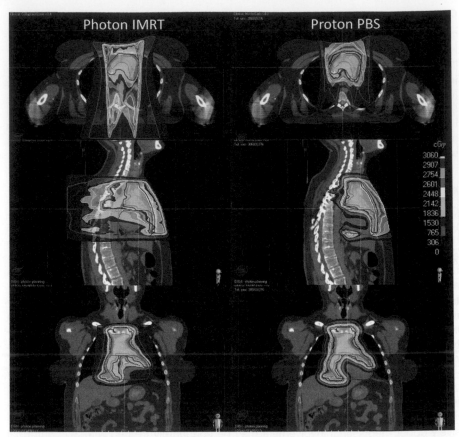

Fig. 1. Photon IMRT (*left*) and PBS proton plans (*right*) for a 36-year-old woman with primary mediastinal B-cell lymphoma.

Although PT's physical dose distribution make it an attractive radiation technique, PT has unique treatment planning considerations. Range calculation uncertainties need to be accounted for, from inaccuracies in Hounsfield units to proton stopping power and setup variation. Strategies to ensure a robust PT plan include either adding a margin along the beam path both distally and proximally to the target volume, or planning to a larger volume than the internal target volume or CTV. Historically, pencil-beam analytical (PBA) algorithms have been used to calculate PT dose, although emerging evidence suggests that PBA may not calculate proton dose in thoracic tumors accurately given the heterogeneous tissue interfaces that the proton beam must traverse through.[66] Because of this, Monte Carlo dose algorithms, which are now commercially available, are preferred to ensure appropriate coverage of the target volume and accurate physical dose estimates to adjacent organs at risk. In addition to physical dose distribution, there may be uncertainty with the relative biological effectiveness (RBE) of protons, especially at the end of the beam path. Although a constant RBE = 1.1 is used for treatment planning, the RBE may be greater than 1.1 just distal to the Bragg peak.[67] This possibility is a potential consideration because, for anterior mediastinal targets, anterior or anterior oblique beams are preferably used, but may end in the heart.

Table 3
Summary of available proton therapy delivery techniques

	Passive Scattering	Uniform Scanning	PBS
Delivery of RT Field	Dose for a field delivered all at one time	Dose delivered on a layer-by-layer basis by switching energy between layers	Magnets steer beam in a rasterlike pattern to deposit dose along the x and y axis of one layer, then switches energy to deliver dose to next layer
Speed of Delivery	Nearly instantaneous	Slower	Slowest
Patient-specific Hardware	• Brass apertures (lateral beam shaping) • Wax/acrylic compensators (distal beam shaping)	• Brass apertures (lateral beam shaping) • Wax/acrylic compensators (distal beam shaping)	None

Abbreviation: RT, radiotherapy.

In addition, given intrafractional mediastinal motion, additional strategies are tailored to specific PT delivery techniques to minimize the risk of interplay. PBS is the least robust PT technique and, when used, several strategies are used, including larger spots, multiple beams or volumetric repainting if a single beam is used, and single field optimization, in which all beams contribute dose to the entire target volume. Another strategy is 4D robust optimization, in which the PT plan is optimized across all phases of respiration.

Intensity-modulated radiation therapy/volumetric modulated arc therapy for mediastinal lymphoma
Compared with 3D conformal techniques, IMRT and VMAT spare more heart and lung (mean and V20).[68,69] Butterfly IMRT or VMAT techniques restrict beams to anteriorly and posteriorly oblique entry angles to avoid entering or exiting through the breast tissue.[69,70] Given increasing availability of volumetric image guidance (eg, cone-beam CT) with most LINACs, DIBH may be incorporated as motion management.

Intensity-modulated radiation therapy/volumetric modulated arc therapy versus proton therapy for mediastinal lymphoma
Deciding between IMRT/VMAT and PT is based on availability of technique, comfort and experience, insurance coverage, and dosimetric superiority. Contemporary dosimetric studies suggest that IMRT with DIBH produces similar heart and lung sparing compared with PT with free breathing.[65] However, among patients with exclusively lower mediastinal involvement, 1 study of 21 patients found lower doses to the heart, breast, and lungs with PT compared with IMRT, with or without DIBH.[71] Guidelines from ILROG highlight consideration of PT for patients with lower mediastinal involvement, young female patients, and/or heavily pretreated patients who are at higher risk of radiation-related toxicity to the bone marrow, heart, and lungs.[72]

Cranial Spinal Irradiation for Central Nervous System Leukemia
Photons or PT may be used for CSI. With PT CSI, dose to the spine enters the patient posteriorly with minimal to no exit dose to the thorax, abdomen, and pelvic midline structures (**Figs. 2** and **3**). Among hematologic patients, PT is associated with lower acute toxicity, including mucositis.[73]

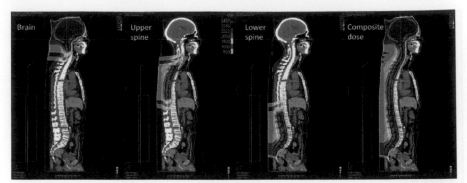

Fig. 2. Proton PBS CSI treatment plan for an adult with relapsed acute myelogenous leukemia with CNS involvement. Three posterior fields are used for the brain, upper spine, and lower spine. A junction of several centimeters is used in which dose from the brain slowly decreases from the prescription dose (*blue*; 2340 cGy [RBE]) to 0 cGy over the same region where the upper spine dose is increasing from 0 cGy to the prescription dose. This process creates a composite dose, as shown on the far right without hot or cold spots. In adults, the anterior vertebral bodies are spared to minimize myelosuppression.

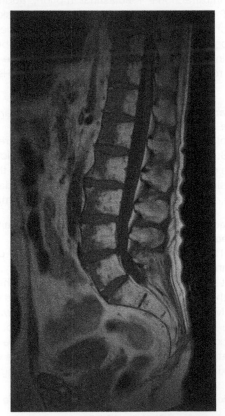

Fig. 3. Sagittal T2-weighted MRI of the thoracic and lumbar spine from the same patient in **Fig. 2**, 1 year from CSI treatment with protons. There is well-demarcated posterior fatty replacement of the posterior vertebral bodies from CSI that corresponds to the proton dose distribution.

Table 4
Cranial spinal irradiation treatment planning by proton therapy delivery technique

	Passive Scattering and Uniform Scanning	PBS
Whole-brain Treatment	2 slight posterior oblique fields (15° off lateral) to ensure nondiverging dose to upper spine	Single posterior field
Spine Treatment	2 posterior fields (adults)	2 posterior fields (adults)
Junctions	• In general 1 cm between whole-brain, upper, and lower spine fields • 3 match lines, corresponding with 3 separate plans	• Gradient junction with 1 plan

CSI treatment planning differs by PT technique, which is summarized in **Table 4**. The availability of PBS has facilitated CSI treatment planning, notably given the ability to create gradient junctions (see **Fig. 2**). Gradient junctions allow the whole brain and upper and lower spine fields to overlap. The same 3 fields are delivered on all days of treatment. Dose at the junction, which spans several centimeters in length, is delivered by the 2 overlapping fields, in which 1 field gradually increases from 0% to 100% whereas the dose from the other overlapping field gradually decreases from 100% to 0%. Because of this gradient, these CSI plans are more forgiving with patient setup errors, faster for treatment planning because no patient-specific hardware needs to be created, and faster for patient delivery because apertures and compensators do not need to be changed for each field.

SUMMARY

Radiation therapy continues to play an extensive role in the management of patients with hematologic malignancies. Advances in radiation therapy technology have allowed more precise dose delivery to sites with high disease burden or high risk for disease involvement, while sparing normal tissue. Future directions include further development of novel techniques to improve the therapeutic ratio and determining the optimal integration of modern radiation therapy with the rapidly evolving systemic therapies in hematologic malignancies.

REFERENCES

1. Eich HT, Diehl V, Gorgen H, et al. Intensified chemotherapy and dose-reduced involved-field radiotherapy in patients with early unfavorable Hodgkin's lymphoma: final analysis of the German Hodgkin Study Group HD11 trial. J Clin Oncol 2010;28:4199–206.
2. Engert A, Plütschow A, Eich HT, et al. Reduced treatment intensity in patients with early-stage Hodgkin's lymphoma. N Engl J Med 2010;363:640–52.
3. Sasse S, Brockelmann PJ, Goergen H, et al. Long-term follow-up of contemporary treatment in early-stage hodgkin lymphoma: updated analyses of the German Hodgkin Study Group HD7, HD8, HD10, and HD11 Trials. J Clin Oncol 2017;35:1999–2007.
4. Thomas J, Ferme C, Noordijk EM, et al. Comparison of 36 Gy, 20 Gy, or no radiation therapy after 6 cycles of EBVP chemotherapy and complete remission in

early-stage Hodgkin lymphoma without risk factors: results of the EORT-GELA H9-F Intergroup Randomized Trial. Int J Radiat Oncol Biol Phys 2018;100: 1133–45.

5. Radford J, Illidge T, Counsell N, et al. Results of a trial of PET-directed therapy for early-stage Hodgkin's lymphoma. N Engl J Med 2015;372:1598–607.

6. Andre MPE, Girinsky T, Federico M, et al. Early positron emission tomography response-adapted treatment in stage I and II Hodgkin lymphoma: final results of the randomized EORTC/LYSA/FIL H10 trial. J Clin Oncol 2017;35:1786–94.

7. Fuchs M, Goergen H, Kobe C, et al. PET-guided treatment of early-stage favorable Hodgkin lymphoma: final results of the International, Randomized Phase 3 Trial HD16 By the German Hodgkin Study Group. Blood 2018;132:925.

8. Maraldo MV, Aznar MC, Vogelius IR, et al. Involved node radiation therapy: an effective alternative in early-stage hodgkin lymphoma. Int J Radiat Oncol Biol Phys 2013;85:1057–65.

9. Specht L, Yahalom J, Illidge T, et al. Modern radiation therapy for Hodgkin lymphoma: field and dose guidelines from the International Lymphoma Radiation Oncology Group (ILROG). Int J Radiat Oncol Biol Phys 2014;89(4):854–62.

10. Borchmann P, Haverkamp H, Diehl V, et al. Eight cycles of escalated-dose BEACOPP compared with four cycles of escalated-dose BEACOPP followed by four cycles of baseline-dose BEACOPP with or without radiotherapy in patients with advanced-stage hodgkin's lymphoma: final analysis of the HD12 trial of the German Hodgkin Study Group. J Clin Oncol 2011;29:4234–42.

11. Kreissl S, von Tresckow BG H, Haverkamp H, et al. BEACOPP-escalated followed by radiotherapy of initial bulk or residual disease in advanced stage Hodgkin lymphoma: long-term follow up of the HD9 and HD12 trials of the German Hodgkin Study Group. Blood 2016;128:923.

12. Engert A, Haverkamp H, Kobe C, et al. Reduced-intensity chemotherapy and PET-guided radiotherapy in patients with advanced stage Hodgkin's lymphoma (HD15 trial): a randomised, open-label, phase 3 non-inferiority trial. Lancet 2012;379:1791–9.

13. Johnson P, Federico M, Kirkwood A, et al. Adapted treatment guided by interim PET-CT scan in advanced Hodgkin's lymphoma. N Engl J Med 2016;374: 2419–29.

14. Gallamini A, Tarella C, Viviani S, et al. Early chemotherapy intensification with escalated BEACOPP in patients with advanced-stage hodgkin lymphoma with a positive interim positron emission tomography/computed tomography scan after two ABVD cycles: long-term results of the GITIL/FIL HD 0607 trial. J Clin Oncol 2018;36:454–62.

15. Hartmann S, Eichenauer DA, Plutschow A, et al. Histopathological features and their prognostic impact in nodular lymphocyte-predominant Hodgkin lymphoma–a matched pair analysis from the German Hodgkin Study Group (GHSG). Br J Haematol 2014;167:238–42.

16. King MT, Donaldson SS, Link MP, et al. Management of nodular lymphocyte predominant Hodgkin lymphoma in the modern era. Int J Radiat Oncol Biol Phys 2015;92:67–75.

17. Lazarovici J, Dartigues P, Brice P, et al. Nodular lymphocyte predominant Hodgkin lymphoma: a Lymphoma Study Association retrospective study. Haematologica 2015;100:1579–86.

18. Chen RC, Chin MS, Ng AK, et al. Early-stage, lymphocyte-predominant Hodgkin's lymphoma: patient outcomes from a large, single-institution series with long follow-up. J Clin Oncol 2010;28:136–41.

19. Horning SJ, Weller E, Kim K, et al. Chemotherapy with or without radiotherapy in limited-stage diffuse aggressive non-Hodgkin's lymphoma: Eastern Cooperative Oncology Group study 1484. J Clin Oncol 2004;22:3032–8.
20. Reyes F, Lepage E, Munck J, et al. Chemotherapy alone with the ACVBP regimen is superior to three cycles of CHOP plus radiotherapy for treatment of low risk localized aggressive lymphoma: the LNH93-1 GELA study. Blood 2003;100:93a.
21. Bonnet C, Fillet G, Mounier N, et al. CHOP alone compared with CHOP plus radiotherapy for localized aggressive lymphoma in elderly patients: a study by the Groupe d'Etude des Lymphomes de l'Adulte. J Clin Oncol 2007;25:787–92.
22. Miller TP, Dahlberg S, Cassady JR, et al. Chemotherapy alone compared with chemotherapy plus radiotherapy for localized intermediate- and high-grade non-Hodgkin's lymphoma. N Engl J Med 1998;339:21–6.
23. Stephens DM, Li H, LeBlanc ML, et al. Continued risk of relapse independent of treatment modality in limited-stage diffuse large B-cell lymphoma: final and long-term analysis of Southwest Oncology Group Study S8736. J Clin Oncol 2016;34: 2997–3004.
24. Pinnix CC, Andraos TY, Dabaja B, et al. Diffuse large B-cell lymphoma in very elderly patients over 80 years old: incorporating consolidative radiation therapy into management decisions. Adv Radiat Oncol 2017;2:370–80.
25. Odejide OO, Cronin AM, Davidoff AJ, et al. Limited stage diffuse large B-cell lymphoma: comparative effectiveness of treatment strategies in a large cohort of elderly patients. Leuk Lymphoma 2015;56:716–24.
26. Held G, Zeynalova S, Murawski N, et al. Impact of rituximab and radiotherapy on outcome of patients with aggressive B-cell lymphoma and skeletal involvement. J Clin Oncol 2013;31:4115–22.
27. Held G, Murawski N, Ziepert M, et al. Role of radiotherapy to bulky disease in elderly patients with aggressive B-cell lymphoma. J Clin Oncol 2014;32:1112–8.
28. Pfreundschuh M, Murawski N, Ziepert M, et al. Radiotherapy to bulky and extra-lymphatic disease in combination with 6×R-CHOP-14 or R-CHOP-21 in young good-prognosis DLBCL patients: results of the 2×2 randomized UNFOLDER trial of the DSHNHL/GLA. J Clin Oncol 2018;36 [abstract: 7574].
29. Lamy T, Damaj G, Soubeyran P, et al. R-CHOP 14 with or without radiotherapy in nonbulky limited-stage diffuse large B-cell lymphoma. Blood 2018;131:174–81.
30. Lowry L, Smith P, Qian W, et al. Reduced dose radiotherapy for local control in non-Hodgkin lymphoma: a randomised phase III trial. Radiother Oncol 2011; 100:86–92.
31. Campbell BA, Connors JM, Gascoyne RD, et al. Limited-stage diffuse large B-cell lymphoma treated with abbreviated systemic therapy and consolidation radiotherapy: involved-field versus involved-node radiotherapy. Cancer 2012;118: 4156–65.
32. Verhappen MH, Poortmans PM, Raaijmakers E, et al. Reduction of the treated volume to involved node radiation therapy as part of combined modality treatment for early stage aggressive non-Hodgkin's lymphoma. Radiother Oncol 2013; 109:133–9.
33. Yahalom J, Illidge T, Specht L, et al. Modern radiation therapy for extranodal lymphomas: field and dose guidelines from the International Lymphoma Radiation Oncology Group. Int J Radiat Oncol Biol Phys 2015;92:11–31.
34. Illidge T, Specht L, Yahalom J, et al. Modern radiation therapy for nodal non-Hodgkin lymphoma-target definition and dose guidelines from the International Lymphoma Radiation Oncology Group. Int J Radiat Oncol Biol Phys 2014;89: 49–58.

35. Brady JL, Binkley MS, Hajj C, et al. Definitive radiotherapy for localized follicular lymphoma staged by (18)F-FDG PET-CT: a collaborative study by ILROG. Blood 2019;133:237–45.
36. Binkley MS, Brady JL, Hajj C, et al. Salvage treatment and survival for relapsed follicular lymphoma following primary radiation therapy: a collaborative study on behalf of ILROG. Int J Radiat Oncol Biol Phys 2019;104(3):522–9.
37. Campbell BA, Voss N, Woods R, et al. Long-term outcomes for patients with limited stage follicular lymphoma: involved regional radiotherapy versus involved node radiotherapy. Cancer 2010;116:3797–806.
38. Ruella M, Filippi AR, Bruna R, et al. Addition of rituximab to involved-field radiation therapy prolongs progression-free survival in stage I-II follicular lymphoma: results of a multicenter study. Int J Radiat Oncol Biol Phys 2016;94:783–91.
39. MacManus M, Fisher R, Roos D, et al. Randomized trial of systemic therapy after involved-field radiotherapy in patients with early-stage follicular lymphoma: TROG 99.03. J Clin Oncol 2018;36(29):2918–25.
40. Martin NE, Ng AK. Good things come in small packages: low-dose radiation as palliation for indolent non-Hodgkin lymphomas. Leuk Lymphoma 2009;50: 1765–72.
41. Ganem G, Lambin P, Socie G, et al. Potential role for low dose limited-field radiation therapy (2 x 2 grays) in advanced low-grade non-Hodgkin's lymphomas. Hematol Oncol 1994;12:1–8.
42. Girinsky T, Guillot-Vals D, Koscielny S, et al. A high and sustained response rate in refractory or relapsing low-grade lymphoma masses after low-dose radiation: analysis of predictive parameters of response to treatment. Int J Radiat Oncol Biol Phys 2001;51:148–55.
43. Haas RL, Poortmans P, de Jong D, et al. High response rates and lasting remissions after low-dose involved field radiotherapy in indolent lymphomas. J Clin Oncol 2003;21:2474–80.
44. Sawyer EJ, Timothy AR. Low dose palliative radiotherapy in low grade non-Hodgkin's lymphoma. Radiother Oncol 1997;42:49–51.
45. Luthy SK, Ng AK, Silver B, et al. Response to low-dose involved-field radiotherapy in patients with non-Hodgkin's lymphoma. Ann Oncol 2008;19:2043–7.
46. Russo AL, Chen YH, Martin NE, et al. Low-dose involved-field radiation in the treatment of non-hodgkin lymphoma: predictors of response and treatment failure. Int J Radiat Oncol Biol Phys 2013;86:121–7.
47. Hoskin PJ, Kirkwood AA, Popova B, et al. 4 Gy versus 24 Gy radiotherapy for patients with indolent lymphoma (FORT): a randomised phase 3 non-inferiority trial. Lancet Oncol 2014;15:457–63.
48. Schechter NR, Portlock CS, Yahalom J. Treatment of mucosa-associated lymphoid tissue lymphoma of the stomach with radiation alone. J Clin Oncol 1998;16:1916–21.
49. Pinnix CC, Gunther JR, Milgrom SA, et al. Outcomes after reduced-dose intensity modulated radiation therapy for gastric mucosa-associated lymphoid tissue (MALT) lymphoma. Int J Radiat Oncol Biol Phys 2019;104(2):447–55.
50. Goda JS, Massey C, Kuruvilla J, et al. Role of salvage radiation therapy for patients with relapsed or refractory hodgkin lymphoma who failed autologous stem cell transplant. Int J Radiat Oncol Biol Phys 2012;84:e329–35.
51. Hiniker SM, Agarwal R, Modlin LA, et al. Survival and neurocognitive outcomes after cranial or craniospinal irradiation plus total-body irradiation before stem cell transplantation in pediatric leukemia patients with central nervous system involvement. Int J Radiat Oncol Biol Phys 2014;89:67–74.

52. Pinnix CC, Yahalom J, Specht L, et al. Radiation in central nervous system leukemia: guidelines from the International Lymphoma Radiation Oncology Group. Int J Radiat Oncol Biol Phys 2018;102:53–8.
53. Bakst RL, Tallman MS, Douer D, et al. How I treat extramedullary acute myeloid leukemia. Blood 2011;118:3785–93.
54. Bakst RL, Dabaja BS, Specht LK, et al. Use of radiation in extramedullary leukemia/chloroma: guidelines from the International Lymphoma Radiation Oncology Group. Int J Radiat Oncol Biol Phys 2018;102:314–9.
55. Tsang RW, Campbell BA, Goda JS, et al. Radiation therapy for solitary plasmacytoma and multiple myeloma: guidelines from the International Lymphoma Radiation Oncology Group. Int J Radiat Oncol Biol Phys 2018;101:794–808.
56. Wax MK, Yun KJ, Omar RA. Extramedullary plasmacytomas of the head and neck. Otolaryngol Head Neck Surg 1993;109:877–85.
57. Liebross RH, Ha CS, Cox JD, et al. Clinical course of solitary extramedullary plasmacytoma. Radiother Oncol 1999;52:245–9.
58. Michalaki VJ, Hall J, Henk JM, et al. Definitive radiotherapy for extramedullary plasmacytomas of the head and neck. Br J Radiol 2003;76:738–41.
59. Dagan R, Morris CG, Kirwan J, et al. Solitary plasmacytoma. Am J Clin Oncol 2009;32:612–7.
60. Ozsahin M, Tsang RW, Poortmans P, et al. Outcomes and patterns of failure in solitary plasmacytoma: a multicenter Rare Cancer Network study of 258 patients. Int J Radiat Oncol Biol Phys 2006;64:210–7.
61. Tseng YD, Cutter DJ, Plastaras JP, et al. Evidence-based review on the use of proton therapy in lymphoma from the Particle Therapy Cooperative Group (PTCOG) Lymphoma Subcommittee. Int J Radiat Oncol Biol Phys 2017;99: 825–42.
62. Denniston KA, Verma V, Bhirud AR, et al. Effect of akimbo versus raised arm positioning on breast and cardiopulmonary dosimetry in pediatric Hodgkin lymphoma. Front Oncol 2016;6:176.
63. Aznar MC, Maraldo MV, Schut DA, et al. Minimizing late effects for patients with mediastinal Hodgkin lymphoma: deep inspiration breath-hold, IMRT, or both? Int J Radiat Oncol Biol Phys 2015;92:169–74.
64. Paumier A, Ghalibafian M, Gilmore J, et al. Dosimetric benefits of intensity-modulated radiotherapy combined with the deep-inspiration breath-hold technique in patients with mediastinal Hodgkin's lymphoma. Int J Radiat Oncol Biol Phys 2012;82:1522–7.
65. Rechner LA, Maraldo MV, Vogelius IR, et al. Life years lost attributable to late effects after radiotherapy for early stage Hodgkin lymphoma: the impact of proton therapy and/or deep inspiration breath hold. Radiother Oncol 2017;125:41–7.
66. Taylor PA, Kry SF, Followill DS. Pencil beam algorithms are unsuitable for proton dose calculations in lung. Int J Radiat Oncol Biol Phys 2017;99:750–6.
67. Paganetti H, Niemierko A, Ancukiewicz M, et al. Relative biological effectiveness (RBE) values for proton beam therapy. Int J Radiat Oncol Biol Phys 2002;53: 407–21.
68. Fiandra C, Filippi AR, Catuzzo P, et al. Different IMRT solutions vs. 3D-conformal radiotherapy in early stage Hodgkin's lymphoma: dosimetric comparison and clinical considerations. Radiat Oncol 2012;7:186.
69. Voong KR, McSpadden K, Pinnix CC, et al. Dosimetric advantages of a "butterfly" technique for intensity-modulated radiation therapy for young female patients with mediastinal Hodgkin's lymphoma. Radiat Oncol 2014;9:94.

70. Starke A, Bowden J, Lynn R, et al. Comparison of butterfly volumetric modulated arc therapy to full arc with or without deep inspiration breath hold for the treatment of mediastinal lymphoma. Radiother Oncol 2018;129(3):449–55.
71. Everett A, Flampouri S, Louis D, et al. Comparison of radiation techniques in lower mediastinal lymphoma. Int J Radiat Oncol Biol Phys 2018;102:S190–1.
72. Dabaja BS, Hoppe BS, Plastaras JP, et al. Proton therapy for adults with mediastinal lymphomas: the International Lymphoma Radiation Oncology Group guidelines. Blood 2018;132:1635.
73. Gunther JR, Rahman AR, Dong W, et al. Craniospinal irradiation prior to stem cell transplant for hematologic malignancies with CNS involvement: effectiveness and toxicity after photon or proton treatment. Pract Radiat Oncol 2017;7:e401–8.
74. Feng M, Moran JH, Koeling T, et al. Int J Radiat Oncol Biol Phys 2011;79(1):10–8.

Pediatric Cancer

Sujith Baliga, MD[a], Torunn I. Yock, MD, MCH[b,c],*

KEYWORDS

- Pediatric cancer • Proton beam therapy • Survivorship

KEY POINTS

- For patients with medulloblastoma, concurrent and adjuvant chemotherapy with reduced volume radiotherapy (RT) is the new treatment paradigm.
- The use of proton beam therapy in pediatric brain tumors has been shown to have equivalent disease control outcomes with promising data demonstrating reduction dose to critical organs at risk.
- RT continues to play an important role for loco-regional control in extracranial pediatric tumors. In rhabdomyosarcoma, tumors larger than 5 cm have increased loco-regional recurrence and likely require higher RT dose.
- The use of proton therapy in extracranial central nervous system tumors can provide a novel strategy to address dose to critical organs, such as the kidney and liver.

INTRODUCTION

Pediatric cancer continues to be the second leading cause of death in children (0–14 years), with an estimated incidence of 11,060 cases and 1190 deaths in 2018.[1] The 3 leading causes of pediatric cancer have remained constant over the past decade, and include hematological malignancies (leukemias), brain tumors, and lymphomas (**Fig. 1**A). Although the incidence of childhood cancers continues to increase, significant advances in chemotherapy, technological advances in radiotherapy, and refinements in surgical techniques have led to a dramatic increase in cure rates for these malignancies. Five-year overall survival (OS) for pediatric cancers has increased from 58% between 1975 and 1979 to 83% from 2003 to 2009.[2] Given the excellent survival, the late effects of the various therapies, including radiation therapy and chemotherapy, have become an important issue for these childhood cancer survivors and therapeutic goals have been altered to include both improving cures but also importantly to mitigate late toxicity.

Conflicts of Interest: None.
[a] Department of Radiation Oncology, Massachusetts General Hospital/Harvard Medical School, Francis H. Burr Proton Therapy Center, 30 Fruit Street, Boston, MA 02114, USA; [b] Francis H. Burr Proton Therapy Center, 30 Fruit Street, Boston, MA 02114, USA; [c] Department of Radiation Oncology, Massachusetts General Hospital/Harvard Medical School, 55 Fruit Street, Boston, MA 02114, USA
* Corresponding author.
E-mail address: tyock@partners.org

Hematol Oncol Clin N Am 34 (2020) 143–159
https://doi.org/10.1016/j.hoc.2019.08.021

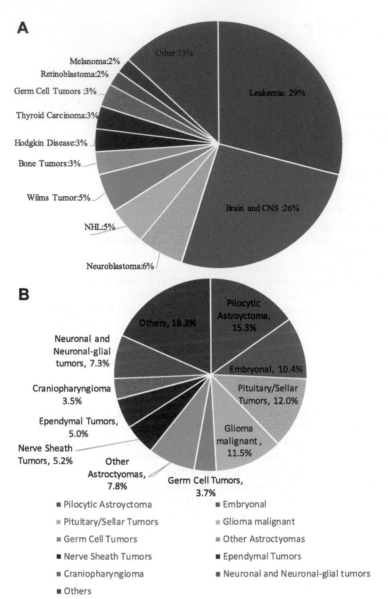

Fig. 1. (*A*) Overall incidence of pediatric tumors by histology and type; diagnoses per year; age 0 to 19 years. (*B*). Most common pediatric CNS tumors in children 0 to 19 years (annual average). NHL, non-Hodgkin lymphoma. ([*A*] *Data from* Siegel RL, Miller KD, Jemal A. Cancer statistics, 2018. CA Cancer J Clin 2018;68(1):7-30; [*B*] *Adapted from* Ostrom QT, Gittleman H, Truitt G, et al. CBTRUS Statistical Report: Primary Brain and Other Central Nervous System Tumors Diagnosed in the United States in 2011-2015. Neuro Oncol 2018;20(suppl_4):iv17; with permission.)

This review focuses on the more common tumors of childhood requiring radiation therapy, including central nervous system (CNS) and non-CNS tumors.

PEDIATRIC BRAIN TUMORS
Background

Pediatric CNS tumors remain the most common solid tumor of childhood and account for most cancer deaths in this group. In aggregate, more than 1000 children are diagnosed with a brain tumor every year, the most common of which are the low-grade astrocytomas.[3] Management of pediatric brain tumors often requires a multidisciplinary approach, but specific therapy is dependent on the histology and whether the tumor is localized or metastatic within the CNS. The most common pediatric CNS tumors are shown in **Fig. 1B**. In the subsequent sections, we discuss the management of both neuro-epithelial and embryonal CNS tumors, with emphasis on the optimal treatment strategies and the latest clinical approaches to these malignancies.

MEDULLOBLASTOMA

Medulloblastoma remains the most common embryonal tumor of childhood and is primarily confined to the posterior fossa. Optimal management in children ≥3 years consists of a combination of surgical resection, cranio-spinal irradiation (CSI) with involved field boost, and concurrent/adjuvant chemotherapy. With this approach, 5-year OS approaches more than 80%.

In the past, surgical resection has been shown to be an important prognosticator of survival in several studies[4-7] and, therefore, patients with a postoperative residual greater than 1.5 cm^2 are generally categorized into high-risk treatment strata. However, a recently published study evaluating the effect of residual disease on outcomes by molecular subgroups (winged [WNT], sonic hedgehog [SHH], Group 3, and Group 4)[7,8] has shown that extent of resection may not be as prognostic as previously thought.[9] Aggressive surgical resection may be associated with posterior fossa syndrome, classically characterized by the triad of emotional lability, ataxia, and impaired language capacity. A recent study of 36 pediatric patients with medulloblastoma with posterior fossa syndrome demonstrated lower mean scores of intellectual, processing speeds, working memory, and spatial domains compared with matched patients who did not have posterior fossa syndrome.[10] Posterior fossa syndrome is much more common in patients with medulloblastoma than in other histologies such as ependymoma or low-grade gliomas of the posterior fossa and its cause remains elusive.

The current standard of care for medulloblastoma in children 3 years and older remains CSI with chemotherapy, given the propensity for this tumor to seed the neuro-axis. The dose of CSI is determined after risk stratification of patients by resection status (≥ or <1.5 cm^2 residual) and the presence of metastatic disease in the brain or spine. Patients who are average risk typically have a gross total resection (GTR) or near total resection with less than 1.5 cm^2 residual and do not have evidence of metastatic disease in the brain or spine. These patients typically receive 23.4 Gy CSI followed by a tumor bed boost to 54 Gy and this treatment paradigm was established by 2 studies lead by the Children's Oncology Group (COG) that demonstrated excellent outcomes for average-risk patients treated with reduced-dose CSI (23.4 Gy) and adjuvant chemotherapy, with a 5-year event-free survival (EFS) of approximately 80%.[11,12] For patients with high-risk medulloblastoma, the optimal management has not been clearly elucidated, but currently involves a combination of 36 Gy CSI with a boost to the tumor bed or whole posterior fossa of 54 Gy. This is delivered with concurrent chemotherapy, typically weekly vincristine, although daily carboplatin has also been used to intensify the therapy and demonstrated a 5-year EFS of 59% to 71% in a COG pilot study.[13] Adjuvant chemotherapy with cisplatin, vincristine, and cyclophosphamide typically follows the radiation. A St Jude's study demonstrated a 5-year OS of 70% for high-risk patients treated with CSI to 36.0 to 39.6 Gy combined with high-dose chemotherapy and stem cell rescue.[14] Sequential chemotherapy followed by hyper-fractionated accelerated radiotherapy (39 Gy in 1.3 Gy twice a day, followed by PF boost to 60 Gy in 1.5 Gy twice a day), dubbed the Milan Strategy, has also been investigated in patients with metastatic medulloblastoma, and has demonstrated a similar 5-year EFS as has been previously reported of 70%.[15] However, the UK experience of this similar strategy resulted in poorer outcomes with a 3-year PFS of 56%[16] with reports of increased rates of neural toxicity.

In the era of modern MRI and computed tomography (CT)-based planning, COG has evaluated the use of a tumor bed boost instead of the historically used whole posterior fossa boost to reduce toxicity. COG's study, ACNS 0331, has been presented at national meetings and in abstract form and demonstrates that the smaller involved field tumor bed boost demonstrates comparable local control and OS compared with a whole posterior fossa volume.[17] Importantly, this same study found that deescalation of CSI dose to 18.0 Gy versus 23.4 Gy for average-risk patients 3 to 7 years of age was inferior with regard to EFS by approximately 10%. However, 18 Gy of CSI with reduced chemotherapy, without concurrent vincristine, is currently being evaluated by COG (ACNS 1422) in the WNT pathway standard risk cohort, as these patients have done very well on retrospective analyses with EFS at 5 years in excess of 95%.[18]

The importance of quality of life in pediatric brain tumor survivors is highlighted by a recent study that demonstrated that only 60% of survivors were able to achieve independence as adults.[19] In an analysis of the Childhood Cancer Survivor Study, more than 50% of medulloblastoma survivors treated in the 1990s were more likely to develop severe life-threating chronic health conditions, including grade 3 to 5 endocrine, hearing, visual, pulmonary, cardiovascular, and neurologic deficits. However, the introduction of low-dose CSI with chemotherapy demonstrated that this standard risk cohort was less likely to use special education services compared with high-risk survivors.[20]

The increasing use of proton radiotherapy may help mitigate some of the late effects associated with treatment, as proton radiotherapy typically irradiates fewer normal tissues in the process of treating patients. A recent prospective Phase II study of proton therapy in pediatric medulloblastoma at the Massachusetts General Hospital demonstrated favorable neurocognitive and ototoxicity outcomes compared with historical photon-treated cohorts, with comparable EFS and OS.[21] Other late effects, such as cardiac disease, were notably absent in the proton cohort, suggesting the dosimetric superiority of this treatment modality. A recent analysis of the Childhood Cancer Survivor study showed a low, albeit not negligible, rate of 5% incidence of cardiac disease in survivors. Interestingly, low to moderate RT doses to large volumes of the heart were associated with a 1.6 times increased risk of cardiac disease.[22]

Integrative genomics studies over the past decade have shown the presence of distinct molecular subgroups of medulloblastoma, with WNT tumors having the most favorable prognosis and Group 3 the worst.[23,24] Current studies are evaluating deescalation of treatment for WNT tumors and should provide further guidance regarding the predictive nature of molecular subgrouping (**Table 1**).

EPENDYMOMA

For patients with intracranial ependymoma, surgery followed by postoperative focal radiotherapy remains the mainstay of therapy for M0 patients. Surgical resection

Table 1
Molecular subclassification of medulloblastoma in pediatric tumors

Subgroup	Proportion, %	Clinical Characteristics	Mutations	Outcomes (10-y OS), %
WNT	10	Age >4, unlikely to metastasize; classic histology	CTNBB1 (exon 3)	~95–100
SHH	10–15	Age <3 and >16; desmoplastic/nodular histology	PTCH1(43%)/SMO (9%)/SuFu (10%) mutation. MYCN amplification (7%)	~65–70
Group 3	25	Infant; 2:1 male-to-female ratio; likely to metastasize; classic/LCA	SMARCA4(9%); MYC amplification (17%);OTX2 (2%)	~50
Group 4	35–40	50% are adolescent patients; 3:1 male-to-female ratio; classic/LCA	CDK6 amplification, MYCN amplification	~55–60

Abbreviations: LCA, large cell/anaplastic; OS, overall survival; SHH, sonic hedgehog; WNT, winged. *Data from* Refs.[18,78,79]

should be performed with the aim of obtaining a GTR, which has been found to be the most important predictor of EFS and OS.[25–27] The use of adjuvant RT, to doses of 50.4 to 59.4 Gy, in the postoperative setting, has been associated with a 5-year EFS of approximately 65% to 70%, based on multiple retrospective and prospective single-institution studies.[28–31] Recently published data from ACNS 0121 demonstrates the importance of RT in nearly all clinical and molecular subgroups of ependymoma. For example, in patients with classic supratentorial ependymoma, 5-year EFS was only 61% with GTR alone. Outcomes remained poor for patients who had an subtotal resection (STR), with a 5-year EFS of 37%, despite the addition of chemotherapy before a second-look surgery and definitive radiotherapy.[32] Radiotherapy volumes should incorporate the extent of postoperative disease and the tumor bed with a 5-mm margin to account for microscopic spread of disease, as defined in the most recent ACNS 0831 protocol. Careful radiation treatment planning requires the registration of both the preoperative and postoperative MRIs. Radiation-related brainstem injury can occur irrespective of radiation modality (protons or photon-based), but the data seem to indicate that the brainstem may be more susceptible to injury at lower doses with proton radiotherapy. ACNS 0831 uses more conservative brainstem dose constraints for protons based on an important dosimetric study from the University of Florida.[33,34]

ATYPICAL TERATOID RHABDOID TUMOR

Atypical teratoid rhabdoid tumor (ATRT) is a malignant embryonal tumor typically seen in very young patients, in both the supratentorial and infratentorial brain and characterized molecularly by loss of INI-1 and bi-allelic loss of SMARCB1. There is no clear treatment consensus for ATRT but management typically consists of maximal safe resection followed by intensive chemotherapy and radiotherapy. Several studies have evaluated the role of GTR and demonstrated improved survival outcomes compared with STR.[35–37] Although there is no standard adjuvant treatment paradigm for ATRT, several studies have evaluated the role of intensive chemotherapy and involved field radiotherapy. Investigators at Dana Farber Cancer Institute pioneered an intensive multimodality adjuvant regimen consisting of pre-irradiation and post-irradiation chemotherapy followed by maintenance chemotherapy. RT consisted of focal RT to 54 Gy in 30 fractions for M0 patients. Outcomes were encouraging with a 2-year PFS of 53% and median OS was not reached. Once again, GTR was found to be the most important predictor of OS, with 2-year OS of 91% in patients able to have complete resection of their tumor.[38] The most recent ATRT protocol, ACNS 0333, incorporates surgery followed by 2 cycles of induction chemotherapy, consideration of a second-look surgery, focal irradiation, and consolidative chemotherapy. Radiation is sequenced at the end for the youngest children (<6–12 months at diagnosis.) Although not yet published, preliminary results have been reported with a 2-year EFS of 43% and OS of 52% for the entire cohort.[39] The COG study demonstrates that disease control is equivalent in the early versus late radiation arms, but that toxicity may be less in the children treated with radiation after the high-dose chemotherapy (COG fall progress report; personal communication with Dr Alyssa Reddy and Anita Mahajan, 2019.)

CENTRAL NERVOUS SYSTEM GERM CELL TUMORS

Intracranial germ cell tumors account for 3.7% of all CNS tumors in patients 0 to 19 years of age and typically peak during the second decade of life.[3] The tumors are often classified as either pure germinomas or non-germinomatous germ cell tumors (NGGCTs). The distinction between these groups is based on the presence of a malignant germ cell component elucidated by biopsy or sometimes by tumor markers. An elevation of alpha feto-protein (AFP) always indicates a nongerminomatous germ cell tumor. A very high beta-Human chorionic gonadotropin (HCG) (in the thousands) usually means a component of choriocarcinoma, although an elevation in the hundreds could indicate a syncytial trophoblastic variant of germinoma and a biopsy should be considered if feasible. Pure germinomas carry a more favorable prognosis than NGGCTs. The most frequent locations of these tumors include the pineal or posterior third ventricular sites (50%–60%) or the suprasellar region (30%–35%).[40] Pure germinomas are more likely to present as bifocal or multiple midline tumors with concurrent lesions in the pineal and suprasellar region, although occasionally NGGCTs also present this way.[41] Although biopsy is generally recommended for all patients with intracranial germ cell tumors, it is particularly important for patients who do not have elevation of cerebrospinal fluid or serum AFP or beta-HCG and with modern surgical technique is safer now than it has been in previous years.

The current standard of care for intracranial germinoma is whole ventricular radiotherapy (WVRT) or chemotherapy followed by reduced-dose WVRT. Several studies have shown that WVRT does not compromise control rates compared with whole-brain radiation or CSI.[42,43] When WVRT is given alone, RT doses of 21–24 Gy to the ventricular axis, followed by a boost to 45 Gy is needed for disease control. A more recent treatment paradigm involves the use of neoadjuvant chemotherapy followed by reduced-dose WVRT. Several studies have shown excellent outcomes with an excellent progression-free survival greater than 90% with this approach.[44,45] The most current COG trial ACNS 1123 aims to determine if a dose reduction in both WVRT to 18 Gy and the tumor bed to 12 Gy would result in similar disease control. Typically 1.5 Gy per fraction is given instead of 1.8 because disease control is the same.

For patients with NGGCTs, the most accepted treatment approach remains neoadjuvant chemotherapy followed by CSI. In COG ACNS 0122, neoadjuvant chemotherapy with 6 cycles of carboplatin/etoposide alternating with ifosfamide/etoposide followed by 36 Gy CSI and tumor bed boost to 54 Gy resulted in an excellent 5-year PFS of 84%. Importantly, serum AFP was found to be a negative prognostic factor in this study.[46] For NGGCTs, COG ACNS 1123 evaluated whether patients who achieve a complete response after chemotherapy or chemotherapy with second-look surgery could omit CSI in substation for WVRT with a boost. An interim analysis of the study demonstrated higher recurrence rates and this arm was closed. Some centers have used less than 36 Gy CSI for patients with nondisseminated NGGCT, but the precise CSI dose in the nondisseminated cases is not known with certainty.[47]

GLIOMAS

Gliomas account for 52.1% of all pediatric tumors, of which most are low-grade gliomas (LGG).[1] For pediatric LGG, the primary goal of treatment is to obtain a GTR with surgery when feasible without undue morbidity. The COG reported patients treated with a GTR and observation to have 8-year OS and PFS of 96% and 78%, respectively, whereas patients with residual disease fared worse, with a 5-year PFS of 56%.[48] Although these patients can be effectively salvaged with RT, chemotherapy has been traditionally used to delay radiotherapy in young patients (typically <10 years of age) in an attempt to spare late side effects. Many regimens can be effective, but typically carboplatin and vincristine are used as first-line therapy due to its more acceptable toxicity profile despite a COG trial showing that TPCV (thioguanine, procarbazine, CCNU, vincristine) appeared to have more favorable 5-year EFS of 52% compared with 39% for carboplatin and vincristine.[49] This study also demonstrated that patients with thalamic tumors had worse PFS and OS. Radiation, when judiciously used, has been shown to be associated with excellent long-term progression-free survival ranging from 60% to 80% in several single-institution studies.[50,51] COG's ACNS 0221 demonstrates a 5-year PFS of 71% with margins of 5 mm for clinical target volume expansion around gross tumor visualized on MRI and inclusive of the resected tumor bed.[52] Reports of pediatric patients treated with proton radiotherapy show good control rates of greater than 80% at 5 years.[53,54]

RHABDOMYOSARCOMA

Rhabdomyosarcoma (RMS) is a rare malignant tumor of striated muscle and the most common soft tissue sarcoma of childhood, accounting for nearly 300 to 400 cases per year in the United States.[55] The standard treatment approach involves systemic chemotherapy with vincristine, dactinomycin, and cyclophosphamide (VAC) with local control consisting of surgery, RT, or both. The intensity of treatment is driven by risk stratification of patients into low, intermediate, and high-risk subgroups. The presence of PAX3/FOXO-1 fusion has been shown to be associated with poorer outcomes[56] in RMS and typically tracks with alveolar histology in contrast to the more favorable embryonal histology. Fusion status is more indicative of prognosis than histologic subtype.[57] **Tables 2** and **3** provide a simplified framework for categorizing patients based on stage, group, and the required dose.

For intermediate-risk patients, a recent publication from COG failed to show an EFS benefit to escalating treatment with VAC/VI (Vincristine and irinotecan) compared with VAC.[58] Nevertheless, the lower hematological toxicity has established this as standard chemotherapy for intermediate-risk RMS. The most recent ARST 1431 trial is currently evaluating whether the addition of a biologic mammalian target of rapamycin inhibitor, temsirolimus, may improve EFS compared with VAC/VI alone. However, recent data presented at American Society of Clinical Oncology in 2018 shows an EFS

Table 2
Clinical grouping

Group	A or B	Extent of Disease/Surgical Result
I	A	Localized tumor, confined to site of origin, completely resected
	B	Localized tumor, beyond site of origin, completely resected
II (microscopic positive)	A	Localized tumor, gross total resection, with microscopic residual disease
	B	Spread to regional lymph nodes, completely resected
	C	Spread to regional lymph nodes and microscopic residual
III (gross disease)	A	Gross residual after biopsy only
	B	Gross residual disease after major resection (50% debulking)
IV (metastatic disease)		Distant metastases

Adapted from Lawrence W, Gehan EA, Hays DM, et al. Prognostic significance of staging factors of the UICC staging system in childhood rhabdomyosarcoma: a report from the Intergroup Rhabdomyosarcoma Study (IRS-II). J Clin Oncol 1987;5(1):46-54; and Crist WM, Garnsey L, Beltangady MS, et al. Prognosis in children with rhabdomyosarcoma: a report of the intergroup rhabdomyosarcoma studies I and II. Intergroup Rhabdomyosarcoma Committee. J Clin Oncol 1990;8(3):443-452.

improvement for patients randomized to maintenance low-dose cyclophosphamide and vinorelbine.[59] ARST 1431 has recently been amended to add maintenance chemotherapy. For patients with metastatic RMS (high risk), the use of interval compressed chemotherapy was associated with improved 3-year EFS compared with historical controls.[60]

Radiotherapy dose varies from 36 to 59.4 Gy depending on the location, stage, and group of the tumor. Typically for patients with fusion positive tumor (often alveolar) and group I disease (GTR with negative microscopic margins), a dose of 36 Gy is used. Children who have group I disease and fusion negative tumors do not receive radiotherapy. Patients with lymph node involvement and resected tumors receive 41.4 Gy and gross residual is given 50.4 Gy if initial size is <5 cm, and 59.4 Gy if the tumor is ≥5 cm. It was only recently that doses more than 50.4 Gy were recommended for larger tumors secondary to an analysis from the COG D9803 study indicating a higher risk of local failure (LF) for patients with tumors 5 cm or larger (25% LF compared with 10% LF). For patients with intermediate-risk RMS, tumor size ≥5 cm

Table 3
Radiotherapy (RT) dose guidelines

RT Dose, Gy	Indications
0	Group I embryonal
36	Alveolar resected node negative disease, delayed primary excision embryonal, or Group IIA with positive margins
41.4	Resected node-positive disease
45–50.4	Gross disease to orbit; 45 Gy if CR to chemotherapy, 50.4 Gy if PR
50.4	Gross disease, <5 cm at diagnosis
59.4	Gross disease, >5 cm at diagnosis

Abbreviations: CR, Complete Response; PR, Partial Response.
   Data from Wolden SL, Lyden ER, Arndt CA, et al. Local Control for Intermediate-Risk Rhabdomyosarcoma: Results From D9803 According to Histology, Group, Site, and Size: A Report From the Children's Oncology Group. Int J Radiat Oncol Biol Phys 2015;93(5):1071-1076.

A   B   C

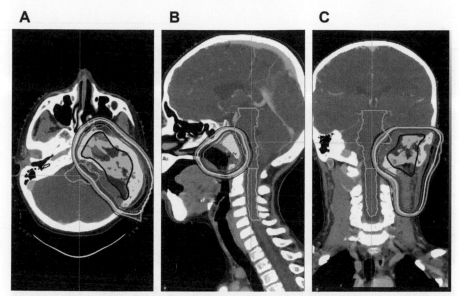

Fig. 2. An 8-year-old patient with a Stage III, Group III intermediate-risk parameningeal embryonal rhabdomyosarcoma of the left skull base (temporal/petrous bone) treated with IMPT. (*A*), (*B*), and (*C*) represent axial, sagittal, and coronal CT sequences of the radiation plan, respectively. IMPT is particularly advantageous in parameningeal tumors of the head and neck, as they allow sculpting of dose around the brainstem, spinal cord, and oral mucosa. Purple: 59.4 Gy line, Orange: 50.4 Gy line, Red: 45 Gy line, Yellow: 40 Gy line, Green: 35 Gy line, and Dark Blue: 30 Gy line.

was associated with increased LF compared with less than 5 cm on the COG D9803 trial.[61] For patients with orbital RMS, combined results of the last 2 COG studies for low-risk RMS indicate that 45 Gy is insufficient in the setting of lower doses of cyclophosphamide used and therefore the recommended dose is now 50.4 Gy for patients who have not had a complete response to the chemotherapy.[62] Proton beam RT in RMS has been shown to be associated with similar local control compared with photon-treated patients, with minimal late grade 3 toxicities (5.3%).[63] Intensity-modulated proton therapy (IMPT) is particularly advantageous in parameningeal head and neck tumors and allows for excellent dose sparing of the brainstem, spinal cord, and oral mucosa (**Fig. 2**).

NEUROBLASTOMA

Neuroblastoma (NB) is a tumor that arises from neural crest cells and is generally found in very young patients. Risk stratification is based on the recently proposed International Neuroblastoma Risk Group classification system and driven by image-defined risk factors.[64] Outcomes for patients with low-risk and intermediate-risk NB remain excellent, and RT is seldomly used. For patients with high-risk NB, outcomes remain poor and treatment consists of induction chemotherapy, surgery, high-dose myeloablative chemotherapy, RT, and then immunotherapy. Immunotherapy with anti-GD2 has been associated with improved EFS and OS compared with isotretinoin alone.[65] For patients with high-risk disease, a dose response has been shown to be associated with improved local control.[66] The most recent ANBL1531 protocol directs 21.6 Gy to the postinduction chemotherapy presurgical volume followed by a boost to

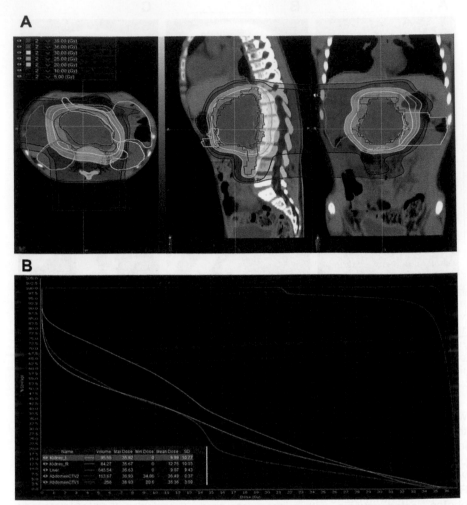

Fig. 3. Patient with high-risk NB treated with IMPT for kidney sparing. (*A*) CTV1 is magenta and CTV2 is purple. IMPT allows for excellent sparing of dose to the kidneys and liver. (*B*): Dose volume histogram of the target structures, kidneys and liver.

36 Gy to gross residual disease, although the utility of the dose escalation to 36 Gy has been questioned and whether to push this high is now somewhat controversial.[67] All persistently metaiodobenzylguanidine (MIBG)-positive metastatic sites after induction chemotherapy typically receive 21.6 Gy. The use of proton beam therapy, particularly with intensity modulation and pencil beam scanning, allows excellent sparing of kidney dose (**Fig. 3**).

WILMS TUMOR

Wilms tumor is the most common pediatric embryonal neoplasm of the kidney, and accounts for approximately 5% of all childhood cancers.[1] The results of multiple cooperative group studies from the National Wilms Tumor Study and the International Society of Pediatric Oncology have led to a reduction in the use of adjuvant RT, particularly for patients with Stage I and II favorable histology (FH) tumors.[68,69]

Table 4
Description of radiotherapy target and dose by clinical indication in patients with Wilms tumor

Target Irradiated	Indication	Dose, Gy
Flank	Stage III favorable histology Stage I-III focal anaplasia Stage I-II diffuse anaplasia Stage II-III clear cell Stage I-III rhabdoid (≤12 mo)	10.8 Gy
Flank	Stage III diffuse anaplasia Stage I-III rhabdoid (>12 mo)	19.8 Gy 19.8 Gy
Tumor boost	Gross disease	10.8 Gy
Lymph node irradiation	Resected lymph node Unresected lymph node	10.8 Gy 19.8 Gy
Whole-abdomen irradiation	Stage III: diffuse spillage. Peritoneal seeding, ascites, preoperative tumor rupture	10.5 Gy
Whole-abdomen irradiation	Stage III: Diffuse peritoneal implants	21 Gy
Whole lung irradiation	Lung metastases with LOH 1p and 16q No CR at week 6 with chemotherapy	10.5 Gy if <12 mo 12 Gy if ≥12 mo
Liver irradiation	Diffuse metastases or focal metastases not resected	19.8 Gy
Bone irradiation	Bone metastases	25.2 Gy if <16 y; 30.6 Gy if ≥16 y
Whole brain	Brain metastases	21.6 Gy if <16 y and 30.6 Gy if ≥16 y

Abbreviations: LOH, Loss of Heterozygosity; CR, Complete Response.

The NWTS-5 trial demonstrated the importance of loss of heterozygosity for 1p/16q, which predicted for increased risk of relapse and death[70]; 1q gain was subsequently found to be associated with inferior OS in FH Wilms.[71]

For patients with Stage III FH, flank RT is given to 10.8 Gy and residual disease is given an additional dose of 10.8 Gy. Whole-abdomen RT is usually given at a dose of 10.5 Gy in 1.5 Gy per fraction. For patients with rhabdoid histology, Stage I-III typically gets escalation of flank RT to 19.8 Gy. For patients with lung metastases and FH, AREN 0533 demonstrated excellent EFS and OS for patients in whom lung RT was omitted after complete response to 6 weeks of vincristine, dactinomycin, and doxorubicin.[72] For patients who have bilateral Wilms (Stage V), AREN 0534 showed an excellent 4-year EFS of 82% with a regimen consisting of induction chemotherapy followed by surgery and further chemotherapy/RT depending on histology.[73] A detailed description of the target irradiated and the dose indicated by each clinical scenario is shown in **Table 4**.

EWING SARCOMA

Ewing sarcoma is the second most common bone tumor in childhood, behind osteosarcoma. Management typically consists of induction chemotherapy followed by local control at week 12, and consolidative chemotherapy. Compressed chemotherapy given every 2 weeks, with vincristine-doxorubicin-cyclophosphamide alternating with ifosfamide-etoposide has been shown to be associated with improved EFS.[74] Local control with either surgery or RT is acceptable and no one modality was shown to be superior in the INT-0091 trial.[75] Other trials have shown higher rates of LF with RT alone with no decrement in EFS or OS.[76,77] RT is typically directed to the anatomically constrained prechemotherapy bone and soft tissue extent for the primary course followed by volume reduction to the prechemotherapy bone and post chemotherapy soft tissue extent. The most recent COG trial, AEWS1031, mandates 55.8 Gy for gross disease, 50.4 Gy for microscopic residual, and 50.4 Gy for vertebral body lesions to respect spinal cord tolerance.

SUMMARY

In summary, survival rates in pediatric oncology have dramatically improved over the past 3 decades, directly due to improvement and refinement in surgical techniques, chemotherapy optimization, and RT delivery. Regardless, RT continues to play a critical role in the treatment of CNS and non-CNS pediatric malignancies and its future use will likely be guided and tailored to the molecular features and genomics of the various tumor types. The advent of intensity modulation in both photon and proton radiation modalities has allowed us to deliver RT in a highly conformal and precise manner with the promise of reduced toxicity and improved quality of life for pediatric cancer survivors. The improvements in radiation techniques and targeting has dramatically improved the quality of radiotherapy and normal tissue sparing. These improvements are starting to show real clinical benefits in both the quality of life and quality of survivorship of our pediatric patients.

REFERENCES

1. Siegel RL, Miller KD, Jemal A. Cancer statistics, 2019. CA Cancer J Clin 2019; 69(1):7–34.
2. DeSantis CE, Lin CC, Mariotto AB, et al. Cancer treatment and survivorship statistics, 2014. CA Cancer J Clin 2014;64(4):252–71.
3. Ostrom QT, Gittleman H, Truitt G, et al. CBTRUS statistical report: primary brain and other central nervous system tumors diagnosed in the United States in 2011-2015. Neuro Oncol 2018;20(suppl_4):iv1–86.
4. Rieken S, Mohr A, Habermehl D, et al. Outcome and prognostic factors of radiation therapy for medulloblastoma. Int J Radiat Oncol Biol Phys 2011;81(3):e7–13.
5. Rutkowski S, Bode U, Deinlein F, et al. Treatment of early childhood medulloblastoma by postoperative chemotherapy alone. N Engl J Med 2005;352(10):978–86.
6. Stavrou T, Bromley CM, Nicholson HS, et al. Prognostic factors and secondary malignancies in childhood medulloblastoma. J Pediatr Hematol Oncol 2001; 23(7):431–6.
7. Cavalli FMG, Remke M, Rampasek L, et al. Intertumoral heterogeneity within medulloblastoma subgroups. Cancer Cell 2017;31(6):737–54.e6.
8. Schwalbe EC, Lindsey JC, Nakjang S, et al. Novel molecular subgroups for clinical classification and outcome prediction in childhood medulloblastoma: a cohort study. Lancet Oncol 2017;18(7):958–71.
9. Thompson EM, Hielscher T, Bouffet E, et al. Prognostic value of medulloblastoma extent of resection after accounting for molecular subgroup: a retrospective integrated clinical and molecular analysis. Lancet Oncol 2016;17(4):484–95.
10. Schreiber JE, Palmer SL, Conklin HM, et al. Posterior fossa syndrome and long-term neuropsychological outcomes among children treated for medulloblastoma on a multi-institutional, prospective study. Neuro Oncol 2017;19(12):1673–82.

11. Packer RJ, Gajjar A, Vezina G, et al. Phase III study of craniospinal radiation therapy followed by adjuvant chemotherapy for newly diagnosed average-risk medulloblastoma. J Clin Oncol 2006;24(25):4202–8.

12. Packer RJ, Zhou T, Holmes E, et al. Survival and secondary tumors in children with medulloblastoma receiving radiotherapy and adjuvant chemotherapy: results of Children's Oncology Group trial A9961. Neuro Oncol 2013;15(1):97–103.

13. Jakacki RI, Burger PC, Zhou T, et al. Outcome of children with metastatic medulloblastoma treated with carboplatin during craniospinal radiotherapy: a Children's Oncology Group Phase I/II study. J Clin Oncol 2012;30(21):2648–53.

14. Gajjar A, Chintagumpala M, Ashley D, et al. Risk-adapted craniospinal radiotherapy followed by high-dose chemotherapy and stem-cell rescue in children with newly diagnosed medulloblastoma (St Jude Medulloblastoma-96): long-term results from a prospective, multicentre trial. Lancet Oncol 2006;7(10): 813–20.

15. Gandola L, Massimino M, Cefalo G, et al. Hyperfractionated accelerated radiotherapy in the Milan strategy for metastatic medulloblastoma. J Clin Oncol 2009;27(4):566–71.

16. Vivekanandan S, Breene R, Ramanujachar R, et al. The UK experience of a treatment strategy for pediatric metastatic medulloblastoma comprising intensive induction chemotherapy, hyperfractionated accelerated radiotherapy and response directed high dose myeloablative chemotherapy or maintenance chemotherapy (Milan strategy). Pediatr Blood Cancer 2015;62(12):2132–9.

17. Michalski JM, Janss A, Vezina G, et al. Results of COG ACNS0331: a phase III trial of involved-field radiotherapy (IFRT) and low dose craniospinal irradiation (LD-CSI) with chemotherapy in average-risk medulloblastoma: a report from the Children's Oncology Group. Int J Radiat Oncol Biol Phys 2016;96(5):937–8.

18. Kool M, Korshunov A, Remke M, et al. Molecular subgroups of medulloblastoma: an international meta-analysis of transcriptome, genetic aberrations, and clinical data of WNT, SHH, Group 3, and Group 4 medulloblastomas. Acta Neuropathol 2012;123(4):473–84.

19. Brinkman TM, Ness KK, Li Z, et al. Attainment of functional and social independence in adult survivors of pediatric CNS tumors: a report from the St Jude Lifetime Cohort Study. J Clin Oncol 2018;36(27):2762–9.

20. Salloum R, Chen Y, Yasui Y, et al. Late morbidity and mortality among medulloblastoma survivors diagnosed across three decades: a report from the childhood cancer survivor study. J Clin Oncol 2019;37(9):731–40.

21. Yock TI, Yeap BY, Ebb DH, et al. Long-term toxic effects of proton radiotherapy for paediatric medulloblastoma: a phase 2 single-arm study. Lancet Oncol 2016;17(3):287–98.

22. Bates JE, Howell RM, Liu Q, et al. Therapy-related cardiac risk in childhood cancer survivors: an analysis of the childhood cancer survivor study. J Clin Oncol 2019;37(13):1090–101.

23. Northcott PA, Korshunov A, Witt H, et al. Medulloblastoma comprises four distinct molecular variants. J Clin Oncol 2011;29(11):1408–14.

24. Rutkowski S, von Hoff K, Emser A, et al. Survival and prognostic factors of early childhood medulloblastoma: an international meta-analysis. J Clin Oncol 2010; 28(33):4961–8.

25. Cage TA, Clark AJ, Aranda D, et al. A systematic review of treatment outcomes in pediatric patients with intracranial ependymomas. J Neurosurg Pediatr 2013; 11(6):673–81.

26. Timmermann B, Kortmann RD, Kuhl J, et al. Combined postoperative irradiation and chemotherapy for anaplastic ependymomas in childhood: results of the German prospective trials HIT 88/89 and HIT 91. Int J Radiat Oncol Biol Phys 2000;46(2):287–95.
27. Aizer AA, Ancukiewicz M, Nguyen PL, et al. Natural history and role of radiation in patients with supratentorial and infratentorial WHO grade II ependymomas: results from a population-based study. J Neurooncol 2013;115(3):411–9.
28. Indelicato DJ, Bradley JA, Rotondo RL, et al. Outcomes following proton therapy for pediatric ependymoma. Acta Oncol 2018;57(5):644–8.
29. Merchant TE, Li C, Xiong X, et al. Conformal radiotherapy after surgery for paediatric ependymoma: a prospective study. Lancet Oncol 2009;10(3):258–66.
30. Macdonald SM, Sethi R, Lavally B, et al. Proton radiotherapy for pediatric central nervous system ependymoma: clinical outcomes for 70 patients. Neuro Oncol 2013;15(11):1552–9.
31. Massimino M, Miceli R, Giangaspero F, et al. Final results of the second prospective AIEOP protocol for pediatric intracranial ependymoma. Neuro Oncol 2016; 18(10):1451–60.
32. Merchant TE, Bendel AE, Sabin ND, et al. Conformal radiation therapy for pediatric ependymoma, chemotherapy for incompletely resected ependymoma, and observation for completely resected, supratentorial ependymoma. J Clin Oncol 2019;37(12):974–83.
33. Indelicato DJ, Flampouri S, Rotondo RL, et al. Incidence and dosimetric parameters of pediatric brainstem toxicity following proton therapy. Acta Oncol 2014; 53(10):1298–304.
34. Yock TI, Constine LS, Mahajan A. Protons, the brainstem, and toxicity: ingredients for an emerging dialectic. Acta Oncol 2014;53(10):1279–82.
35. Hilden JM, Meerbaum S, Burger P, et al. Central nervous system atypical teratoid/ rhabdoid tumor: results of therapy in children enrolled in a registry. J Clin Oncol 2004;22(14):2877–84.
36. Tekautz TM, Fuller CE, Blaney S, et al. Atypical teratoid/rhabdoid tumors (ATRT): improved survival in children 3 years of age and older with radiation therapy and high-dose alkylator-based chemotherapy. J Clin Oncol 2005;23(7):1491–9.
37. Woehrer A, Slavc I, Waldhoer T, et al. Incidence of atypical teratoid/rhabdoid tumors in children: a population-based study by the Austrian Brain Tumor Registry, 1996-2006. Cancer 2010;116(24):5725–32.
38. Chi SN, Zimmerman MA, Yao X, et al. Intensive multimodality treatment for children with newly diagnosed CNS atypical teratoid rhabdoid tumor. J Clin Oncol 2009;27(3):385–9.
39. Reddy A, Strother D, Judkins A, et al. AT-09TREATMENT of atypical teratoid rhabdoid tumors (ATRT) of the central nervous system with surgery, intensive chemotherapy, and 3-D conformal radiation (ACNS0333). A report from the Children's Oncology Group 2016;Vol 18:1–21.
40. Echevarria ME, Fangusaro J, Goldman S. Pediatric central nervous system germ cell tumors: a review. Oncologist 2008;13(6):690–9.
41. Aizer AA, Sethi RV, Hedley-Whyte ET, et al. Bifocal intracranial tumors of nongerminomatous germ cell etiology: diagnostic and therapeutic implications. Neuro Oncol 2013;15(7):955–60.
42. Haas-Kogan DA, Missett BT, Wara WM, et al. Radiation therapy for intracranial germ cell tumors. Int J Radiat Oncol Biol Phys 2003;56(2):511–8.
43. Rogers SJ, Mosleh-Shirazi MA, Saran FH. Radiotherapy of localised intracranial germinoma: time to sever historical ties? Lancet Oncol 2005;6(7):509–19.

44. Buckner JC, Peethambaram PP, Smithson WA, et al. Phase II trial of primary chemotherapy followed by reduced-dose radiation for CNS germ cell tumors. J Clin Oncol 1999;17(3):933–40.

45. Cheng S, Kilday JP, Laperriere N, et al. Outcomes of children with central nervous system germinoma treated with multi-agent chemotherapy followed by reduced radiation. J Neurooncol 2016;127(1):173–80.

46. Goldman S, Bouffet E, Fisher PG, et al. Phase II trial assessing the ability of neo-adjuvant chemotherapy with or without second-look surgery to eliminate measurable disease for nongerminomatous germ cell tumors: a Children's Oncology Group Study. J Clin Oncol 2015;33(22):2464–71.

47. MacDonald SM, Trofimov A, Safai S, et al. Proton radiotherapy for pediatric central nervous system germ cell tumors: early clinical outcomes. Int J Radiat Oncol Biol Phys 2011;79(1):121–9.

48. Wisoff JH, Sanford RA, Heier LA, et al. Primary neurosurgery for pediatric low-grade gliomas: a prospective multi-institutional study from the Children's Oncology Group. Neurosurgery 2011;68(6):1548–54 [discussion: 1554–5].

49. Ater JL, Zhou T, Holmes E, et al. Randomized study of two chemotherapy regimens for treatment of low-grade glioma in young children: a report from the Children's Oncology Group. J Clin Oncol 2012;30(21):2641–7.

50. Merchant TE, Kun LE, Wu S, et al. Phase II trial of conformal radiation therapy for pediatric low-grade glioma. J Clin Oncol 2009;27(22):3598–604.

51. Paulino AC, Mazloom A, Terashima K, et al. Intensity-modulated radiotherapy (IMRT) in pediatric low-grade glioma. Cancer 2013;119(14):2654–9.

52. Cherlow JM, Shaw DWW, Margraf LR, et al. Conformal radiation therapy for pediatric patients with low-grade glioma: results from the Children's Oncology Group Phase 2 Study ACNS0221. Int J Radiat Oncol Biol Phys 2019;103(4):861–8.

53. Indelicato DJ, Rotondo RL, Uezono H, et al. Outcomes following proton therapy for pediatric low-grade glioma. Int J Radiat Oncol Biol Phys 2019;104(1):149–56.

54. Greenberger BA, Pulsifer MB, Ebb DH, et al. Clinical outcomes and late endocrine, neurocognitive, and visual profiles of proton radiation for pediatric low-grade gliomas. Int J Radiat Oncol Biol Phys 2014;89(5):1060–8.

55. Sultan I, Qaddoumi I, Yaser S, et al. Comparing adult and pediatric rhabdomyosarcoma in the surveillance, epidemiology and end results program, 1973 to 2005: an analysis of 2,600 patients. J Clin Oncol 2009;27(20):3391–7.

56. Missiaglia E, Williamson D, Chisholm J, et al. PAX3/FOXO1 fusion gene status is the key prognostic molecular marker in rhabdomyosarcoma and significantly improves current risk stratification. J Clin Oncol 2012;30(14):1670–7.

57. Williamson D, Missiaglia E, de Reynies A, et al. Fusion gene-negative alveolar rhabdomyosarcoma is clinically and molecularly indistinguishable from embryonal rhabdomyosarcoma. J Clin Oncol 2010;28(13):2151–8.

58. Hawkins DS, Chi YY, Anderson JR, et al. Addition of vincristine and irinotecan to vincristine, dactinomycin, and cyclophosphamide does not improve outcome for intermediate-risk rhabdomyosarcoma: a report from the Children's Oncology Group. J Clin Oncol 2018;36(27):2770–7.

59. Bisogno G, Salvo GLD, Bergeron C, et al. Maintenance low-dose chemotherapy in patients with high-risk (HR) rhabdomyosarcoma (RMS): a report from the European Paediatric Soft Tissue Sarcoma Study Group (EpSSG). J Clin Oncol 2018; 36(18_suppl):LBA2.

60. Weigel BJ, Lyden E, Anderson JR, et al. Intensive multiagent therapy, including dose-compressed cycles of ifosfamide/etoposide and vincristine/doxorubicin/cyclophosphamide, irinotecan, and radiation, in patients with high-risk

rhabdomyosarcoma: a report from the Children's Oncology Group. J Clin Oncol 2016;34(2):117–22.

61. Wolden SL, Lyden ER, Arndt CA, et al. Local control for intermediate-risk rhabdomyosarcoma: results from d9803 according to histology, group, site, and size: a report from the Children's Oncology Group. Int J Radiat Oncol Biol Phys 2015; 93(5):1071–6.

62. Ermoian RP, Breneman J, Walterhouse DO, et al. 45 Gy is not sufficient radiotherapy dose for Group III orbital embryonal rhabdomyosarcoma after less than complete response to 12 weeks of ARST0331 chemotherapy: a report from the Soft Tissue Sarcoma Committee of the Children's Oncology Group. Pediatr Blood Cancer 2017;64(9):1–11.

63. Ladra MM, Szymonifka JD, Mahajan A, et al. Preliminary results of a phase II trial of proton radiotherapy for pediatric rhabdomyosarcoma. J Clin Oncol 2014; 32(33):3762–70.

64. Cohn SL, Pearson AD, London WB, et al. The International Neuroblastoma Risk Group (INRG) classification system: an INRG Task Force report. J Clin Oncol 2009;27(2):289–97.

65. Yu AL, Gilman AL, Ozkaynak MF, et al. Anti-GD2 antibody with GM-CSF, interleukin-2, and isotretinoin for neuroblastoma. N Engl J Med 2010;363(14): 1324–34.

66. Haas-Kogan DA, Swift PS, Selch M, et al. Impact of radiotherapy for high-risk neuroblastoma: a Children's Cancer Group study. Int J Radiat Oncol Biol Phys 2003;56(1):28–39.

67. COG Neuroblastoma Committee. Change in radiation therapy to the primary tumor site in patients with high-risk neuroblastoma 2019.

68. D'Angio GJ, Evans A, Breslow N, et al. The treatment of Wilms' tumor: results of the Second National Wilms' Tumor Study. Cancer 1981;47(9):2302–11.

69. D'Angio GJ, Breslow N, Beckwith JB, et al. Treatment of Wilms' tumor. Results of the Third National Wilms' Tumor Study. Cancer 1989;64(2):349–60.

70. Grundy PE, Breslow NE, Li S, et al. Loss of heterozygosity for chromosomes 1p and 16q is an adverse prognostic factor in favorable-histology Wilms tumor: a report from the National Wilms Tumor Study Group. J Clin Oncol 2005;23(29): 7312–21.

71. Gratias EJ, Dome JS, Jennings LJ, et al. Association of chromosome 1q gain with inferior survival in favorable-histology Wilms tumor: a report from the Children's Oncology Group. J Clin Oncol 2016;34(26):3189–94.

72. Dix DB, Seibel NL, Chi YY, et al. Treatment of stage IV favorable histology Wilms tumor with lung metastases: a report from the Children's Oncology Group AREN0533 Study. J Clin Oncol 2018;36(16):1564–70.

73. Ehrlich P, Chi YY, Chintagumpala MM, et al. Results of the first prospective multiinstitutional treatment study in children with bilateral Wilms tumor (AREN0534): a report from the Children's Oncology Group. Ann Surg 2017;266(3):470–8.

74. Womer RB, West DC, Krailo MD, et al. Randomized controlled trial of intervalcompressed chemotherapy for the treatment of localized Ewing sarcoma: a report from the Children's Oncology Group. J Clin Oncol 2012;30(33):4148–54.

75. Yock TI, Krailo M, Fryer CJ, et al. Local control in pelvic Ewing sarcoma: analysis from INT-0091–a report from the Children's Oncology Group. J Clin Oncol 2006; 24(24):3838–43.

76. DuBois SG, Krailo MD, Gebhardt MC, et al. Comparative evaluation of local control strategies in localized Ewing sarcoma of bone: a report from the Children's Oncology Group. Cancer 2015;121(3):467–75.

77. Schuck A, Ahrens S, Paulussen M, et al. Local therapy in localized Ewing tumors: results of 1058 patients treated in the CESS 81, CESS 86, and EICESS 92 trials. Int J Radiat Oncol Biol Phys 2003;55(1):168–77.

78. Taylor MD, Northcott PA, Korshunov A, et al. Molecular subgroups of medullo-blastoma: the current consensus. Acta Neuropathol 2012;123(4):465–72.

79. Northcott PA, Robinson GW, Kratz CP, et al. Medulloblastoma. Nat Rev Dis Primers 2019;5(1):11.

Malignant Soft-Tissue Sarcomas

Jeremy M. Brownstein, MD[a], Thomas F. DeLaney, MD[b],*

KEYWORDS

- Soft-tissue sarcoma • Retroperitoneal sarcoma • Extremity sarcoma
- Radiation therapy

KEY POINTS

- Soft-tissue sarcomas are rare tumors arising primarily from fat, muscle, and other connective tissues.
- Although ideal management varies by histology, location, extent of disease, and functional status, appropriate strategies frequently include a combination of surgery, radiation, and/or chemotherapy.
- Sarcomas that are treated with a suboptimal approach are more prone to recurrence, thus treatment should only be attempted by an experienced multidisciplinary team.

INTRODUCTION

Sarcomas are malignant tumors that arise from skeletal and extraskeletal connective tissues, including the peripheral nervous system. Although ectodermal in origin, the malignant tumors of the peripheral nerves are included because of the similarities in clinical behavior, management, and outcome. Sarcomas are rare, with an estimated incidence in the United States of approximately 16,250 diagnosed annually, representing about 0.92% of the 1,762,450 new malignant tumors. Bone sarcomas are rarer still, compromising only 14.5% of all sarcomas.[1,2]

Because of the rarity and gravity of these tumors, one might predict a clinical advantage for evaluation and management in a center with a team of dedicated subspecialists including clinicians in surgical, orthopedic, medical, pediatric, and radiation oncology. The gain in outcome provided by this multidisciplinary expertise was illustrated in 1 study that examined the outcome in 375 patients with soft-tissue sarcoma (STS) of the extremities and torso according to the time of referral

Disclosure: The authors have nothing to disclose.
[a] Francis H. Burr Proton Beam Therapy Center, Massachusetts General Hospital, 30 Fruit Street, Boston, MA 02114, USA; [b] Department of Radiation Oncology, Francis H. Burr Proton Beam Therapy Center, Massachusetts General Hospital, Harvard Medical School, 30 Fruit Street, Boston, MA 02114, USA
* Corresponding author.
E-mail address: tdelaney@partners.org

to a tumor center in the South Sweden Health Care Region.[3] Compared with patients referred preoperatively, local recurrence rates were increased in patients not referred at any time (2.4 times higher), and in patients referred after surgery (1.3 times higher).

PATHOGENETIC FACTORS

Although there is no clearly defined cause in most cases of STS, some associated or predisposing factors have been identified. They include a genetic predisposition, oncogenic viruses, immunodeficiency, radiation, chemotherapy, chemical carcinogens, chronic irritation, and lymphedema.[4] Several well-characterized genetic syndromes that portend a higher risk for malignant sarcoma development include Beckwith-Wiedemann syndrome, Bloom syndrome, hereditary retinoblastoma, Li-Fraumeni syndrome, and neurofibromatosis type 1, among others; lastly familial adenomatous polyposis is associated with development of benign desmoids.[5] However, a genetic review of 1162 patients with STS found that of the 911 families with informative pedigrees, only 17% fit a known hereditary germline cancer syndrome.[6] Nevertheless, recent findings from a large kindred study demonstrated that about half of patients with sarcoma have putatively pathogenic monogenic and polygenic variation in known and novel cancer genes, with implications for risk management and treatment.[6]

CLASSIFICATION

Most sarcomas are classified according to their differentiation characteristics and, therefore, their presumed tissue of origin (eg, liposarcoma, leiomyosarcoma, rhabdomyosarcoma [RMS], fibrosarcoma, and angiosarcoma). For other sarcomas, the designation reflects the histologic pattern (eg, alveolar sarcoma of soft parts, epithelioid sarcoma, and clear cell sarcoma). There are also benign soft-tissue tumors. Although the prevalence of benign tumors is difficult to quantify because most are not biopsied, their incidence is likely significantly higher than their malignant counterparts.[4] Examples include desmoids, atypical lipoma, and neuroma. In addition, there are nonneoplastic lesions that may be confused with a benign or a low-grade mesenchymal neoplasm, such as Dupuytren contracture and plantar fibromatosis.

CLINICAL PRESENTATION

The patient with a STS of the extremity most often presents with a painless lump of a few weeks or months duration. Less commonly, there is pain or symptoms secondary to pressure effects on nerve or bone from an unappreciated mass. Patients with retroperitoneal sarcomas may have vague abdominal discomfort, gastrointestinal symptoms, or a mass, although many are asymptomatic or minimally symptomatic until the tumors are large enough to produce local symptoms. Metastases at initial presentation are uncommon.[7]

ANATOMIC DISTRIBUTION

Sarcomas of the soft tissue occur at all anatomic sites of the body, most being present in the extremities. The relative frequency was illustrated in a report of 7563 consecutive STSs seen at MD Anderson Cancer center between 1996 and 2006[4]:

- Head and neck: 5%
- Upper extremity: 11%

- Thoracic: 8%
- Visceral: 25%
- Retroperitoneal: 25%
- Lower extremity: 26%

DIAGNOSTIC EVALUATION

A complete history and physical examination should define the anatomic areas of involvement, the patient being evaluated for evidence of skin, major vessel, nerve or bone invasion, the status of regional lymph nodes, and the presence of edema. The following methods are used for the diagnostic evaluation:

- MRI and computed tomography (CT) scan—MRI (**Fig. 1**) is generally used for assessment of the primary site in the extremity, trunk, and head and neck lesion, whereas CT scan is preferred for retroperitoneal and thoracic primaries. CT scan is used to evaluate the lungs for metastatic disease in patients with high-grade lesions.[8–11]
- PET scan—may have a role in evaluating nodal involvement in patients with histologies with potential for nodal involvement (epithelioid sarcoma, clear cell sarcoma, RMS, synovial sarcoma, and angiosarcoma). However, a retrospective review of 109 patients with primarily grade 2 to 3 nonpediatric, trunk and extremity sarcomas staged with PET/CT noted that, when assessing for distant disease, PET improved sensitivity of CT in only 5% of cases.[12]
- Bone scan—is usually *not* helpful for initial staging. In the absence of multiple metastases in other sites, bone metastases are unusual in adults, except for myxoid liposarcoma, in which metastases may involve the marrow without cortical changes and not be detected by bone scan.
- Biopsy—provides the basis for definitive tissue diagnosis, a critical step in management of the patient with STS. Core needle is generally preferred but can also be performed by incisional technique, fine-needle aspiration in some experienced centers, or excision of small lesions. Of note, biopsy should be planned

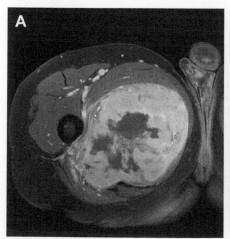
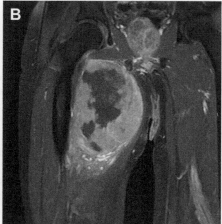

Fig. 1. T1, (A) postgadolinium axial and (B) coronal MRI scans of a 69-year-old man presenting with a 14 × 13 × 11-cm high-grade, undifferentiated pleomorphic sarcoma arising in the adductor magnus muscle in the right medial thigh.

in communication with a multidisciplinary sarcoma team to ensure that uninvolved compartments are avoided and that the track can be resected en bloc with tumor.

- Histologic diagnosis—should be performed by pathologists with expertise in soft tissue pathologic conditions. Distinction between high-grade sarcomas (eg, undifferentiated pleomorphic sarcoma, extraskeletal osteosarcoma), and nonmalignant conditions (eg, nodular fasciitis and myositis ossificans) can be extremely difficult.
- Molecular analysis—molecular genetic testing has played an increasingly important role in classification of STSs. A cohort of 395 patients with STS (of whom 384 met eligibility criteria) underwent both pathologic characterization and molecular characterization. Following review by a panel of experts, the pathologic diagnosis and therapeutic strategy was modified in over an eighth of patients (13.4%) owing to molecular findings. The authors of this article recommend that pathologic analysis is conducted at centers with access and expertise in molecular profiling of STSs.[13]

STAGING

The decision as to the most appropriate treatment strategy is strongly influenced by the stage at initial diagnosis.

American Joint Committee on Cancer (AJCC) staging system incorporates histologic grade (G), tumor size (T), lymph node metastases (N), and distant metastases (M) to characterize 4 stage groupings.[14] Each tumor is assigned a grade of low (1), intermediate (2), or high (3) on the basis of histopathologic characteristics. Stage IV is defined by either regional nodal involvement or evidence of distant metastatic disease. If either of these is present, the lesion is stage IV regardless of grade, size, or site.

For trunk and extremity sarcomas, 5-year overall survival (OS) rates by AJCC 8th edition staging criteria are[15]:

- *1A/1B:* 85.3%/85%
- *II:* 79%
- *IIIA/IIIB:* 62.4%/50.1%
- *IV(N+ M–)/IV(M+):* 33.1%/12.4%

ALTERNATIVE STAGING SYSTEMS

Some orthopedic surgical units use other staging systems such as that of the Musculoskeletal Tumor Society,[16] the Memorial Sloan-Kettering (MSK),[17] and the Swedish SIN (tumor size, vascular invasion, and microscopic tumor necrosis) systems.[18] In the surgical staging system of the Musculoskeletal Tumor Society, the stage is based on grade (a 2-tiered system, low versus high) and compartmentality, that is, confinement to an anatomic compartment. This parameter is important in predicting local control probability for surgery alone, but it is not an accurate predictor of local recurrence with combined surgery and radiation.[19] For localized extremity STS, the AJCC or the MSK staging systems are most predictive of the risk of systemic relapse.[20]

Histologic Grading

To increase the prognostic value of histologic assessment, several grading systems have been developed: 2-tier,[16] 3-tier,[21] and 4-tier[22] grading systems have been used and there is debate among pathologists about which is most predictive.[23] The AJCC 8th edition has adopted a 3-tier grading system that includes scoring based on differentiation, mitotic count and necrosis.

Tumor Size

The standard measurement of tumor size is the largest diameter of the lesion. For almost all types of tumor, the frequency of distant metastasis is related to size and grade.[14,24,25]

Tumor Depth

The pervious iteration of the AJCC staging system (7th edition) incorporated tumor depth into stage,[26] yet this has been omitted from the 8th edition.[14] Historically, many have noted that tumor depth is prognostic for numerous endpoints including survival,[27] postoperative mortality,[28] and local/distant recurrence.[29] However, a recent multivariate analysis demonstrates that depth loses prognostic value when tumor size is a covariate, possibly owing to the relative scarcity of large superficial tumors and small and deep sarcomas.[30] In addition, depth is clearly less relevant when discussing retroperitoneal sarcomas or other visceral sites. Still, there are some who advocate for staging systems that incorporate depth, such as the Vanderbilt staging system.[31]

Other Prognostic Indicators

Cellular DNA content, ploidy, cell proliferation kinetics, gene activation, amplification, deletions, or mutations, are helpful to predict the outcome for the individual patient. The most well-known prognostic gene expression signature is that from Chibon and colleagues,[32] the complexity index in sarcomas (CINSARC), composed of 67 genes related to mitosis and chromosome management.

Proliferative Activity

The proliferative activity of a tumor, which may be an indicator of the potential for distant metastasis can be assessed by several techniques, such as the staining of cells by the monoclonal antibody Ki-67, which reacts with a nuclear antigen present on cells in active cell cycle. Increased nuclear staining for Ki-67 may be an independent prognostic marker in patients with STSs.[33]

MOLECULAR TESTING

There are increasing data demonstrating the importance of molecular testing in the diagnosis of STS. In a meta-analysis of 70 eligible studies, Kandel and colleagues[34] identified 4 molecular assays that provide clinically relevant data with high sensitivity and specificity:

- *MDM2 amplification* (detected via fluorescence in situ hybridization [FISH] or real-time polymerase chain reaction [PCR]) can differentiate atypical/malignant lipomatous histologies (eg, atypical lipomatous tumor, well-differentiated liposarcoma, and de-differentiated liposarcoma) from benign lipoma or other sarcoma histologies.
- *SYT-SSX fusion* (detected real-time PCR) or *SS18 break-apart* (by FISH) can differentiate synovial sarcoma from other sarcoma histologies.
- *CTNNB1 mutation* (detected via PCR/next-generation sequencing/Sanger sequencing) portends a decreased chance of tumor recurrence for desmoid

tumors (see Jeremy M. Brownstein and Thomas F. DeLaney's article, "Bone Sarcomas and Desmoids," in this issue).

Additional prototypical mutations that aid in the diagnosis of STS include:

- EWSR1-FLI1 fusion—highly sensitive and specific for the diagnosis of Ewing sarcoma family tumors[35] (for detailed description of Ewing sarcoma family tumors, see Sujith Baliga and Torunn I. Yock's, "Pediatric Cancer," in this issue).
- FOXO1-PAX fusion—in RMS, the presence or absence of this fusion may be more helpful in predicting more aggressive biology than a histologic classification of alveolar RMS versus embryonal RMS.[36,37] In addition, for RMS a FOXO1-PAX fusion involving PAX3 portends a worse prognosis than a fusion involving PAX7[37] (for detailed description of RMS, see Sujith Baliga and Torunn I. Yock's, "Pediatric Cancer," in this issue).
- FUS-CHOP or EWSR1-CHOP are present in all cases of myxoid/round cell liposarcoma.[38]

SOFT-TISSUE SARCOMA OF THE EXTREMITIES

In treating STS of the extremities, the therapeutic goals are survival, avoidance of a local recurrence, maximizing function, and minimizing morbidity. The treatment requires individual tailoring of the approach, because a variety of clinical situations can arise from a tumor involving a multitude of anatomic sites with a range of histologies of variable grade and size. Surgery is used as the primary local therapy for nearly all patients, with the exception of medically inoperable patients, those who decline surgery, and if resection would result in unacceptable functional loss. Wide, local excision of tumor with an attempt to secure negative margins without violation of the tumor is the predominant surgical approach; amputation is done in a small proportion of patients with massive tumors, extensive involvement of the neurovascular bundle, and nonfunctional limbs at presentation. The use of adjuvant therapy can vary according to the anatomic site, size, and histologic grade. The following can serve as a useful guide.[39]

Patients with superficial low-grade tumors that are less than 5 cm in diameter can generally be treated with surgical resection alone, expecting excellent local control and survival rates approximating 90%. The most important surgical variable that influences local control is the presence or absence of tumor cells at the surgical margins. In series reporting radical resection with clear margins, such as the Scandinavian Sarcoma Group, the local failures are low (8%).[40] In a second study of 559 patients treated with surgery alone from the same group, an inadequate surgical margin led to a 2.9-fold greater risk of local recurrence than did clear surgical margins.[41]

With high-grade sarcomas, wide local excision alone may be insufficient. A histologic analysis of peritumoral edema in 15 patients with high-grade STSs noted malignant cells extending greater than 1 cm beyond the primary tumor in 27% of cases.[42] In patients with high-grade STSs of the extremities, surgical excision with wide negative margins in combination with radiotherapy yields excellent local control (90% at 10 years) and excellent cause-specific survival (84% at 10 years).[43] Conversely, for sarcomas with negative/close margins, surgery alone yields significantly worse local control. In an analysis of 514 patients with resected, mostly high-grade sarcomas from the US Sarcoma Collaborative, Gannon and colleagues[44] report that local recurrence without radiation therapy (RT) versus with RT was 5.7% versus 0% for tumors with a ≤1-mm margin; and was 10.2% versus 1.4% for tumors with a >1-mm margin. Surgical resection alone for high-grade tumors should only be contemplated for small and superficial tumors and should follow consultation with a multidisciplinary sarcoma team.

RT can be delivered either before or after surgery because each strategy has advantages and disadvantages. Preoperative RT is expected to reduce tumor burden before resection, allowing more conservative surgical therapy (**Fig. 2**). Postoperative radiotherapy allows histologic examination of the tumor specimen, especially the margins, aiding in further treatment planning; although it is associated with fewer acute wound healing complications, it is more likely to produce chronic treatment-related toxicity (see below).

The only phase III clinical trial to compare preoperative versus postoperative administration of radiation, was a randomized National Cancer Institute of Canada (NCIC) trial designed to ascertain the incidence of acute wound healing complications in patients with potentially curable extremity STS.[45] Patients were randomized to either 50 Gy preoperative radiation (with a 16- to 20-Gy postoperative boost only for those randomized to this arm having positive margins), or postoperative radiation (50 Gy to the initial field plus a 16- to 20-Gy boost for all patients). The study revealed similar oncologic efficacy with either approach. The rate of acute wound healing complications (generally reversible) was higher in preoperatively treated patients, whereas the rate of irreversible late complications, including grade 3 to 4 fibrosis, was higher in the postoperative radiation arm.

Compared with conventional and 3D radiotherapy, intensity modulated RT (IMRT) is more conformal, and has led to improved toxicity profiles in the treatment of head and neck cancer,[46–48] prostate cancer,[49] and cervical cancer,[50] as well as other malignancies.[51–53] For extremity sarcoma, IMRT allows one to better spare adjacent bone and lymphatics. O'Sullivan and colleagues[45,54] published their institutional experience with preoperative IMRT for lower-extremity sarcoma, noting a numerically improved rate of wound complications and significantly lower rates of tissue transfer compared with NCIC trial. In addition, a recently published retrospective analysis of patients receiving IMRT for extremity sarcoma (14% preoperative, 86% postoperative) reported significantly lower cumulative risk of femoral neck fracture compared with the

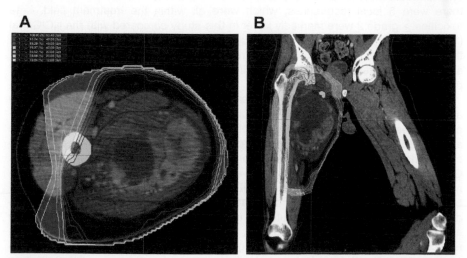

Fig. 2. (*A*) Axial and (*B*) coronal images from preoperative intensity modulated RT plan for the 69-year-old man described in **Fig. 1**, delivering 50.4 Gy in 28 fractions. Laterally, a segment of uninvolved soft tissue is spared to preserve lymphatic drainage.

rates predicted by the Princess Margarete Hospital nomogram of 6.7% versus 25.6%.[55,56] Finally, Folkert and colleagues[57] reported in a retrospective study that, despite a preponderance of higher-risk features (especially close/positive margin) in the IMRT group, IMRT was associated with significantly reduced local recurrence compared with conventional external beam RT for primary STS of the extremity.

Attempts to limit toxicities by decreasing postoperative treatment volume have thus far been unsuccessful. VORTEX was a phase III trial randomizing patients with extremity STS to postoperative RT to 50 Gy to initial tumor with a margin of 5 cm longitudinally and 2 cm radially, followed by a 16-Gy boost volume with a margin of 2 cm both longitudinally and radially (control arm) and a second cohort who received 66 Gy to the single smaller boost volume (experimental arm). The results on the primary outcome of limb function at 2 years were presented at the ASTRO 2016 meeting and demonstrated no significant difference in local control or late grade 2 or higher toxicity between the arms[58]; formal publication is pending.

Image-guided RT (IGRT) has led to significantly improved outcomes and toxicity profiles across many disease sites (summarized by Bujold and colleagues[59]). There have been 2 prospective trials that have attempted to use IGRT and IMRT to limit the toxicities for preoperative RT (as opposed to limiting toxicities from postoperative RT in the VORTEX study discussed above). O'Sullivan and colleagues[45,54] conducted a phase II trial using IG-IMRT to treat 70 patients with lower-extremity sarcomas. The 30.5% incidence of acute wound complications was numerically lower than the 43% risk derived from the NCIC SR2 trial but did not reach statistical significance. Preoperative IG-IMRT significantly diminished the need for tissue transfer. RT chronic morbidities and the need for subsequent secondary operations for wound complications were lowered, although not significantly, whereas good limb function was maintained. Radiation Therapy Oncology Group (RTOG) 0630 sought to reduce late toxicities by using IGRT and decreasing preoperative clinical target treatment volumes. In this study, the gross target volume was expanded 3 cm longitudinally and 1.5 cm radially for high-grade tumors greater than 8 cm; and only 2 cm longitudinally and 1 cm radially for low-grade tumors or those less than 8 cm. IMRT was used in 75% of patients. With a median follow-up of 3.6 years, of the 79 patients available for assessment, there were 5 local recurrences, which were all within the treatment field. Late toxicities $\geq$ grade 2 were markedly lower in this study compared with the NCIC trial (10.5% versus 37% $P<.001$).[45,60] Although longer follow-up is needed to confirm the adequacy and durability of local control, the results of RTOG 0630 are promising and may ultimately alter recommendations for preoperative sarcoma treatment planning.

In patients with high-grade STS greater than 5 cm, excellent local control can be achieved with surgery and radiotherapy, but at least 40% of patients will develop metastatic disease. In this situation, the use of adjuvant chemotherapy may benefit some and should be considered, although its role remains uncertain because randomized clinical trials have not consistently demonstrated a benefit.[61] At the Massachusetts General Hospital, a regimen of *preoperative* chemotherapy consisting of mesna, adriamycin, ifosfamide, and dacarbazine (MAID) interdigitated with radiotherapy followed by resection and postoperative chemotherapy with or without radiotherapy was designed to improve treatment outcome in large (>8 cm) extremity STS.[62] Following aggressive chemoradiation and surgery, the treated patients showed a significant reduction in distant metastases with a highly significant gain in disease-free and OS when compared with historical controls. This was borne out in an updated analysis published in 2012. With a median follow-up of 9.3 years in the MAID group and 13.2 years in historical controls, the MAID group retained significantly higher 7-year disease-specific survival and OS (81% and 79%) compared with controls (50% and 45%).[63] A similar regimen was used in a multi-institution phase II RTOG trial to treat patients with greater than 8-cm sarcomas of the extremity and body wall. Compared with the Massachusetts General Hospital (MGH) experience, the RTOG trial had more modest oncologic outcomes, possibly owing to higher percentage of grade 3 tumors (80% versus 48%); and the RTOG trial had worse toxicity, likely owing to a 25% higher dose of ifosfamide used. Despite high rates or toxicity and noncompliance, outcomes on the RTOG trial compared favorably with historical controls.

Because metastatic tumor to the lung can be resected and metastatic disease is frequently asymptomatic, it is highly recommended to follow-up all patients regularly after therapy. Imaging studies, preferably CT scans of the chest and MRI of the primary tumor site (if not readily assessable by physical examination), should be performed at 6-month intervals for the first 2 to 3 years and then yearly out to 5 years.

RETROPERITONEAL SARCOMA

Retroperitoneal sarcomas account for approximately 13% of STSs in adults,[64] the most common retroperitoneal tumors being the liposarcomas and leiomyosarcomas. Most liposarcomas are low- to intermediate-grade lesions.

Clinical Manifestations

Most patients present with an asymptomatic abdominal mass. Sarcomas of the retroperitoneal tissues have a less satisfactory outcome than STSs at other sites owing to several factors:[65]

- Retroperitoneal sarcomas are often unusually large at diagnosis, and anatomically situated such that resection is difficult in almost all patients.
- Even with complete resection, retroperitoneal liposarcomas tend to do worse than extremity lesions independent of tumor size, grade, or surgical margin.[66]
- The surrounding normal tissues (liver, kidney, gastrointestinal tract, and spinal cord) have relatively low tolerance for radiation. As a result, radiation dose levels must be kept below those typically used for extremity sarcomas.

Numerous retrospective analyses demonstrate that both high-grade and nonlipomatous histology portend diminished survival in retroperitoneal sarcomas; however, unlike extremity sarcomas, tumor size is not prognostic.[66-68]

Primary Treatment

Complete surgical resection at the time of primary presentation is the most important prognostic factor. Resectability rates range from 50% to 100%.[69,70] The addition of adjuvant (postoperative) RT to surgical resection is associated with a reduced risk of local recurrence and a longer recurrence-free interval in nonrandomized, retrospective studies.[69,71,72] In addition, a recent National Cancer Data Base noted significantly improved OS for surgery with either preoperative or postoperative RT compared with surgery alone (hazard ratio = 0.70 and 0.78, respectively).[73]

In the postoperative setting, however, radiation doses to the tumor bed are often limited by the radiation tolerance of surrounding normal issues, most notably small bowel, which falls into the resection bed following surgical removal of the tumor. The delivery of external beam RT before surgery—with or without intraoperative RT (IORT) at the time of surgical resection—may permit safe delivery of higher doses of radiation than is possible in the postoperative setting.[74] These approaches make it possible to maximize the likelihood of disease control while minimizing normal tissue

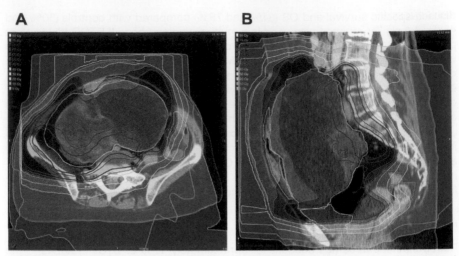

Fig. 3. A 67-year-old woman with a dedifferentiated retroperitoneal sarcoma. (*A*) Axial and (*B*) coronal images from preoperative intensity modulated proton therapy plan, undergoing treatment on protocol. The primary volume received 50.4 Gy with a simultaneous integrated boost to the high-risk retroperitoneal margin to 63 Gy, all delivered in 28 fractions.

toxicity. With preoperative radiation, the tumor can be precisely localized for radiation planning allowing for accurate targeting of the radiation volume around the tumor. Preoperative radiation is administered with the tumor in situ, allowing the tumor itself to displace radiosensitive viscera out of the radiation treatment volume. This results in an improved therapeutic window for external beam RT and satisfactory tumoricidal radiation doses to be administered with relatively little risk of radiation injury to adjacent normal issues.

Because surgical margins are never wide and are often positive, some centers have used a treatment policy of preoperative radiation, resection, and IORT boost to deliver additional dose to areas of positive margin.[75] For patients who have a grossly complete resection, the treatment protocol would be: preoperative radiation (45–50.4 Gy at 1.8 Gy per fraction over a total time of 5–6 weeks), a rest period of approximately 3 to 5 weeks, followed by surgical resection and IORT (10–12 Gy as a single dose to the resection bed).[76] MGH recently published a phase trial 1 trial of preoperative intensity modulated proton RT to 50.4 Gy (1.8 Gy/fraction) with simultaneous integrated boost delivered to the high-risk retroperitoneal margin (up to 63 at 2.25 Gy/fraction). Treatment in all dose cohorts was tolerated without any acute dose-limiting toxicities.[77] This protocol included a similar multi-institutional phase I dose-escalation scheme using IMRT; the multi-institutional phase 2 trial, which has nonrandomized IMRT and intensity modulated proton arms is now accruing, using doses of 50.4 Gy to the average risk clinical target volume with a simultaneous integrated boost of 63 Gy to the high-risk retroperitoneal margin[78] (**Fig. 3**).

SUMMARY

Although STSs are composed of many histologies and can occur throughout the body, management strategies tend to focus on resection with risk-adapted neoadjuvant and/or adjuvant treatment. Given their rarity, sarcomas are best managed by a multidisciplinary team with expertise in sarcoma treatment.

REFERENCES

1. Noone A, Howlader N, Krapcho M, et al. SEER cancer statistics review, 1975-2015. Bethesda (MD): National Cancer Institute; 2018.
2. Siegel RL, Miller KD, Jemal A. Cancer statistics, 2019. CA Cancer J Clin 2019; 69(1):7–34.
3. Gustafson P, Dreinhofer KE, Rydholm A. Soft tissue sarcoma should be treated at a tumor center. A comparison of quality of surgery in 375 patients. Acta Orthop Scand 1994;65(1):47–50.
4. Hoda SA. Enzinger and Weiss's soft tissue tumors, 6th edition. Adv Anat Pathol 2014;21:216.
5. Farid M, Ngeow J. Sarcomas associated with genetic cancer predisposition syndromes: a review. Oncologist 2016;21(8):1002–13.
6. Ballinger ML, Goode DL, Ray-Coquard I, et al. Monogenic and polygenic determinants of sarcoma risk: an international genetic study. Lancet Oncol 2016;17(9): 1261–71.
7. Rydholm A, Berg NO, Gullberg B, et al. Epidemiology of soft-tissue sarcoma in the locomotor system. A retrospective population-based study of the inter-relationships between clinical and morphologic variables. Acta Pathol Microbiol Immunol Scand A 1984;92(5):363–74.
8. Aisen AM, Martel W, Braunstein EM, et al. MRI and CT evaluation of primary bone and soft-tissue tumors. AJR Am J Roentgenol 1986;146(4):749–56.
9. Demas BE, Heelan RT, Lane J, et al. Soft-tissue sarcomas of the extremities: comparison of MR and CT in determining the extent of disease. AJR Am J Roentgenol 1988;150(3):615–20.
10. McKenzie AF. The role of magnetic resonance imaging. Acta orthopaedica Scand 1997;68(sup273):21–4.
11. Panicek DM, Gatsonis C, Rosenthal DI, et al. CT and MR imaging in the local staging of primary malignant musculoskeletal neoplasms: report of the Radiology Diagnostic Oncology Group. Radiology 1997;202(1):237–46.
12. Roberge D, Vakilian S, Alabed YZ, et al. FDG PET/CT in initial staging of adult soft-tissue sarcoma. Sarcoma 2012;2012:960194.
13. Italiano A, Di Mauro I, Rapp J, et al. Clinical effect of molecular methods in sarcoma diagnosis (GENSARC): a prospective, multicentre, observational study. Lancet Oncol 2016;17(4):532–8.
14. American Joint Committee on Cancer. AJCC cancer staging manual. 8th edition. Cham (Switzerland): Springer; 2017.
15. Fisher SB, Chiang Y-J, Feig BW, et al. Comparative performance of the 7th and 8th editions of the American Joint Committee on cancer staging systems for soft tissue sarcoma of the trunk and extremities. Ann Surg Oncol 2018;25(5): 1126–32.
16. Enneking WF, Spanier SS, Goodman MA. A system for the surgical staging of musculoskeletal sarcoma. Clin Orthop Relat Res 1980;(153):106–20.
17. Hajdu SI, Shiu MH, Brennan MF. The role of the pathologist in the management of soft tissue sarcomas. World J Surg 1988;12(3):326–31.
18. Gustafson P, Akerman M, Alvegard TA, et al. Prognostic information in soft tissue sarcoma using tumour size, vascular invasion and microscopic tumour necrosis—the SIN-system. Eur J Cancer 2003;39(11):1568–76.
19. Spiro IJ, Gebhardt MC, Jennings LC, et al. Prognostic factors for local control of sarcomas of the soft tissues managed by radiation and surgery. Semin Oncol 1997;24(5):540–6.

20. Wunder JS, Healey JH, Davis AM, et al. A comparison of staging systems for localized extremity soft tissue sarcoma. Cancer 2000;88(12):2721–30.
21. Guillou L, Coindre JM, Bonichon F, et al. Comparative study of the National Cancer Institute and French Federation of Cancer Centers Sarcoma Group grading systems in a population of 410 adult patients with soft tissue sarcoma. J Clin Oncol 1997;15(1):350–62.
22. Angervall L, Kindblom LG, Rydholm A, et al. The diagnosis and prognosis of soft tissue tumors. Semin Diagn Pathol 1986;3(4):240–58.
23. Kandel RA, Bell RS, Wunder JS, et al. Comparison between a 2- and 3-grade system in predicting metastatic-free survival in extremity soft-tissue sarcoma. J Surg Oncol 1999;72(2):77–82.
24. Gutierrez JC, Perez EA, Franceschi D, et al. Outcomes for soft-tissue sarcoma in 8249 cases from a large state cancer registry. J Surg Res 2007;141(1):105–14.
25. Ferrari A, Miceli R, Meazza C, et al. Soft tissue sarcomas of childhood and adolescence: the prognostic role of tumor size in relation to patient body size. J Clin Oncol 2009;27(3):371–6.
26. American Joint Committee on Cancer. AJCC cancer staging handbook. 7th edition. New York: Springer-Verlag; 2010.
27. Tsujimoto M, Aozasa K, Ueda T, et al. Multivariate analysis for histologic prognostic factors in soft tissue sarcomas. Cancer 1988;62(5):994–8.
28. Kattan MW, Leung DH, Brennan MF. Postoperative nomogram for 12-year sarcoma-specific death. J Clin Oncol 2002;20(3):791–6.
29. Stojadinovic A, Leung DHY, Hoos A, et al. Analysis of the prognostic significance of microscopic margins in 2,084 localized primary adult soft tissue sarcomas. Ann Surg 2002;235(3):424–34.
30. Maki RG, Moraco N, Antonescu CR, et al. Toward better soft tissue sarcoma staging: building on American Joint Committee on cancer staging systems versions 6 and 7. Ann Surg Oncol 2013;20(11):3377–83.
31. Justin MMC. The AJCC 8th edition staging system for soft tissue sarcoma of the extremities or trunk: a cohort study of the SEER database. J Natl Compr Canc Netw 2018;16(2):144–52.
32. Chibon F, Lagarde P, Salas S, et al. Validated prediction of clinical outcome in sarcomas and multiple types of cancer on the basis of a gene expression signature related to genome complexity. Nat Med 2010;16(7):781–7.
33. Kim JR, Moon YJ, Kwon KS, et al. Expression of SIRT1 and DBC1 is associated with poor prognosis of soft tissue sarcomas. PLoS One 2013;8(9):e74738.
34. Kandel RA, Yao X, Dickson BC, et al. Molecular analyses in the diagnosis and prediction of prognosis in non-GIST soft tissue sarcomas: a systematic review and meta-analysis. Cancer Treat Rev 2018;66:74–81.
35. Machado I, Noguera R, Pellin A, et al. Molecular diagnosis of Ewing sarcoma family of tumors: a comparative analysis of 560 cases with FISH and RT-PCR. Diagn Mol Pathol 2009;18(4):189–99.
36. Williamson D, Missiaglia E, de Reynies A, et al. Fusion gene-negative alveolar rhabdomyosarcoma is clinically and molecularly indistinguishable from embryonal rhabdomyosarcoma. J Clin Oncol 2010;28(13):2151–8.
37. Skapek SX, Anderson J, Barr FG, et al. PAX-FOXO1 fusion status drives unfavorable outcome for children with rhabdomyosarcoma: a Children's Oncology Group report. Pediatr Blood Cancer 2013;60(9):1411–7.
38. Crago AM, Dickson MA. Liposarcoma: multimodality management and future targeted therapies. Surg Oncol Clin N Am 2016;25(4):761–73.

39. DeLaney TF, Gebhardt MC, Ryan CW. Overview of multimodality treatment for primary soft tissue sarcoma of the extremities and chest wall. In: Maki R, Pollock RE, editors. UpToDate. 2018. Available at: https://www.uptodate.com/contents/overview-of-multimodality-treatment-for-primary-soft-tissue-sarcoma-of-the-extremities-and-chest-wall. Accessed September 1, 2019.

40. Alvegard TA, Sigurdsson H, Mouridsen H, et al. Adjuvant chemotherapy with doxorubicin in high-grade soft tissue sarcoma: a randomized trial of the Scandinavian Sarcoma Group. J Clin Oncol 1989;7(10):1504–13.

41. Trovik CS, Bauer HCF, Alvegård TA, et al. Surgical margins, local recurrence and metastasis in soft tissue sarcomas: 559 surgically-treated patients from the Scandinavian Sarcoma Group Register. Eur J Cancer 2000;36(6):710–6.

42. White LM, Wunder JS, Bell RS, et al. Histologic assessment of peritumoral edema in soft tissue sarcoma. Int J Radiat Oncol Biol Phys 2005;61(5):1439–45.

43. McGee L, Indelicato DJ, Dagan R, et al. Long-term results following postoperative radiotherapy for soft tissue sarcomas of the extremity. Int J Radiat Oncol Biol Phys 2012;84(4):1003–9.

44. Gannon NP, King DM, Ethun CG, et al. The role of radiation therapy and margin width in localized soft-tissue sarcoma: analysis from the US Sarcoma Collaborative. J Surg Oncol 2019;120(3):325–31.

45. O'Sullivan B, Davis AM, Turcotte R, et al. Preoperative versus postoperative radiotherapy in soft-tissue sarcoma of the limbs: a randomised trial. Lancet 2002;359(9325):2235–41.

46. Lin A, Kim HM, Terrell JE, et al. Quality of life after parotid-sparing IMRT for head-and-neck cancer: a prospective longitudinal study. Int J Radiat Oncol Biol Phys 2003;57(1):61–70.

47. Nutting CM, Morden JP, Harrington KJ, et al. Parotid-sparing intensity modulated versus conventional radiotherapy in head and neck cancer (PARSPORT): a phase 3 multicentre randomised controlled trial. Lancet Oncol 2011;12(2):127–36.

48. Peng G, Wang T, Yang KY, et al. A prospective, randomized study comparing outcomes and toxicities of intensity-modulated radiotherapy vs. conventional two-dimensional radiotherapy for the treatment of nasopharyngeal carcinoma. Radiother Oncol 2012;104(3):286–93.

49. Zelefsky MJ, Levin EJ, Hunt M, et al. Incidence of late rectal and urinary toxicities after three-dimensional conformal radiotherapy and intensity-modulated radiotherapy for localized prostate cancer. Int J Radiat Oncol Biol Phys 2008;70(4):1124–9.

50. Lin Y, Chen K, Lu Z, et al. Intensity-modulated radiation therapy for definitive treatment of cervical cancer: a meta-analysis. Radiat Oncol 2018;13(1):177.

51. Fredman ET, Abdel-Wahab M, Kumar AMS. Influence of radiation treatment technique on outcome and toxicity in anal cancer. J Radiat Oncol 2017;6(4):413–21.

52. Chun SG, Hu C, Choy H, et al. Impact of intensity-modulated radiation therapy technique for locally advanced non-small-cell lung cancer: a secondary analysis of the NRG oncology RTOG 0617 randomized clinical trial. J Clin Oncol 2017;35(1):56–62.

53. Lin SH, Wang L, Myles B, et al. Propensity score-based comparison of long-term outcomes with 3-dimensional conformal radiotherapy vs intensity-modulated radiotherapy for esophageal cancer. Int J Radiat Oncol Biol Phys 2012;84(5):1078–85.

54. O'Sullivan B, Griffin AM, Dickie CI, et al. Phase 2 study of preoperative image-guided intensity-modulated radiation therapy to reduce wound and combined

modality morbidities in lower extremity soft tissue sarcoma. Cancer 2013;119(10): 1878–84.

55. Folkert MR, Casey DL, Berry SL, et al. Femoral fracture in primary soft-tissue sarcoma of the thigh and groin treated with intensity-modulated radiation therapy: observed versus expected risk. Ann Surg Oncol 2019;26(5):1326–31.

56. Gortzak Y, Lockwood GA, Mahendra A, et al. Prediction of pathologic fracture risk of the femur after combined modality treatment of soft tissue sarcoma of the thigh. Cancer 2010;116(6):1553–9.

57. Folkert MR, Singer S, Brennan MF, et al. Comparison of local recurrence with conventional and intensity-modulated radiation therapy for primary soft-tissue sarcomas of the extremity. J Clin Oncol 2014;32(29):3236–41.

58. Robinson MH, Gaunt P, Grimer R, et al. Vortex trial: a randomized controlled multicenter phase 3 trial of volume of postoperative radiation therapy given to adult patients with extremity soft tissue sarcoma (STS). Int J Radiat Oncol Biol Phys 2016;96(2):S1.

59. Bujold A, Craig T, Jaffray D, et al. Image-guided radiotherapy: has it influenced patient outcomes? Semin Radiat Oncol 2012;22(1):50–61.

60. Wang D, Zhang Q, Eisenberg BL, et al. Significant reduction of late toxicities in patients with extremity sarcoma treated with image-guided radiation therapy to a reduced target volume: results of Radiation Therapy Oncology Group RTOG-0630 Trial. J Clin Oncol 2015;33(20):2231–8.

61. Le Cesne A, Ouali M, Leahy MG, et al. Doxorubicin-based adjuvant chemotherapy in soft tissue sarcoma: pooled analysis of two STBSG-EORTC phase III clinical trials. Ann Oncol 2014;25(12):2425–32.

62. DeLaney TF, Spiro IJ, Suit HD, et al. Neoadjuvant chemotherapy and radiotherapy for large extremity soft-tissue sarcomas. Int J Radiat Oncol Biol Phys 2003;56(4):1117–27.

63. Mullen JT, Kobayashi W, Wang JJ, et al. Long-term follow-up of patients treated with neoadjuvant chemotherapy and radiotherapy for large, extremity soft tissue sarcomas. Cancer 2012;118(15):3758–65.

64. Lawrence W Jr, Donegan WL, Natarajan N, et al. Adult soft tissue sarcomas. A pattern of care survey of the American College of Surgeons. Ann Surg 1987; 205(4):349–59.

65. Linehan DC, Lewis JJ, Leung D, et al. Influence of biologic factors and anatomic site in completely resected liposarcoma. J Clin Oncol 2000;18(8):1637–43.

66. Nathan H, Raut CP, Thornton K, et al. Predictors of survival after resection of retroperitoneal sarcoma: a population-based analysis and critical appraisal of the AJCC staging system. Ann Surg 2009;250(6):970–6.

67. Tseng W, Martinez SR, Tamurian RM, et al. Histologic type predicts survival in patients with retroperitoneal soft tissue sarcoma. J Surg Res 2012;172(1):123–30.

68. Abbott AM, Habermann EB, Parsons HM, et al. Prognosis for primary retroperitoneal sarcoma survivors. Cancer 2012;118(13):3321–9.

69. Catton CN, O'Sullivan B, Kotwall C, et al. Outcome and prognosis in retroperitoneal soft tissue sarcoma. Int J Radiat Oncol Biol Phys 1994;29(5):1005–10.

70. Lewis JJ, Leung D, Woodruff JM, et al. Retroperitoneal soft-tissue sarcoma: analysis of 500 patients treated and followed at a single institution. Ann Surg 1998; 228(3):355–65.

71. Heslin MJ, Lewis JJ, Nadler E, et al. Prognostic factors associated with long-term survival for retroperitoneal sarcoma: implications for management. J Clin Oncol 1997;15(8):2832–9.

72. Kelly KJ, Yoon SS, Kuk D, et al. Comparison of perioperative radiation therapy and surgery versus surgery alone in 204 patients with primary retroperitoneal sarcoma: a retrospective 2-institution study. Ann Surg 2015;262(1):156–62.
73. Nussbaum DP, Rushing CN, Lane WO, et al. Preoperative or postoperative radiotherapy versus surgery alone for retroperitoneal sarcoma: a case-control, propensity score-matched analysis of a nationwide clinical oncology database. Lancet Oncol 2016;17(7):966–75.
74. Tzeng C-WD, Fiveash JB, Popple RA, et al. Preoperative radiation therapy with selective dose escalation to the margin at risk for retroperitoneal sarcoma. Cancer 2006;107(2):371–9.
75. Delaney TF, Kepka L, Goldberg SI, et al. Radiation therapy for control of soft-tissue sarcomas resected with positive margins. Int J Radiat Oncol Biol Phys 2007;67(5):1460–9.
76. Gieschen HL, Spiro IJ, Suit HD, et al. Long-term results of intraoperative electron beam radiotherapy for primary and recurrent retroperitoneal soft tissue sarcoma. Int J Radiat Oncol Biol Phys 2001;50(1):127–31.
77. DeLaney TF, Chen Y-L, Baldini EH, et al. Phase 1 trial of preoperative image guided intensity modulated proton radiation therapy with simultaneously integrated boost to the high risk margin for retroperitoneal sarcomas. Adv Radiat Oncol 2017;2(1):85–93.
78. Proton or Photon RT for Retroperitoneal Sarcomas. Available at: https://ClinicalTrials.gov/show/NCT01659203. Accessed September 1, 2019.

Bone Sarcomas and Desmoids

Jeremy M. Brownstein, MD[a,b], Thomas F. DeLaney, MD[c],*

KEYWORDS

- Osteosarcoma • Chondrosarcoma • Chordoma • Desmoid • Radiation therapy

KEY POINTS

- Bone sarcomas are rare mesenchymal tumors arising in bone.
- Although ideal management varies by histology, location, extent of disease, and functional status, appropriate strategies generally include surgery, with chemotherapy for high-grade tumors and adjuvant or neoadjuvant radiation in anatomic sites where adequate surgical margins are difficult to achieve.
- Desmoids are benign but infiltrative neoplasms often requiring multidisciplinary treatment.
- Sarcomas that are treated with a suboptimal approach are more prone to recurrence, thus treatment should only be attempted by an experienced multidisciplinary team.

INTRODUCTION

Primary bone sarcomas are extremely rare, comprising approximately 15% of sarcomas and less than 0.2% of cancers registered in the Surveillance, Epidemiology, and End Results (SEER) database.[1,2] The incidence of osteosarcomas (the most common bone sarcoma) is bimodal, with a primary peak occurring in the second decade followed by a secondary peak occurring in the eighth.[3] In contrast, chondrosarcomas and chordomas rarely occur in children or adolescents. Presentation varies by site and histology. Osteosarcomas typically occur along the metaphyseal region of long bones and may have a painful soft tissue mass, chondrosarcomas are most frequently found within the medullary canals of long bones and less commonly in the pelvis and spine,[4] and chordomas occur exclusively within the axial skeleton along the vestiges of the primitive notochord.

Disclosure: The authors have nothing to disclose.
[a] Francis H. Burr Proton Beam Therapy Center, Massachusetts General Hospital, 30 Fruit Street, Boston, MA 02114, USA; [b] Department of Radiation Oncology, Comprehensive Cancer Center, The Ohio State University, Columbus, Ohio, USA; [c] Department of Radiation Oncology, Harvard Medical School, Francis H. Burr Proton Therapy Center, Massachusetts General Hospital, 30 Fruit Street, Boston, MA 02114, USA
* Corresponding author.
E-mail addresses: tdelaney@partners.org; tdelaney@mgh.Harvard.edu

OSTEOSARCOMA

Osteosarcomas are the most common primary bone tumor among children and adolescents, but are nonetheless rare, with annual US incidence of 5.1 per 1,000,000.[5] Although osteosarcomas among adolescents almost always occur de novo, more than 50% of those occurring in the elderly arise secondarily, typically following a diagnosis of Paget disease or radiation exposure.[6] Before the incorporation of systemic therapy, the prognosis was dismal, with ~ 16% survival observed in patients who received local treatment only, leading many clinicians to believe that osteosarcoma was metastatic at presentation.[7] Supporting this hypothesis is an analysis of bone marrow and blood samples of 49 patients with localized osteosarcoma showing that as many as 63% had tumor cells present in their bone marrow.[8] Multiagent neoadjuvant systemic therapy has led to dramatic improvements in 5-year overall survival (now about 70%[7]).

Neoadjuvant chemotherapy followed by surgery has become the standard approach to patients with osteosarcomas of the extremities. The ideal neoadjuvant systemic regimen has not been determined but data suggest that a 3-drug regimen is superior to a 2-drug regimen.[7] The authors of this article recommend the regimen used in the control arm of the American Osteosarcoma Study Group (AOST) 0331 trial, including methotrexate, doxorubicin, and cisplatin.[9]

Attaining wide surgical margins can present technical challenges in the extremity when chemotherapy response is poor,[10] or when associated with pathologic fractures.[11] In addition, complete resection is often difficult to achieve in the pelvis and is rarely achievable in lesions occurring in the axial skeleton, base of skull, and the head and neck. These factors contribute to the high rates of local recurrence reported at these anatomic sites. Picci and colleagues[10] noted that local recurrences after limb-salvage surgery for high-grade osteosarcoma of the extremities were associated with less than wide surgical margins, suboptimal chemotherapy response, and complications from the biopsy procedure (hematoma, delayed healing). A large review including more than 2500 patients from 10 international collaborations showed that less than 90% response to neoadjuvant chemotherapy was associated with a 2.17 relative risk for local recurrence on multivariate analysis.[12] Scully and colleagues[11] reported local recurrences in 7 of 23 (23%) patients presenting with pathologic fractures who were managed with limb-salvage procedures.

Nonextremity osteosarcomas have much higher local recurrence rates owing to anatomic considerations that make it much more difficult to obtain adequate surgical margins. Local recurrence rates for lesions in the pelvis were noted to be 70% among 67 patients reported by the Cooperative Osteosarcoma Study Group (COSS), 31 of 50 (62%) undergoing resection and 16 of 17 not undergoing operation (94%).[13] Among 22 patients with lesions of the spine reported by COSS, 15 (68%) experienced local failure[14]; among patients with osteosarcoma of the head and neck, local recurrence has been reported to occur in approximately 50% of patients, with mandible being the most favorable site, followed by maxilla, and then by the extragnathic sites (zygoma, orbit, nasoethmoid, cranial bones).[15]

Traditional single-modality, nonsurgical options have not been reliably effective at control of the primary tumor.[16,17] In the prechemotherapy era, Sir Stanford Cade[18] used a technique of irradiation and delayed amputation for those patients who did not develop metastatic disease. The primary tumor was controlled in some patients who refused amputation, but lung metastases occurred early and no patients remained alive at 5 years.[18] A dose-response relationship has been reported with no lesions controlled at doses of 30 Gy in 1 series, whereas all lesions receiving greater than 90 Gy were controlled.[19] Intra-arterial chemotherapy has been similarly ineffective, with only a small number of patients achieving disease control in the experience reported from the MD Anderson Cancer Center.[20]

The additional of chemotherapy (even when delivered with suboptimal intensity) seems to improve outcomes compared with radiation alone. Ciernik and colleagues[21] reviewed the Massachusetts General Hospital experience treating 55 patients with unresectable or incompletely resected osteosarcoma with proton or proton/photon radiotherapy. Most patients had cranial, spine, or pelvic tumors. Most patients (>90%) received doses greater than 60 Gy and half (50.1%) received doses greater than 70 Gy, and most received some chemotherapy (91%); however, only 35% received what they described as full intensive standard chemotherapy with anthracyclines and cisplatin alternating with methotrexate. At 5 years, local control was 72%, distant control was 75%, and overall survival was 67%. Particle therapy seems highly effective for small tumors. In a cohort of 44 medically inoperable patients with trunk osteosarcoma with less than 500 cm^3 of gross disease who were treated with carbon ion therapy in Chiba, Japan, local control was 88% at 5 years.[22]

Although the historical clinical experience with radiation therapy as monotherapy suggested limited efficacy, the data presented earlier suggest that it may contribute to local control when combined with surgery and/or chemotherapy. Similarly, in some series, radiation does seem to be most effective when disease burden is low following gross resection, subtotal resection of tumor (in contrast with biopsy only), or following a good response to chemotherapy. In contrast, the local control using carbon ion radiotherapy in the aforementioned Japanese series for patients with a higher disease burden (ie, >500 cm^3) was 31%, far lower than the 88% observed with less than 500 cm^3 of gross disease.[22] However, Ciernik and colleagues[21] conducted a meta-analysis of published data suggesting that upfront resection was advantageous only in patients receiving less than 70 Gy.

These data lend credence to the use of radiation therapy in situations in which resection is not technically possible without undue morbidity, when surgery is refused, and when the tumor is partially resected or resected with positive margins. In addition, radiation may be helpful in sites at high risk for local failure, such as the spine, pelvis, or head/face/skull, or in the extremity when margins are close with a poor histologic response or when patients present with a pathologic fracture. The optimal radiation dose remains to be determined for these patients. Highly conformal radiation therapy techniques, such as intensity modulated radiation therapy and/or proton beam radiation therapy, are important tools in the management of patients with lesions adjacent to critical radiosensitive structures in the skull, head and neck region, the spine, and the pelvis.

In addition, given the success of Ra-223, an alpha particle–emitting radioisotope, in the treatment of osseous metastases from prostate cancer,[23] there has been growing interest in the use of this agent for other blastic bone tumors.[24] A phase I dose escalation study of Ra-223 for high-risk osteosarcoma showed that this agent was tolerable, although efficacy has not yet been determined.[25]

Principles of Radiation Therapy

For completely resected tumors with negative margins, there is no need for adjuvant radiation. If margins are positive, the authors recommend treating the postoperative field to a total dose of 64.8 to 66 Gy in 1.8-Gy fractions plus or minus concurrent ifosfamide/etoposide. When surgical resection is not feasible, we recommend definitive chemoradiation. Following induction chemotherapy with the AOST 0331 regimen as described earlier, we use a shrinking field technique, treating clinical target volume

(CTV) 1 (gross tumor volume [GTV] + 1–1.5 cm margin) to 45 Gy followed by a sequential boost to the CTV2 = GTV to a total dose of 72 Gy in 1.8-Gy fractions, delivered with concurrent ifosfamide/etoposide (**Fig. 1**).

CHONDROSARCOMA

Chondrosarcoma is a tumor in which the basic neoplastic tissue is cartilaginous; it is the second most frequent malignant bone tumor in adults. Chondrosarcomas develop either de novo in previously normal bone or secondarily in a preexisting benign cartilage tumor, most commonly an enchondroma. By some estimates, as many as 40% of chondrosarcomas may arise from enchondromas,[26] whereas the risk of malignant transformation from a solitary enchondroma is less than 5%.[27] Chondrosarcomas comprise a wide histologic and clinical range, varying from low-grade tumors to high-grade malignancies (dedifferentiated or mesenchymal chondrosarcomas). Isocitrate dehydrogenase 1 (IDH1) and IDH2 mutations are common in cartilaginous tumors (present in 56% of cases of enchondroma/central chondrosarcoma[28]) and the presence of this mutation may help distinguish chondrosarcomas from noncartilaginous

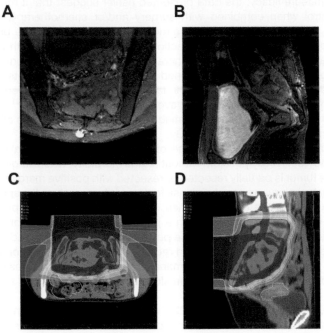

Fig. 1. Unresectable sacral osteosarcoma. An 18-year-old woman with an unresectable sacral osteosarcoma. (*A*) Contrast-enhanced axial and (*B*) sagittal T1 MRI showing a heterogeneously enhancing mass occupying much of the sacrum. She underwent neoadjuvant chemotherapy with doxorubicin/platinum alternating with methotrexate, followed by definitive pure proton beam radiation chemoradiation using ifosfamide and etoposide, treating CTV1 to 45 Gy and GTV to a total dose of 72 Gy followed by 4 months of additional adjuvant chemotherapy. Additional adjuvant chemotherapy was given (*C*) Axial and (*D*) sagittal views of radiation treatment plan show sharp dose decrease anteriorly, allowing sparing of the uterus (maximum dose, 3.2 Gy; mean dose, 0.05 Gy), left ovary (maximum dose, 1 Gy; mean dose, 0.04 Gy), and right ovary (maximum dose, 0.2 Gy; mean dose, 0.03 Gy). The patient remains free of disease over 11 years after diagnosis, pain-free, fully ambulatory, with normal sacral nerve function; her menses resumed 1 year after completion of chemotherapy.

histologies. Radiation therapy is used for chondrosarcomas when surgical margins are positive, gross residual disease remains after surgery, or lesions cannot be resected (ie, in locations with difficult anatomy, such as the base of the skull, craniofacial region, spine, and pelvis).

Although it has been stated repeatedly that chondrosarcoma is a radioresistant tumor,[29,30] several reports have shown the effectiveness of conventional radiation therapy for this histology.[31–33] Particle radiotherapy has similarly yielded high rates of local control for lesions in the base of skull/cervical spine[34–36] and lower spine and sacrum.[37] Some confusion about the effectiveness of radiation therapy for this histology may exist because the tumors do not shrink after radiation therapy because of their underlying cartilaginous matrix. Nevertheless, after effective radiation therapy treatment, they will permanently cease further growth.

Principles of Radiation Therapy

Similar to osteosarcoma, no adjuvant treatment is required in the case of negative surgical margins. For positive margins, the authors typically prescribe 66.6 to 70.2 Gy in 1.8-Gy fractions. When radiation is prescribed definitively, we similarly use a shrinking field technique with CTV1 (GTV + 1–1.5 cm) receiving 45 to 50 Gy and a sequential boost to CTV2 = GTV to a total dose of 77.4 Gy or 74 Gy in 1.8 Gy or 2 Gy fractions, respectively. Proton beam therapy is typically needed to safely achieve doses this high in the axial skeleton. For osteosarcomas/chondrosarcomas of the pelvis and spine for which resection is feasible but there is a concern that resection margins will be positive, we prescribe 19.8 Gy to gross disease with 1.0–1.5 cm margin preoperatively. If surgical margins are indeed positive at resection, we offer adjuvant radiation, treating to the combined total adjuvant doses described earlier.[38]

CHORDOMAS

Chordoma is a tumor arising from the remnants of the primitive notochord. It can develop from normal products of the notochord, the nuclei pulposi, or from abnormal rests of notochordal tissue.[39] Chordomas are rare (l%–4% of bone tumors) and can arise anywhere in the vertebral column, most commonly in the sacrococcygeal region (50%) and the base of skull (approximately 35%), and less commonly in the mobile vertebral spine (15%).[40] The distinction between chordoma, in particular the chondroid variant, and chondrosarcoma can be difficult on hematoxylin-eosin–stained material. The availability of immunohistochemistry has helped to clarify this issue.[41] Although the metastatic rate is low (~10%–30%),[42,43] achieving local control of these aggressive tumors has been a challenge. Even in small lesions after radical resection, recurrence rates are greater than 50%,[44] with local control and survival curves following a continuous downward slope; salvage treatment after local failure is rarely successful.[44,45] A possible dose-response relationship for conventional radiation treatment has been reported.[46] One of the best results of conventional, postoperative radiation treatment were published by Keisch and colleagues[47] from the Mallinckrodt Institute of Radiology. The rate of actuarial disease-free survival at 5 years was significantly better for patients undergoing surgery and radiotherapy (60%) compared with 7 patients undergoing surgery only (25%). Patients continued to recur beyond 5 years, which emphasizes the need for high doses of radiotherapy and long-term follow-up for these patients.[47]

Hug and colleagues[37] reported 5-year rates of local control and survival for lower spine and sacral chordomas of 53% and 50% respectively, with a mean dose of 74.6 CGE (cobalt gray equivalent). A trend for improved local control was noted for primary lesions compared with recurrent tumors, with radiation doses of at least 77 CGE and less residual tumor burden. In our experience at Massachusetts General Hospital treating 29 primarily sacral chordomas, a high rate of local control was obtained with preoperative/postoperative or definitive radiation treatment greater than 72 CGE. At 5 years, local control was significantly lower for those with recurrent disease than for those treated primarily (0% vs 50%); of note, there were no local recurrences at 5 years for the 7 out of 23 primary chordomas that underwent biopsy followed by definitive radiation therapy, suggesting that definitive radiation should be considered as an alternative to an incomplete resection.[48] Kabolizadeh and colleagues[49] reported 5-year local control of 85% among 40 patients with unresected chordomas treated with definitive, proton-based radiation therapy.

At present, there are no highly effective systemic therapies for chordoma.[43] Imatinib has been investigated in a multicentric, nonrandomized, phase II trial in patients with progressive advanced chordoma. The objective response rate by RECIST (Response Evaluation Criteria in Solid Tumors) criteria[50] was only 2%, although 64% of patients had clinical benefit as defined as response or stable disease for greater than 6 months.[51] Some investigators have advocated the use of immune therapy in chordoma,[52] and there is currently a phase II trial underway for patients with advanced chordoma using a vaccine that targets brachyury,[53] a protein that is expressed in chordoma but is not typically observed in other adult tissues.[54]

Given the high rates of disease control when primary chordoma is treated with appropriate local therapies, and given that nononcologic resection and/or resection without radiotherapy results in high rates of recurrence for which there are minimal effective treatments, the authors argue that this rare disease is best managed by a multidisciplinary team with significant experience treating chordoma.

Principles of Radiation Therapy

Given the high rate of local recurrence, the authors routinely use radiotherapy in the treatment of localized chordoma. For resectable chordomas, the authors administer 50.4 Gy preoperatively followed by a course of adjuvant radiation. If the tumor is resected en bloc with negative margins, without intralesional incisions, and without any violation of the capsule, we find a combined dose of 64.8 Gy in 1.8-Gy fractions provides excellent control. However, for cases that involve 1 or several of these risk factors, we typically treat to a total dose of 70.2 to 73.8 Gy in 1.8-Gy fractions, depending on the adverse features present. For unresectable chordomas, we typically treat to a total dose of 77.4 to 79.2 Gy in 1.8-Gy fractions (**Fig. 2**). To achieve these doses, we allow the surface of the spinal cord (when in the field) to reach a maximum dose of 67 Gy for cervical lesions and 63 Gy for thoracolumbar lesions while constraining the central cord to maximum dose of 55 Gy and 54 Gy respectively[33,48] (**Fig. 3**).

DESMOID TUMORS

Desmoid tumors are benign, slow-growing fibroblastic neoplasms arising from fibroblastic stromal elements. (See Tony Y. Eng and colleagues' article, "Radiation Therapy for Benign Disease: Arteriovenous Malformations, Desmoid Tumor, Dupuytren Contracture, Graves Ophthalmopathy, Gynecomastia, Heterotopic Ossification, Histiocytosis," in this issue.) Despite being neoplastic and locally aggressive, they do not have the capacity to metastasize. On histology, the lesions are characterized by a small number of slender, bland fibroblasts in an abundant fibrous stroma that locally infiltrate adjacent tissue and structures. Usually, necrosis is absent and only few mitotic figures are present.

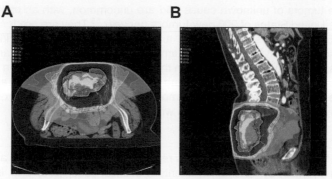

Fig. 2. Unresectable sacral chordoma. A 77-year-old woman with an unresectable sacral chordoma. She underwent definitive radiation therapy with a mixture of protons (57.6 Gy) and photons (19.8 Gy) with an initial primary volume treated to 50.4 Gy and gross disease receiving 77.4 Gy. (*A*) Axial and (*B*) sagittal views. Of note, in cases in which doses are greater than 70 Gy and when maintenance of fertility is not a concern, the authors routinely administer part of the treatment with photons to better spare the skin.

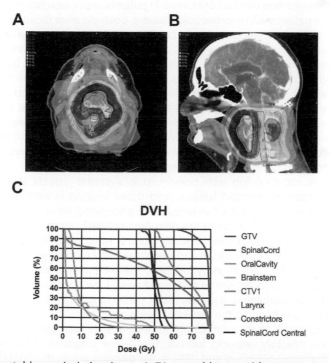

Fig. 3. Unresectable cervical chordoma. A 71-year-old man with an unresectable cervical chordoma following cervical fusion and stabilization. He underwent definitive radiation therapy with a mixture of protons (57.6 Gy) and photons (19.8 Gy) with an initial primary volume treated to 50.4 Gy and gross disease receiving 77.4 Gy. (*A*) Axial and (*B*) sagittal views, and the (*C*) dose-volume histogram (DVH) shows that it was not possible to completely cover the GTV to the prescription dose to meet spinal cord constraints (spinal cord maximum, 60.56<65 Gy; and central spinal cord, 54.5<55 Gy).

These are tumors of unknown cause and are uncommon, with an estimated incidence in the United States of 900 new tumors per year.[55] They are predominant in individuals 15 to 60 years of age, with a slightly higher prevalence in women.[56] An association has been found between familial adenomatous polyposis and desmoid tumors. Desmoids can occur anywhere in the body but are most common in the torso (shoulder girdle and hip-buttock region) and the extremities. They usually arise deep in the muscles or along fascial planes. Desmoids have an unpredictable growth pattern and 30% to 92% spontaneously regress without treatment.[57,58]

Treatment

Because of the high rate of spontaneous regression,[57] desmoid tumors are currently managed in minimally symptomatic patients with initial observation and, in some patients, nonsteroidal medication such as sulindac. If there is tumor progression, persistence of symptoms, an imminent risk to adjacent structures, or a significant cosmetic concern, surgery is then indicated. Ideally, desmoids should be treated by surgical resection with a wide margin whenever medically and technically feasible. Nonetheless, avoidance of functional or cosmetic morbidity should be prioritized given that the tumor is benign and effective function-sparing treatment using radiation is available.[59,60] With surgery alone, desmoids have a high rate of recurrence (25%–50%), depending on margin status.

Postoperative radiation can be considered in patients with macroscopic residual disease. For those patients with microscopic disease, postoperative radiation therapy can be deferred, because only about 50% of patients with a positive margin experience a local recurrence. There is currently no role for radiation therapy in the treatment of completely resected primary disease. Radiation therapy is effective as a primary therapeutic option for patients who are not good surgical candidates, decline surgery, or for whom surgical morbidity would be excessive. In several reports, radiation therapy alone (50–60 Gy), or combined with surgery in patients with positive margins, achieves permanent control in 70% to 80% of desmoids.[61–67] When treating definitively, the authors commonly treat to a total dose of 56 Gy. We do not routinely offer adjuvant treatment except after debulking of multiply recurrent disease. In that instance, we prescribe 50 to 56 Gy, depending on the presence of gross residual disease.

Experience is accumulating with noncytotoxic systemic agents in patients with advanced or recurrent desmoid tumors, and those located in intra-abdominal and abdominal wall sites. Therapy is often begun with a hormonal agent such as tamoxifen, or progestational agents.[68–72] There are also documented responses to nonsteroidal antiinflammatory drugs (most often sulindac), alone or often in combination with tamoxifen.[71–76] Regression is usually partial and may take many months after an initial period of tumor enlargement. Chemotherapy can be offered to patients with unresectable tumors that are refractory to tamoxifen and/or sulindac. Low doses of methotrexate and vinblastine produce worthwhile response rates, particularly in children.[72,77,78] However, targeted agents have become the preferred systemic therapy. In a recently published phase 3 randomized study comparing sorafenib with placebo for treatment of advanced and refractory desmoid tumors, the 2-year progression-free survival rate was 81% in the sorafenib group and 36% in the placebo group (P<.001).[79]

SUMMARY

Bone sarcomas are rare entities that are managed primarily through surgery and medical therapies (where applicable). With the exception of chordomas, radiation is generally reserved for instances in which a margin-negative resection is difficult to attain.

Desmoids are similarly a surgical disease, with radiation reserved for those cases that are inoperable or refractory to medical and surgical therapies. Given the rarity of bone sarcomas, management is best handled by clinicians who have experience.

REFERENCES

1. Fletcher CDM, World Health Organization, International Agency for Research on Cancer. WHO classification of tumours of soft tissue and bone. 4th edition. Lyon (France): IARC Press; 2013.
2. Hauben EI, Hogendoorn PCW. Chapter 1 - Epidemiology of primary bone tumors and economical aspects of bone metastases. In: Heymann D, editor. Bone cancer. 2nd edition. San Diego (CA): Academic Press; 2015. p. 5–10.
3. Mirabello L, Troisi RJ, Savage SA. Osteosarcoma incidence and survival rates from 1973 to 2004: data from the Surveillance, Epidemiology, and End Results Program. Cancer 2009;115(7):1531–43.
4. Lin PP. Bone sarcoma: MD Anderson cancer care series. New York: Springer; 2012.
5. Surveillance, Epidemiology, and End Results (SEER) Program Populations (1969-2016). Available at: www.seer.cancer.gov/popdata. Accessed April 14, 2019.
6. Huvos AG. Osteogenic sarcoma of bones and soft tissues in older persons. A clinicopathologic analysis of 117 patients older than 60 years. Cancer 1986; 57(7):1442–9.
7. Anninga JK, Gelderblom H, Fiocco M, et al. Chemotherapeutic adjuvant treatment for osteosarcoma: where do we stand? Eur J Cancer 2011;47(16):2431–45.
8. Bruland OS, Hoifodt H, Saeter G, et al. Hematogenous micrometastases in osteosarcoma patients. Clin Cancer Res 2005;11(13):4666–73.
9. Whelan JS, Bielack SS, Marina N, et al. EURAMOS-1, an international randomised study for osteosarcoma: results from pre-randomisation treatment. Ann Oncol 2015;26(2):407–14.
10. Picci P, Sangiorgi L, Bahamonde L, et al. Risk factors for local recurrences after limb-salvage surgery for high-grade osteosarcoma of the extremities. Ann Oncol 1997;8(9):899–903.
11. Scully SP, Ghert MA, Zurakowski D, et al. Pathologic fracture in osteosarcoma : prognostic importance and treatment implications. J Bone Joint Surg Am 2002; 84-a(1):49–57.
12. Pakos EE, Nearchou AD, Grimer RJ, et al. Prognostic factors and outcomes for osteosarcoma: an international collaboration. Eur J Cancer 2009;45(13): 2367–75.
13. Ozaki T, Flege S, Kevric M, et al. Osteosarcoma of the pelvis: experience of the Cooperative Osteosarcoma Study Group. J Clin Oncol 2003;21(2):334–41.
14. Ozaki T, Flege S, Liljenqvist U, et al. Osteosarcoma of the spine: experience of the Cooperative Osteosarcoma Study Group. Cancer 2002;94(4):1069–77.
15. Kassir RR, Rassekh CH, Kinsella JB, et al. Osteosarcoma of the head and neck: meta-analysis of nonrandomized studies. Laryngoscope 1997;107(1):56–61.
16. Jenkin R, Allt W, Fitzpatrick P. Osteosarcoma. An assessment of management with particular reference to primary irradiation and selective delayed amputation. Cancer 1972;30(2):393–400.
17. Beck JC, Wara WM, Bovill EG Jr, et al. The role of radiation therapy in the treatment of osteosarcoma. Radiology 1976;120(1):163–5.
18. Cade S. Osteogenic sarcoma; a study based on 133 patients. J R Coll Surg Edinb 1955;1(2):79–111.

19. Gaitan-Yanguas M. A study of the response of osteogenic sarcoma and adjacent normal tissues to radiation. Int J Radiat Oncol Biol Phys 1981;7(5):593–5.

20. Jaffe N, Carrasco H, Raymond K, et al. Can cure in patients with osteosarcoma be achieved exclusively with chemotherapy and abrogation of surgery? Cancer 2002;95(10):2202–10.

21. Ciernik IF, Niemierko A, Harmon DC, et al. Proton-based radiotherapy for unresectable or incompletely resected osteosarcoma. Cancer 2011;117(19):4522–30.

22. Matsunobu A, Imai R, Kamada T, et al. Impact of carbon ion radiotherapy for unresectable osteosarcoma of the trunk. Cancer 2012;118(18):4555–63.

23. Parker C, Nilsson S, Heinrich D, et al. Alpha emitter radium-223 and survival in metastatic prostate cancer. N Engl J Med 2013;369(3):213–23.

24. Humm JL, Sartor O, Parker C, et al. Radium-223 in the treatment of osteoblastic metastases: a critical clinical review. Int J Radiat Oncol Biol Phys 2015;91(5): 898–906.

25. Subbiah V, Anderson PM, Kairemo K, et al. Alpha particle Radium 223 dichloride in high-risk osteosarcoma: a phase I dose escalation trial. Clin Cancer Res 2019; 25:3802–10.

26. Brien EW, Mirra JM, Kerr R. Benign and malignant cartilage tumors of bone and joint: their anatomic and theoretical basis with an emphasis on radiology, pathology and clinical biology. I. The intramedullary cartilage tumors. Skeletal Radiol 1997;26(6):325–53.

27. Altay M, Bayrakci K, Yildiz Y, et al. Secondary chondrosarcoma in cartilage bone tumors: report of 32 patients. J Orthop Sci 2007;12(5):415–23.

28. Amary MF, Bacsi K, Maggiani F, et al. IDH1 and IDH2 mutations are frequent events in central chondrosarcoma and central and periosteal chondromas but not in other mesenchymal tumours. J Pathol 2011;224(3):334–43.

29. Onishi AC, Hincker AM, Lee FY. Surmounting chemotherapy and radioresistance in chondrosarcoma: molecular mechanisms and therapeutic targets. Sarcoma 2010;2011:381564.

30. Moussavi-Harami F, Mollano A, Martin JA, et al. Intrinsic radiation resistance in human chondrosarcoma cells. Biochem Biophys Res Commun 2006;346(2):379–85.

31. Harwood AR, Krajbich JI, Fornasier VL. Radiotherapy of chondrosarcoma of bone. Cancer 1980;45(11):2769–77.

32. McNaney D, Lindberg RD, Ayala AG, et al. Fifteen year radiotherapy experience with chondrosarcoma of bone. Int J Radiat Oncol Biol Phys 1982;8(2):187–90.

33. De Amorim Bernstein K, DeLaney T. Chordomas and chondrosarcomas-The role of radiation therapy. J Surg Oncol 2016;114(5):564–9.

34. Munzenrider JE, Liebsch NJ. Proton therapy for tumors of the skull base. Strahlenther Onkol 1999;175(Suppl 2):57–63.

35. Uhl M, Mattke M, Welzel T, et al. High control rate in patients with chondrosarcoma of the skull base after carbon ion therapy: first report of long-term results. Cancer 2014;120(10):1579–85.

36. Austin-Seymour M, Munzenrider J, Goitein M, et al. Fractionated proton radiation therapy of chordoma and low-grade chondrosarcoma of the base of the skull. J Neurosurg 1989;70(1):13–7.

37. Hug EB, Fitzek MM, Liebsch NJ, et al. Locally challenging osteo- and chondrogenic tumors of the axial skeleton: results of combined proton and photon radiation therapy using three-dimensional treatment planning. Int J Radiat Oncol Biol Phys 1995;31(3):467–76.

38. Wagner TD, Kobayashi W, Dean S, et al. Combination short-course preoperative irradiation, surgical resection, and reduced-field high-dose postoperative

irradiation in the treatment of tumors involving the bone. Int J Radiat Oncol Biol Phys 2009;73(1):259–66.

39. Brian JW, Daniel MSR, Erin G, et al. Diagnosis and treatment of chordoma. J Natl Compr Canc Netw 2013;11(6):726–31.
40. Rich TA, Schiller A, Suit HD, et al. Clinical and pathologic review of 48 cases of chordoma. Cancer 1985;56(1):182–7.
41. Wojno KJ, Hruban RH, Garin-Chesa P, et al. Chondroid chordomas and low-grade chondrosarcomas of the craniospinal axis. An immunohistochemical analysis of 17 cases. Am J Surg Pathol 1992;16(12):1144–52.
42. Catton C, O'Sullivan B, Bell R, et al. Chordoma: long-term follow-up after radical photon irradiation. Radiother Oncol 1996;41(1):67–72.
43. Stacchiotti S, Casali PG. Systemic therapy options for unresectable and metastatic chordomas. Curr Oncol Rep 2011;13(4):323–30.
44. Hanna SA, Aston WJS, Briggs TWR, et al. Sacral chordoma: can local recurrence after sacrectomy be predicted? Clin Orthop Relat Res 2008;466(9):2217–23.
45. Higinbotham NL, Phillips RF, Farr HW, et al. Chordoma. Thirty-five-year study at Memorial Hospital. Cancer 1967;20(11):1841–50.
46. Cummings BJ, Hodson DI, Bush RS. Chordoma: the results of megavoltage radiation therapy. Int J Radiat Oncol Biol Phys 1983;9(5):633–42.
47. Keisch ME, Garcia DM, Shibuya RB. Retrospective long-term follow-up analysis in 21 patients with chordomas of various sites treated at a single institution. J Neurosurg 1991;75(3):374–7.
48. DeLaney TF, Liebsch NJ, Pedlow FX, et al. Phase II study of high-dose photon/proton radiotherapy in the management of spine sarcomas. Int J Radiat Oncol Biol Phys 2009;74(3):732–9.
49. Kabolizadeh P, Chen YL, Liebsch N, et al. Updated outcome and analysis of tumor response in mobile spine and sacral chordoma treated with definitive high-dose photon/proton radiation therapy. Int J Radiat Oncol Biol Phys 2017;97(2):254–62.
50. Therasse P, Arbuck SG, Eisenhauer EA, et al. New guidelines to evaluate the response to treatment in solid tumors. European Organization for Research and Treatment of Cancer, National Cancer Institute of the United States, National Cancer Institute of Canada. J Natl Cancer Inst 2000;92(3):205–16.
51. Stacchiotti S, Longhi A, Ferraresi V, et al. Phase II study of imatinib in advanced chordoma. J Clin Oncol 2012;30(9):914–20.
52. Patel SS, Schwab JH. Immunotherapy as a potential treatment for chordoma: a review. Curr Oncol Rep 2016;18(9):55.
53. Colia V, Stacchiotti S. Medical treatment of advanced chordomas. Eur J Cancer 2017;83:220–8.
54. Heery CR. Chordoma: the quest for better treatment options. Oncol Ther 2016;4(1):35–51.
55. Reitamo JJ, Hayry P, Nykyri E, et al. The desmoid tumor. I. Incidence, sex-, age- and anatomical distribution in the Finnish population. Am J Clin Pathol 1982;77(6):665–73.
56. Hoda SA. Enzinger and Weiss's soft tissue tumors, 6th edition. Adv Anat Pathol 2014;21:216.
57. Bonvalot S, Ternes N, Fiore M, et al. Spontaneous regression of primary abdominal wall desmoid tumors: more common than previously thought. Ann Surg Oncol 2013;20(13):4096–102.
58. Burtenshaw SM, Cannell AJ, McAlister ED, et al. Toward observation as first-line management in abdominal desmoid tumors. Ann Surg Oncol 2016;23(7):2212–9.

59. Ballo MT, Zagars GK, Pollack A, et al. Desmoid tumor: prognostic factors and outcome after surgery, radiation therapy, or combined surgery and radiation therapy. J Clin Oncol 1999;17(1):158–67.
60. Abbas AE, Deschamps C, Cassivi SD, et al. Chest-wall desmoid tumors: results of surgical intervention. Ann Thorac Surg 2004;78(4):1219–23 [discussion: 1219–23].
61. Plukker JT, van Oort I, Vermey A, et al. Aggressive fibromatosis (non-familial desmoid tumour): therapeutic problems and the role of adjuvant radiotherapy. Br J Surg 1995;82(4):510–4.
62. Nuyttens JJ, Rust PF, Thomas CR Jr, et al. Surgery versus radiation therapy for patients with aggressive fibromatosis or desmoid tumors: a comparative review of 22 articles. Cancer 2000;88(7):1517–23.
63. Ballo MT, Zagars GK, Pollack A. Radiation therapy in the management of desmoid tumors. Int J Radiat Oncol Biol Phys 1998;42(5):1007–14.
64. Acker JC, Bossen EH, Halperin EC. The management of desmoid tumors. Int J Radiat Oncol Biol Phys 1993;26(5):851–8.
65. Zlotecki RA, Scarborough MT, Morris CG, et al. External beam radiotherapy for primary and adjuvant management of aggressive fibromatosis. Int J Radiat Oncol Biol Phys 2002;54(1):177–81.
66. Spear MA, Jennings LC, Mankin HJ, et al. Individualizing management of aggressive fibromatoses. Int J Radiat Oncol Biol Phys 1998;40(3):637–45.
67. Goy BW, Lee SP, Eilber F, et al. The role of adjuvant radiotherapy in the treatment of resectable desmoid tumors. Int J Radiat Oncol Biol Phys 1997;39(3):659–65.
68. Thomas S, Datta-Gupta S, Kapur BM. Treatment of recurrent desmoid tumour with tamoxifen. Aust N Z J Surg 1990;60(11):919–21.
69. Wilcken N, Tattersall MH. Endocrine therapy for desmoid tumors. Cancer 1991; 68(6):1384–8.
70. Gelmann EP. Tamoxifen for the treatment of malignancies other than breast and endometrial carcinoma. Semin Oncol 1997;24(1 Suppl 1):S1-65-1-70.
71. Tsukada K, Church JM, Jagelman DG, et al. Noncytotoxic drug therapy for intra-abdominal desmoid tumor in patients with familial adenomatous polyposis. Dis Colon Rectum 1992;35(1):29–33.
72. Izes JK, Zinman LN, Larsen CR. Regression of large pelvic desmoid tumor by tamoxifen and sulindac. Urology 1996;47(5):756–9.
73. Bauernhofer T, Stoger H, Schmid M, et al. Sequential treatment of recurrent mesenteric desmoid tumor. Cancer 1996;77(6):1061–5.
74. Clark SK, Phillips RK. Desmoids in familial adenomatous polyposis. Br J Surg 1996;83(11):1494–504.
75. Lackner H, Urban C, Kerbl R, et al. Noncytotoxic drug therapy in children with unresectable desmoid tumors. Cancer 1997;80(2):334–40.
76. Hansmann A, Adolph C, Vogel T, et al. High-dose tamoxifen and sulindac as first-line treatment for desmoid tumors. Cancer 2004;100(3):612–20.
77. Azzarelli A, Gronchi A, Bertulli R, et al. Low-dose chemotherapy with methotrexate and vinblastine for patients with advanced aggressive fibromatosis. Cancer 2001;92(5):1259–64.
78. Shkalim Zemer V, Toledano H, Kornreich L, et al. Sporadic desmoid tumors in the pediatric population: a single center experience and review of the literature. J Pediatr Surg 2017;52(10):1637–41.
79. Gounder MM, Mahoney MR, Van Tine BA, et al. Sorafenib for advanced and refractory desmoid tumors. N Engl J Med 2018;379(25):2417–28.

Contemporary Topics in Radiation Medicine
Skin Cancer

Sarah J. Gao, MD*, Roy H. Decker, MD, PhD

KEYWORDS

- Squamous cell carcinoma • Basal cell carcinoma • Merkel cell carcinoma
- Melanoma • Mycosis fungoides • Primary cutaneous B-cell lymphoma

KEY POINTS

- Postoperative radiation should be considered in the presence of positive margins or significant adverse risk factors in squamous and basal cell carcinoma of the skin.
- Postoperative radiation to the surgical site or regional lymph nodes is not indicated in patients with melanoma unless there are high-risk factors present.
- For Merkel cell carcinoma, postoperative radiation to the surgical site is typically indicated given the high rates of local recurrence and nodal metastases.
- Total skin electron beam therapy plays a key role in the palliation of patients with mycosis fungoides.
- Local radiation provides excellent local control for most patients with primary cutaneous B-cell lymphoma.

INTRODUCTION

Skin cancer is a heterogenous group of diseases that collectively forms the most common malignancy in the United States.[1] Worldwide, the incidence of both melanomatous and nonmelanomatous skin cancers is increasing, partly due to increased occupational and recreational ultra violet (UV) exposure.[1,2] As such, the proper diagnosis and treatment of skin cancer is more important than ever.

This article examines the management of squamous cell carcinoma (SCC), basal cell carcinoma (BCC), melanoma, Merkel cell carcinoma (MCC), cutaneous T-cell lymphoma (CTCL), and primary cutaneous B-cell lymphoma (PCBCL), with a focus on the role of radiotherapy in the treatment of these diseases.

Disclosure: The authors have nothing to disclose.
Department of Therapeutic Radiology, Smilow Cancer Center, Yale University, 35 Park Street, Lower Lobby, New Haven, CT 06510, USA
* Corresponding author.
E-mail address: sarah.gao@yale.edu

Hematol Oncol Clin N Am 34 (2020) 189–203
https://doi.org/10.1016/j.hoc.2019.09.008
hemonc.theclinics.com

SQUAMOUS CELL AND BASAL CELL CARCINOMA
Basal Cell Carcinoma

BCC is an indolent disease with a less than 0.01% rate of metastases.[3] UV exposure is a major risk factor for the development of BCC, which typically presents on sun-exposed areas. Of all BCC cases, 70% to 80% occur in the head or neck region, whereas 15% occur on the trunk.[4]

Tumor location is also a risk factor for recurrence. BCC occurring in area H (central face, eyebrows, eyelids, periorbital, nose, lips, chin, mandible, preauricular and post-auricular skin, temple, ear, genitalia, hands, or feet) have a higher recurrence rates after surgery and are classified as high-risk lesions regardless of size. Lesions in area M (cheeks, forehead, scalp, neck, and pretibial) are considered high risk by the National Comprehensive Cancer Network if they are larger than 10 mm, whereas lesions in area L (trunk and extremities) are considered high risk if they are larger than 20 mm.[5]

Other high-risk factors for recurrence include histologic subtype (eg, morpheaform, basosquamous, infiltrative, and micronodular), immunosuppression, poorly defined borders, recurrent tumors, prior radiation, and perineural invasion (PNI) or lymphovascular invasion (LVI).[5]

Squamous Cell Carcinoma

Approximately 60% of SCC cases arise from premalignant macules called actinic keratoses, which develop as a result of UV damage and are often erythematous and scaly in appearance.[6] Physical examination findings concerning for transformation to SCC include pain at the site of the lesion, bleeding, or increase in thickness and size, all of which are indications for biopsy. SCC also develops from areas of chronic inflammation, such as chronic wounds or ulcers (Marjolin tumor). Tumors arising from areas of chronic inflammation are thought to have a higher risk of recurrence following surgical excision.[7]

Unsurprisingly, poorly differentiated SCC has a greater risk of local recurrence and metastases compared with well-differentiated tumors. High-risk histologic subtypes, including adenoid, adenosquamous, metaplastic, and desmoplastic tumors, are also associated with worse outcomes, with the desmoplastic subtype being particularly aggressive.[8–10]

Staging

BCC and SCC are staged according to the American Joint Committee on Cancer (AJCC), 8th edition, staging system, which applies only to tumors of the head and neck.

Treatment

Cutaneous SCC and BCC can be treated using various modalities, including superficial therapies, surgery, and radiation. When selecting a treatment, it is important to take into account the general fitness of the patient, as well as cosmetic goals.

Superficial therapies include cryotherapy, topical imiquimod and 5-fluorouracil, and photodynamic therapy. These treatments have lower cure rates compared with surgery and should be limited to the treatment of SCC in situ.[11,12]

Upfront surgery is the treatment of choice for most SCC and BCC lesions due to its high local control rates. Standard surgical excision is an acceptable option for low-risk tumors. Margins of at least 4 to 6 mm should be removed; larger tumors require wider margin excision to ensure complete resection.[5,13] Conversely, Mohs micrographic surgery allows for detailed examination of surgical margins and, as such, is the treatment of choice for high-risk lesions.[14]

Postoperative radiation therapy (PORT) should be considered when negative margins cannot be achieved or in the presence of significant adverse risk factors for recurrence after surgery. One such risk factor is PNI, which is associated with higher rates of recurrence and metastases, even with surgical margin clearance.[8] PORT should always be considered in cases of clinically evident PNI because these patients have worse local control rates compared with those with microscopic PNI.[15,16] As such, careful assessment for neurologic symptoms suggestive of PNI, including burning, numbness, or paralysis, should be conducted. In the case of microscopic PNI, PORT should be considered if there is extensive disease (involving >2 nerves) or if the diameter of the involved nerve is greater than 0.1 mm.[17]

Other risk factors associated with worse local control that should prompt consideration of PORT include large tumor size ($\geq$4 cm), recurrent tumors, deep tumor invasion (>6 mm deep or invasion into bone, skull base neural foramina, or soft tissue), immunosuppression, and aggressive histology, particularly of the desmoplastic subtype in SCC.[13]

In cases in which margin interpretation after Mohs is difficult owing to poorly differentiated histology or highly infiltrative behavior, additional cytokeratin immunohistochemical staining may help with the detection of tumor cells. If margin status remains unclear, the decision to administer PORT will rely on clinical judgment, and should be strongly considered in the presence of high-risk factors, particularly when there is extensive or clinically evident PNI, in-transit metastasis, or a high suspicion for residual disease.

A variety of radiation treatment regimens are used in the postoperative setting. Dosing typically ranges from 50 to 66 Gy in 1.8 to 2.5 Gy fractions, with target biological equivalent dose $(BED)_{10}$ values ranging from 62.5 to 79.2.[5,13,18]

Definitive radiation is recommended for patients who are ineligible for upfront surgery, as well as patients with tumors in areas such as the midface area where surgery could lead to cosmetically unfavorable results. For optimization of cosmetic outcomes, lower fractional doses (1.8–2 Gy) should be given to a total dose of 60 to 70 Gy and BED_{10} value of 70.8 to 84, with larger tumors typically receiving higher doses.[5,13,19] Acceptable moderately hypofractionated regimens include 55 Gy in 2.75 Gy fractions or 50 Gy in 3.33 fractions.[18] Extreme hypofractionated dose fractionation schemes, such as 30 Gy in 5 fractions given over 2 weeks, can be used for smaller (<2 cm) tumors.[13] Patients who are in particularly poor condition with tumors causing symptoms such as pain, bleeding, or drainage can elect to have palliative radiation to 10 to 15 Gy in a single fraction or 20 to 30 Gy in 5 to 10 fractions.[19]

Radiation can be delivered using a variety of modalities, such as megavoltage (MV) photons and electrons, brachytherapy, and electronically generated low-energy sources (ELSs).

ELSs encompass several different lower energy therapies, such as orthovoltage, superficial X-ray therapy, and electronic brachytherapy. It is generally used to treat early-stage superficial SCC and BCC with depths of up to 0.5 cm. A margin of 1 cm should be added to the gross total volume (GTV) to account for microscopic spread, although this margin may be reduced to spare nearby critical organs. Three-dimensional (3-D) planning is generally unnecessary when using ELS.

Both superficial and deeper lesions can be treated with megaelectronvolt (MeV) electrons. Electrons with energies in the range of 6 to 20 MeV characteristically have steep dose fall-off curves laterally and distally.[20] As such, this modality is particularly useful for minimizing toxicity to deeper underlying structures. When using electrons, the 90% isodose line should be a few millimeters deeper than the base of the tumor **(Fig. 1)**.[19]

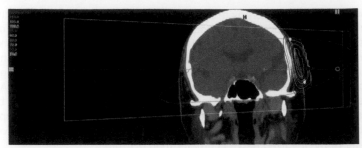

Fig. 1. Treatment plan for a patient with stage I T1N0M0 SCC (1.0 × 1.0 cm) of the left temple status post Mohs excision treated postoperatively to 60 Gy in 2 Gy fractions using electrons. A 1 cm bolus was used, and the treatment area, which consisted of the postoperative bed plus 1.5 cm margins, was delineated with wiring.

On the other hand, MV photon beams are more suitable for the treatment of deeper lesions or lesions with bone or cartilage involvement. No significant differences in local control have been observed between treatments with MeV electrons versus MV photons.[21]

For both MeV electron and MV photon therapy, 3-D planning should be used to ensure complete coverage of the lesion.[19] Treatment margins of at least 1 to 2 cm around the GTV should be used to ensure adequate coverage of microscopic disease.[22] For patients with head and neck tumors with clinically or radiographically evident PNI or extensive microscopic PNI (involving >2 nerves), the target volume should track the involved nerves to their ganglia proximal to the base of skull.[15,23]

High dose rate (HDR) brachytherapy using radioactive isotopes has been shown to have similar short term local control rates compared with external beam radiation, as well as excellent cosmetic results.[24] HDR brachytherapy is performed using a variety of applicators tailored to treat different anatomic locations. Surface brachytherapy is used to treat superficial lesions less than 0.5 cm deep and is performed using a variety of applicators, including conical applicators and surface molds (**Fig. 2**).[25] Interstitial HDR can be used to treat deeper lesions and may require 3-D planning to ensure adequate tumor coverage and sparing of normal tissues. Adequate margins around the gross target volume should be included in the treatment field, though this can be customized depending on the proximity of critical structures.[26]

For treatment of nodal disease, radiation is indicated after resection of the involved nodes in most cases. The exception includes patients with only 1 involved node less than 3 cm, for whom observation after surgery may be considered.[5,13] Five-year overall survival (OS) rates range from 70% to 75% for patients with nodal disease treated with surgery and PORT. Patients with negative margins without ECE found on pathologic assessment should be treated to 50 to 60 Gy in 1.8 to 2 Gy fractions. Patients with positive resection margins or ECE should be treated with a dose 60 Gy or higher. Similarly, node-positive patients who cannot undergo resection should be treated with definitive radiation to 60 Gy or higher.

Given the limited data on elective nodal basin radiation, the low rate of regional nodal metastases in patients with SCC or BCC, and the adverse effects associated with nodal basin radiation (eg, lymphedema and dermatitis), routine elective lymph node basin irradiation in high-risk patients is not recommended. However, elective

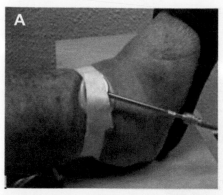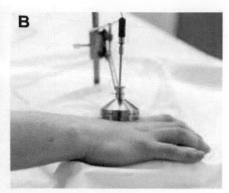

Fig. 2. Surface applicators are used during brachytherapy treatment of superficial skin lesions and are directly in contact with skin. Two commonly used surface applicators are (A) Elekta Valencia and (B) Varian Leipzig. (From Ouhib Z, Kasper M, Perez Calatayud J, et al. Aspects of dosimetry and clinical practice of skin brachytherapy: The American Brachytherapy Society working group report. Brachytherapy 2015;14(6):850; with permission; and Varian Medical Systems, Inc. All rights reserved.)

nodal radiation may be considered in patients with high-risk disease who are not candidates for nodal dissection in the event of nodal metastases.

MELANOMA

Melanomas begin as indolent tumors that undergo radial growth in the epidermis, often for several years (**Fig. 3**).[27] Once the lesion enters a vertical growth phase and infiltrates the dermis, the risk of metastases is much higher. Tumor thickness is one of the most important predictive factors for lymph node metastases, followed by ulceration and mitotic index.[28]

Historically, invasive melanomas have been classified into 4 major pathologic subtypes: superficial spreading, lentigo maligna, acral lentiginous, and nodular melanoma, with nodular and acral lentiginous exhibiting more aggressive behavior.[29] With the development of targeted therapies, melanoma is increasingly being categorized based on mutational signatures. Importantly, BRAF mutations are present in 40% to 60% of unresectable or metastatic melanomas, with data suggesting that BRAF mutations are associated with more aggressive behavior.[30] For patients with activating BRAF mutations, BRAF inhibitors, such as vemurafenib and dabrafenib, have been shown to have considerable antitumor activity, with phase III trials reporting significantly prolonged OS and progression-free survival. MEK inhibitors are commonly used with BRAF inhibitors, and the combination has been shown to achieve radiologic responses in up to 70% of patients with BRAF V600 mutations. Of note, the use of radiation is contraindicated in patients receiving BRAF or MEK inhibitors because this can lead to severe toxicity, including severe dermatitis and visceral toxicity.

Staging

Melanoma is staged according to the *AJCC*, 8th edition, staging system.

Treatment

Wide local excision of the primary lesion is the treatment of choice for nonmetastatic melanoma. Sentinel lymph node biopsies (SLNBs) are not required for patients with

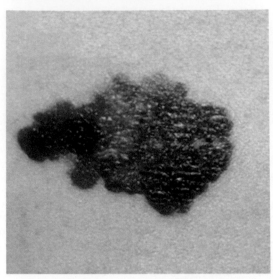

Fig. 3. Melanomatous lesion of the skin. Lesions suspicious for melanoma may exhibit one or more features of the ABCDE criteria: asymmetry, irregular borders, variegated color, a diameter greater than 6 mm, and evolution of appearance. (*From* National Cancer Institute. Common Moles, Dysplastic Nevi, and Risk of Melanoma. Available at: http://www.cancer. gov/types/skin/moles-fact-sheet. Accessed Sept 4 2019.)

tumors less than 0.8 mm in thickness without other risk factors because the risk of nodal metastases is less than 5% in these patients.[31] SLNB should be considered in cases in which the tumor thickness is 0.8 to 1 cm and cases in which the tumor thickness is less than 0.8 mm but there are other risk factors such as ulceration, LVI, or high mitotic index. In all other cases, SLNB is indicated. A PET scan should be ordered in node-positive cases to further assess the extent of disease.[32] Patients with nodal metastases should undergo complete lymph node dissection.[33]

Patients with facial lentigo maligna melanomas may consider definitive radiation compared with surgery because resection of these tumors may result in severe disfiguration. Although there is no standard dosing scheme, larger tumors can be treated to 50 to 70 Gy in 1.8 to 2.5 Gy fractions for target BED_{10} values of 59.0 to 87.5, with fraction size depending on skin health and cosmetic outcomes. Hypofractionated regimens, such as 35 Gy in 5 fractions, may be considered for smaller (<3 cm) lesions.[31]

For invasive disease, PORT to the primary site is not routinely indicated because local recurrence rates following wide local excision are low (approximately 10%). However, adjuvant radiation may be considered for cases with high-risk factors, including desmoplastic histology or tumor thickness greater than 4 mm associated with ulceration. Appropriate treatment doses for PORT include 60 to 66 Gy in 30 to 33 fractions (BED_{10} 72–79.2) or 48 Gy in 20 Gy fractions (BED_{10} 59.5). The surgical scar should be included in the tumor volume, as well as a 3 to 4 cm margin, which may be adjusted depending on proximity to critical structures.[31]

Elective lymph node radiation is generally not recommended. However, patients with positive lymph nodes who undergo lymph node dissection may consider PORT to the nodal basin if there are high-risk features, such as ECE, involvement of multiple nodes (ie, ≥1 parotid node, ≥2 cervical or axillary nodes, or ≥3 inguinofemoral nodes), and enlarged (≥3 cm in diameter) nodes. A randomized trial examining subjects with these high-risk features found a significant improvement in 5-year local control with the addition of PORT (77% vs 60%, $P = .023$) but no benefit in OS.[34] Appropriate radiation doses include 48 Gy in 20 fractions and 50 to 66 Gy in 25 to 33 fractions.[31]

Patients with oligometastatic disease can be treated palliatively with radiation if they are refractory to or unable to tolerate immunotherapy or targeted therapy. The addition of radiation in combination with immunotherapy in patients with oligometastatic disease in an effort to achieve a synergistic response via the abscopal effect remains controversial, although preclinical data are increasingly supportive of this approach. Currently, there are several ongoing trials investigating the combination of radiation and immunotherapy. In the meantime, the decision to use radiation in conjunction with immunotherapy should be made in a multidisciplinary setting.

MERKEL CELL CARCINOMA

MCC of the skin is a rare neuroendocrine malignancy associated with high rates of local recurrence and nodal metastases. Immunosuppression is a significant risk factor, with the incidence of MCC found to be 24 times greater in transplant patients compared with immunocompetent patients. Interestingly, Merkel cell polyomavirus, which is found on normal skin flora, is detected in 80% of MCC tumors, and virus-positive and virus-negative tumors are thought to have different mechanisms of tumor development.[35]

Clinically, MCC often presents on sun-exposed skin as a fast-growing red or purple painless nodule with a shiny surface, though flesh-colored nodules or plaque-like lesions can also be seen. Owing to its ambiguous appearance, an MCC lesion is commonly missed or misdiagnosed as a benign lesion.[36]

At diagnosis, approximately 65% of patients with MCC have disease localized to skin, 26% have involvement of lymph nodes, and 8% have distant metastatic disease. Regional lymph nodes are the most common site of metastases, followed by lung, bone, brain, and distant skin sites.[37,38]

Staging

MCC is staged according to the *AJCC*, 8th edition, staging system.

Treatment

Following biopsy, upfront wide local excision of the primary lesion with 1 to 2 cm margins is the recommended treatment.[39] LVI is associated with worse prognosis and should be pathologically assessed.[40] Patients with clinically node-negative disease should undergo SLNB with immunohistochemistry staining. Of note, the rate of false-negative results from SLNBs are considerably higher for patients with head and neck lesions compared with other sites owing to variable lymphatic drainage of the head and neck.[41]

Patients with small primary tumors (ie, <1 cm in diameter), negative surgical margins, and no other risk factors may be considered for observation following surgery.[39] Otherwise, adjuvant PORT to the primary site is recommended.[42] A treatment dose of 50 to 56 Gy, 56 to 60 Gy, and 60 to 66 Gy in 1.8 to 2 Gy fractions should be given to patients with negative margins, microscopic margins, and positive margins, respectively. The target volume should include the surgical bed with wide margins.[39,43]

Patients found to have node-negative disease after SLNB can typically forego radiation to the draining lymph node basin. However, lymph node irradiation should be considered for patients at a high risk of having a false-negative SLNB, such as immunosuppressed individuals or patients with head and neck lesions.[44]

Patients with microscopic nodal involvement found on SLNB should undergo full-body imaging, preferably with PET-computed tomography, to assess extent of disease. Lymph node dissection or radiation to the affected lymph node basin are reasonable treatment options. Appropriate radiation dosing ranges between 50 and 56 Gy in 2 Gy fractions.[39]

For clinically positive nodes, node dissection is the recommended treatment. Adjuvant radiation is generally recommended for patients with high-risk features such as multiple nodes involved or ECE. The appropriate radiation dose following lymph node dissection is 50 to 60 Gy in 2 Gy fractions.[39]

Patients who cannot undergo surgery should receive definitive radiation to 60 to 66 Gy in 2 Gy fractions. Similarly, patients with clinically positive nodes who cannot undergo lymph node dissection should receive radiation to the nodal basin to a dose of 60 to 66 Gy in 2 Gy fractions.[39]

Metastatic MCC was historically treated with chemotherapy agents typically used in small cell lung cancer, such as carboplatin or cisplatin-etoposide. Now, checkpoint inhibitor immunotherapy is the first-line systemic treatment. Avelumab (an anti-PDL-1 [Programmed death-ligand 1] agent), pembrolizumab, and nivolumab (anti-PD1 antibodies) have demonstrated promising antitumor activity and are approved for the treatment of metastatic MCC.[39,45,46] Various targeting agents are being investigated, particularly for virus-negative tumors with a high mutational burden.

MYCOSIS FUNGOIDES AND SÉZARY SYNDROME

Mycosis fungoides (MF) is a rare non-Hodgkin lymphoma that accounts for approximately 70% of CTCL.[47] Although the disease may remain in an indolent state for many years, the advanced stage is associated with a substantial mortality rate.[48]

Sézary syndrome is an aggressive form of CTCL that is closely related to MF and involves circulating malignant T cells and erythroderma.[49] Compared with MF, patients with Sézary syndrome have worse prognosis, with a median survival of 2 to 4 years following diagnosis compared with a median survival of 11 years for MF across all stages.[49]

MF typically arises from skin-tropic CD4+ T cells that cluster in the basement membrane of the epidermis. Very-early-stage disease typically begins with the development of ring-like erythematous macules on non–sun-exposed skin. The disease may remain in this stage, termed the premycotic phase, for several years.[50]

The premycotic phase is followed by a patch or plaque phase characterized by the development of eczematous, scaling patches and plaques that can affect both sun-shielded and sun-exposed skin, though a truncal distribution is the most common. Left untreated, plaques develop into tumors, although very few cases enter the tumor-phase de novo. Finally, erythroderma, defined as an area of erythema covering more than 80% of the skin, is an advanced manifestation of the disease and can develop from previous stages or occur de novo.[51]

In advanced stages of the disease, there may be involvement of regional lymph nodes, as well as visceral organs, most commonly in the lungs, central nervous system, oral cavity, and pharynx.[52] Approximately 40% of patients will undergo large cell transformation, which is associated with aggressive behavior akin to high-grade lymphoma.[51,53]

Sézary syndrome is defined as erythroderma caused by malignant T cells (Sézary cells) along with at least 1 of the 3 following criteria: (1) an absolute Sézary cell count of at least 1000 cells/μL; (2) a CD4 to CD8 ratio of 10 or more by flow cytometry, and (3) increased proportion of CD4+ cells with an abnormal immunophenotype (eg, CD4+ to CD7− ratio ≥40%). Sézary syndrome is thought to be closely related to but distinct from MF, and both diseases share a common staging system.[54,55]

Staging

MF and Sézary syndrome are staged using the tumor, node, metastases, and blood (TNMB) staging system.

Treatment

In the patch or plaque stage, skin-directed therapies are the preferred options, including psoralen and ultraviolet A (PUIVA), ultraviolet B (UVB), topical corticosteroids, topical carmustine, and topical nitrogen mustard agents, as well as localized radiotherapy. For patients with unilesional disease, local radiation to doses between 24 and 30 Gy are considered reasonable and curative, with local recurrences rarely occurring in patients who receive greater than or equal to 24 Gy.[56] The target volume should cover the lesion of concern and margins of 1 to 2 cm, depending on the size and location of the lesions.

Patients with multiple lesions requiring palliative radiation are typically treated with doses ranging from 8 to 12 Gy, with doses greater than 8 Gy reported to achieve complete response rates greater than 90%.[57] Dose fractionation ultimately depends on the patient's history of prior RT, size of the proposed treatment area, and future consideration of total skin electron beam therapy (TSEBT). Eight Gy in 1 fraction has been shown to yield good results, although reirradiation cases would benefit from smaller fraction sizes.

Patients with more advanced disease (stage IIB or greater) should consider a combination of systemic therapy and TSEBT for palliative treatment. TSEBT dose ranges from 8 to 36 Gy. Although higher complete response rates are correlated with higher doses, the response is typically not durable. Considering that patients have a significant risk of relapse requiring reirradiation, lower doses (10–12 Gy) that allow for retreatment are increasingly favored, especially because several studies have shown that these lower doses are associated with excellent response rates.[58]

The goal of TSEBT is irradiate the entire skin surface with less than 10% dose inhomogeneity at treatment distance in the coronal plane. The most common technique aims to expose as much body surface area as possible by having the patient assume 6 positions (**Fig. 4**). Patients stand approximately 3 m from the source and a dual-field configuration is used to ensure coverage of the patient's entire body. A Lucite plate placed in front of the patient serves to scatter electrons and reduce photon contamination. Areas that typically require supplemental treatment include the top of the scalp, perineum, soles of the foot, and areas under the breast. Maximum dose (D_{max}) should be set at the skin surface and the 80% isodose line should be at least 4 mm deep to the skin surface to ensure adequate coverage to the dermis and epidermis.[51,56,59]

TSEBT is well-tolerated, though toxicities may include dermatitis, pruritus, alopecia, loss of fingernails and toenails, and edema to the hands and feet. To reduce toxicity, lead shields over the eyes, lips, ears, hands and feet should be used during treatment.

Following TSEBT, adjuvant systemic therapy is strongly recommended to improve the durability of the response. Patients with particularly poor prognosis may consider allogeneic stem cell transplant for long-term local control.

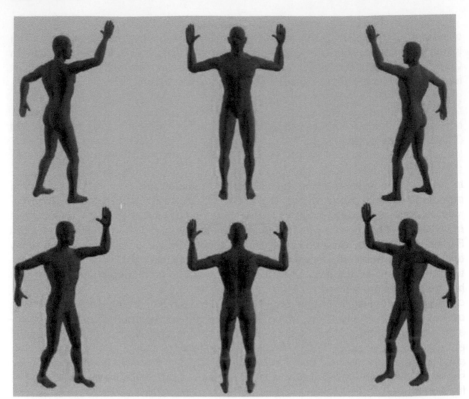

Fig. 4. Treatment positions for TSEBT. Top row (from left to right): right posterior oblique, straight anterior, left posterior oblique. Bottom row (from left to right): right anterior oblique, straight posterior, and left anterior oblique. (*From* Specht L, Dabaja B, Illidge T, et al. Modern radiation therapy for primary cutaneous lymphomas: field and dose guidelines from the International Lymphoma Radiation Oncology Group. Int J Radiat Oncol Biol Phys 2015;92(1):37; with permission.)

PRIMARY CUTANEOUS B-CELL LYMPHOMA

PCBCLs are a form of non-Hodgkin lymphoma that occur in the skin without evidence of extracutaneous disease at diagnosis. PCBCL consists of 3 main subtypes: primary cutaneous marginal zone lymphoma (PCMZL), primary cutaneous follicular center lymphoma (PCFCL), and primary cutaneous large B cell lymphoma, leg type (PCLBCL, leg type).[60] PCLBCL, leg type, often characterized by the expression of BCL-2, BCL-6, MUM1, MYC, and FOXP1, is more aggressive compared with PCMZL and PCFCL, and frequently spreads to extracutaneous sites. The 5-year OS rates for PCLBCL, leg type, are estimated to range from 41% to 60% in patients treated without rituximab and more than 74% in patients treated with rituximab.[61–63]

Staging

PCBCL is staged using the EORTC and International Society for Cutaneous Lymphomas tumor, node, and metastases (TNM) staging system for primary cutaneous lymphomas other than MF and Sézary syndrome.

Treatment

PCMZL and PCFCL are indolent lymphomas with a low frequency of spreading to extracutaneous sites. Lesions that can fit within a radiation field should be treated with local radiation to a dose of 24 Gy. Radiation provides excellent local control with minor side effects and is preferred to surgery due to its noninvasive nature. The target volume should cover the area of disease along with lateral margins of 1 to 1.5 cm. Tumor thickness must be considered, and an additional margin of 1 to 1.5 cm beyond the depth of the tumor should be treated to ensure adequate coverage. A bolus is often required to avoid skin-sparing. Although electrons are sufficient for most lesions, bulky disease may require treatment with photons.[56]

Due to the indolent nature of these diseases, patients with asymptomatic multifocal lesions are recommended for observation. Symptomatic patients can receive intralesional triamcinolone or palliative radiation to 4 Gy in 2 fractions, which has been shown to have complete remission rates of 72%. The use of chemotherapy is discouraged due to the indolent nature of PCMZL and PCFCL.[64]

In contrast to PCMZL and PCFCL, PCLBCL, leg type, has a tendency to spread to extracutaneous sites. Patients with localized disease are initially treated with R-CHOP (rituximab, cyclophosphamide, Adriamycin, vincristine, and prednisone) followed with radiation. The radiation volume should include the prechemotherapy tumor volume with margins of 1 to 2 cm. Again, electrons are generally sufficient, but bulkier tumors may require photons to ensure complete coverage of the base of the tumor. Owing to the more aggressive nature of this disease, patients are treated to 36 to 40 Gy.[56]

SUMMARY

Radiation plays an important role in the treatment of a wide range of cutaneous malignancies. Definitive radiation has been shown to be associated with good local control for cutaneous SCC and BCC, which is important for patients wishing to avoid disfiguring surgeries. Additionally, definitive radiation is a curative option for early-stage MF and PCBCL. In the postoperative setting, radiation is commonly delivered to the tumor bed to improve local control in high-risk SCC, BCC, melanoma, and MCC. Both photons and electrons are commonly used treatment modalities for external beam radiotherapy. Although photons are preferred for deeper lesions, electrons are suitable for superficial lesions and are useful for sparing the dose to underlying structures.

The role of radiation in patients with skin cancer with metastatic disease is an exciting and unresolved area of study. Currently, there are several ongoing trials investigating whether radiation and immunotherapy can be used together to produce a synergistic treatment effect. The results of these trials will shed light on the proimmunogenic effects of radiation and guide further treatment decisions.

REFERENCES

1. Leiter U, Eigentler T, Garbe C. Epidemiology of skin cancer. Adv Exp Med Biol 2014;810:120–40.

2. Apalla Z, et al. Skin cancer: epidemiology, disease burden, pathophysiology, diagnosis, and therapeutic approaches. Dermatol Ther 2017;7(Suppl 1):5–19.

3. Awad R, Andrade JCB, Mousa H, et al. Invasive basal cell carcinoma of the skin treated successfully with vismodegib: a case report. Perm J 2018;22:17–181.

4. Wang YJ, Tang TY, Wang JY, et al. Genital basal cell carcinoma, a different pathogenesis from sun-exposed basal cell carcinoma? A case-control study of 30 cases. J Cutan Pathol 2018. https://doi.org/10.1111/cup.13304.

5. Network, N.C.C. Basal cell skin cancer (Version 1.2019). 2019. Available at: https://www.nccn.org/professionals/physician_gls/pdf/nmsc.pdf. Accessed March 24, 2019.

6. Marks R, Rennie G, Selwood TS. Malignant transformation of solar keratoses to squamous cell carcinoma. Lancet 1988;1(8589):795–7.

7. Pekarek B, Buck S, Osher L. A comprehensive review on Marjolin's ulcers: diagnosis and treatment. J Am Col Certif Wound Spec 2011;3(3):60–4.

8. Jennings L, Schmults CD. Management of high-risk cutaneous squamous cell carcinoma. J Clin Aesthet Dermatol 2010;3(4):39–48.

9. Eigentler TK, Leiter U, Häfner HM, et al. Survival of patients with cutaneous squamous cell carcinoma: results of a prospective cohort study. J Invest Dermatol 2017;137(11):2309–15.

10. AJCC cancer staging manual. In Amin MB, Edge S, Greene F, et al, Editors, 8th edition, New York: Springer Publishing.

11. Ahmed I, Berth-Jones J, Charles-Holmes S, et al. Comparison of cryotherapy with curettage in the treatment of Bowen's disease: a prospective study. Br J Dermatol 2000;143(4):759–66.

12. Overmark M, Koskenmies S, Pitkanen S. A retrospective study of treatment of squamous cell carcinoma in situ. Acta Derm Venereol 2016;96(1):64–7.

13. Network, N.C.C., Squamous Cell Skin Cancer (Version 2.2019). 2019.

14. Nehal KS, Bichakjian CK. Update on keratinocyte carcinomas. N Engl J Med 2018;379(4):363–74.

15. Jackson JE, Dickie GJ, Wiltshire KL, et al. Radiotherapy for perineural invasion in cutaneous head and neck carcinomas: toward a risk-adapted treatment approach. Head Neck 2009;31(5):604–10.

16. Reule RB, Golda NJ, Wheeland RG. Treatment of cutaneous squamous cell carcinoma with perineural invasion using Mohs micrographic surgery: report of two cases and review of the literature. Dermatol Surg 2009;35(10):1559–66.

17. Han A, Ratner D. What is the role of adjuvant radiotherapy in the treatment of cutaneous squamous cell carcinoma with perineural invasion? Cancer 2007; 109(6):1053–9.

18. Manyam BV, Nikhil J, Koyfman SA. A review of the role of external-beam radiation therapy in nonmelanomatous skin cancer. Appl Rad Oncol 2017;6:6–10.

19. Howle J, Veness M. Cutaneous carcinomas. In: Leonard Gunderson JT, editor. Clinical radiation oncology. Elsevier; 2015. p. 763–77.

20. Hogstrom KR, Almond PR. Review of electron beam therapy physics. Phys Med Biol 2006;51(13):R455–89.

21. van Hezewijk M, Creutzberg CL, Putter H, et al. Efficacy of a hypofractionated schedule in electron beam radiotherapy for epithelial skin cancer: analysis of 434 cases. Radiother Oncol 2010;95(2):245–9.

22. Khan L, Choo R, Breen D, et al. Recommendations for CTV margins in radiotherapy planning for non melanoma skin cancer. Radiother Oncol 2012;104(2): 263–6.

23. Gluck I, Ibrahim M, Popovtzer A, et al. Skin cancer of the head and neck with perineural invasion: defining the clinical target volumes based on the pattern of failure. Int J Radiat Oncol Biol Phys 2009;74(1):38–46.

24. Zaorsky NG, Lee CT, Zhang E, et al. Skin CanceR Brachytherapy vs External beam radiation therapy (SCRiBE) meta-analysis. Radiother Oncol 2018;126(3): 386–93.

25. Ouhib Z, Kasper M, Perez Calatayud J, et al. Aspects of dosimetry and clinical practice of skin brachytherapy: the American Brachytherapy Society working group report. Brachytherapy 2015;14(6):840–58.
26. Skowronek J. Brachytherapy in the treatment of skin cancer: an overview. Postepy Dermatol Alergol 2015;32(5):362–7.
27. Available at: http://www.cancer.gov/types/skin/moles-fact-sheet. Accessed March 24, 2019.
28. Breslow A. Thickness, cross-sectional areas and depth of invasion in the prognosis of cutaneous melanoma. Ann Surg 1970;172(5):902–8.
29. Lasithiotakis KG, Leiter U, Gorkievicz R, et al. The incidence and mortality of cutaneous melanoma in Southern Germany: trends by anatomic site and pathologic characteristics, 1976 to 2003. Cancer 2006;107(6):1331–9.
30. Long GV, Menzies AM, Nagrial AM, et al. Prognostic and clinicopathologic associations of oncogenic BRAF in metastatic melanoma. J Clin Oncol 2011;29(10): 1239–46.
31. Network, N.C.C. Cutaneous melanoma (Version 2.2019). 2019. Available at: https://www.nccn.org/professionals/physician_gls/pdf/cutaneous_melanoma.pdf. Accessed March 24, 2019.
32. Marsden JR, Newton-Bishop JA, Burrows L, et al. Revised U.K. guidelines for the management of cutaneous melanoma 2010. Br J Dermatol 2010;163(2):238–56.
33. Voit CA, van Akkooi AC, Schäfer-Hesterberg G, et al. Rotterdam criteria for sentinel node (SN) tumor burden and the accuracy of ultrasound (US)-guided fine-needle aspiration cytology (FNAC): can US-guided FNAC replace SN staging in patients with melanoma? J Clin Oncol 2009;27(30):4994–5000.
34. Henderson MA, Burmeister BH, Ainslie J, et al. Adjuvant lymph-node field radiotherapy versus observation only in patients with melanoma at high risk of further lymph-node field relapse after lymphadenectomy (ANZMTG 01.02/TROG 02.01): 6-year follow-up of a phase 3, randomised controlled trial. Lancet Oncol 2015; 16(9):1049–60.
35. Leroux-Kozal V, Lévêque N, Brodard V, et al. Merkel cell carcinoma: histopathologic and prognostic features according to the immunohistochemical expression of Merkel cell polyomavirus large T antigen correlated with viral load. Hum Pathol 2015;46(3):443–53.
36. Heath M, Jaimes N, Lemos B, et al. Clinical characteristics of Merkel cell carcinoma at diagnosis in 195 patients: the AEIOU features. J Am Acad Dermatol 2008;58(3):375–81.
37. Haymerle G, Fochtmann A, Kunstfeld R, et al. Management of Merkel cell carcinoma of unknown primary origin: the Vienna Medical School experience. Eur Arch Otorhinolaryngol 2015;272(2):425–9.
38. Asgari MM, Sokil MM, Warton EM, et al. Effect of host, tumor, diagnostic, and treatment variables on outcomes in a large cohort with Merkel cell carcinoma. JAMA Dermatol 2014;150(7):716–23.
39. Network, N.C.C. Merkel Cell Carcinoma (Version 2.2019). 2019. Available at: https://www.nccn.org/professionals/physician_gls/pdf/mcc.pdf. Accessed March 24, 2019.
40. Andea AA, Coit DG, Amin B, et al. Merkel cell carcinoma: histologic features and prognosis. Cancer 2008;113(9):2549–58.
41. Liu J, Larcos G, Howle J, et al. Lack of clinical impact of (18) F-fluorodeoxyglucose positron emission tomography with simultaneous computed tomography for stage I and II Merkel cell carcinoma with concurrent sentinel lymph node

biopsy staging: a single institutional experience from Westmead Hospital, Sydney. Australas J Dermatol 2017;58(2):99–105.

42. Bhatia S, Storer BE, Iyer JG, et al. Adjuvant radiation therapy and chemotherapy in Merkel cell carcinoma: survival analyses of 6908 cases from the national cancer data base. J Natl Cancer Inst 2016;108(9) [pii:djw042].

43. Rush Z, Fields RC, Lee N, et al. Radiation therapy in the management of Merkel cell carcinoma: current perspectives. Expert Rev Dermatol 2011;6(4):395–404.

44. Arruda EP, Higgins KM. Role of sentinel lymph node biopsy in the management of Merkel cell carcinoma. J Skin Cancer 2012;2012:176173.

45. D'Angelo SP, Russell J, Lebbé C, et al. Efficacy and safety of first-line avelumab treatment in patients with stage IV metastatic Merkel cell carcinoma: a preplanned interim analysis of a clinical trial. JAMA Oncol 2018;4(9):e180077.

46. Nghiem PT, Bhatia S, Lipson EJ, et al. PD-1 blockade with pembrolizumab in advanced Merkel-cell carcinoma. N Engl J Med 2016;374(26):2542–52.

47. Wilcox RA. Cutaneous T-cell lymphoma: 2016 update on diagnosis, risk-stratification, and management. Am J Hematol 2016;91(1):151–65.

48. Weinstock MA, Reynes JF. The changing survival of patients with mycosis fungoides: a population-based assessment of trends in the United States. Cancer 1999;85(1):208–12.

49. Yamashita T, Fernandes Abbade LP, Alencar Marques ME, et al. Mycosis fungoides and Sézary syndrome: clinical, histopathological and immunohistochemical review and update. An Bras Dermatol 2012;87(6):817–30.

50. Hwang ST, Janik JE, Jaffe ES, et al. Mycosis fungoides and Sezary syndrome. Lancet 2008;371(9616):945–57.

51. Grace L, Smith LDW, Dabaja BS. Mycosis fungoides. In: Leonard Gunderson JT, editor. Clinical radiation oncology. Elsevier; 2015. p. 1556–76.

52. de Coninck EC, Kim YH, Varghese A, et al. Clinical characteristics and outcome of patients with extracutaneous mycosis fungoides. J Clin Oncol 2001;19(3):779–84.

53. Diamandidou E, Colome-Grimmer M, Fayad L, et al. Transformation of mycosis fungoides/Sezary syndrome: clinical characteristics and prognosis. Blood 1998;92(4):1150–9.

54. Vonderheid EC, Bernengo MG, Burg G, et al. Update on erythrodermic cutaneous T-cell lymphoma: report of the International Society for Cutaneous Lymphomas. J Am Acad Dermatol 2002;46(1):95–106.

55. Olsen E, Vonderheid E, Pimpinelli N, et al. Revisions to the staging and classification of mycosis fungoides and Sezary syndrome: a proposal of the International Society for Cutaneous Lymphomas (ISCL) and the cutaneous lymphoma task force of the European Organization of Research and Treatment of Cancer (EORTC). Blood 2007;110(6):1713–22.

56. Specht L, Dabaja B, Illidge T, et al. Modern radiation therapy for primary cutaneous lymphomas: field and dose guidelines from the International Lymphoma Radiation Oncology Group. Int J Radiat Oncol Biol Phys 2015;92(1):32–9.

57. Cotter GW, Baglan RJ, Wasserman TH, et al. Palliative radiation treatment of cutaneous mycosis fungoides–a dose response. Int J Radiat Oncol Biol Phys 1983;9(10):1477–80.

58. Harrison C, Young J, Navi D, et al. Revisiting low-dose total skin electron beam therapy in mycosis fungoides. Int J Radiat Oncol Biol Phys 2011;81(4):e651–7.

59. Jones GW, Kacinski BM, Wilson LD, et al. Total skin electron radiation in the management of mycosis fungoides: consensus of the European Organization for

Research and Treatment of Cancer (EORTC) Cutaneous Lymphoma Project Group. J Am Acad Dermatol 2002;47(3):364–70.

60. Senff NJ, Noordijk EM, Kim YH, et al. European Organization for Research and Treatment of Cancer and International Society for Cutaneous Lymphoma consensus recommendations for the management of cutaneous B-cell lymphomas. Blood 2008;112(5):1600–9.

61. Grange F, Beylot-Barry M, Courville P, et al. Primary cutaneous diffuse large B-cell lymphoma, leg type: clinicopathologic features and prognostic analysis in 60 cases. Arch Dermatol 2007;143(9):1144–50.

62. Grange F, Joly P, Barbe C, et al. Improvement of survival in patients with primary cutaneous diffuse large B-cell lymphoma, leg type, in France. JAMA Dermatol 2014;150(5):535–41.

63. Kim YH, Willemze R, Pimpinelli N, et al. TNM classification system for primary cutaneous lymphomas other than mycosis fungoides and Sezary syndrome: a proposal of the International Society for Cutaneous Lymphomas (ISCL) and the Cutaneous Lymphoma Task Force of the European Organization of Research and Treatment of Cancer (EORTC). Blood 2007;110(2):479–84.

64. Neelis KJ, Schimmel EC, Vermeer MH, et al. Low-dose palliative radiotherapy for cutaneous B- and T-cell lymphomas. Int J Radiat Oncol Biol Phys 2009;74(1):154–8.

Radiation Therapy for Benign Disease
Arteriovenous Malformations, Desmoid Tumor, Dupuytren Contracture, Graves Ophthalmopathy, Gynecomastia, Heterotopic Ossification, Histiocytosis

Tony Y. Eng, MD[a],*, Mustafa Abugideiri, MD[a],
Tiffany W. Chen, MD[b], Nicholas Madden, MD[a],
Tiffany Morgan, MD[a], Daniel Tanenbaum, MD[a],
Narine Wandrey, MD[b], Sarah Westergaard, MD[a], Karen Xu, MD[a]

KEYWORDS

- Radiation therapy • Benign disease • Arteriovenous malformations • Gynecomastia
- Heterotopic ossification • Histiocytosis • Desmoid tumor • Dupuytren contracture
- Graves ophthalmopathy

KEY POINTS

- Although the use of ionizing radiation in malignant conditions has been well established, its application in benign conditions has not been fully accepted and has been inadequately recognized by health care providers outside of radiation therapy.
- Radiation therapy has been shown to be effective as one of the treatment modalities for several benign conditions.
- Most patients experience no or few symptomatic side effects while achieving good long-term control and improved quality of life.
- Clinicians must still carefully balance all the potential risks against the benefits before proceeding with radiation therapy, especially in younger patients and children.

This is an update of an article that first appeared in the *Hematology/Oncology Clinics of North America*, Volume 20, Issue 2, April 2006.
Disclosure Statement: All authors have nothing to disclose.
[a] Radiation Oncology Department, Winship Cancer Institute of Emory University, 1365 Clifton Road Northeast, Building C, Atlanta, GA 30322, USA; [b] Department of Radiation Oncology, University of Texas Health Science Center San Antonio, 7979 Wurzbach Road, San Antonio, TX 78229, USA
* Corresponding author.
E-mail address: t.y.eng@emory.edu

INTRODUCTION

Once the imaging capabilities of x-rays were discovered in 1895 by Wilhelm Röntgen, their observed biological effect to create inflammation led other scientists to propose its use in treating medical disease. The first known successful use of x-rays for benign disease was by Leopold Freund in 1896, who demonstrated the effective use of x-rays on a 5-year-old girl suffering from a large hairy nevus on her back.[1] Initial clinical successes in the experimental use of x-rays led to many benign conditions treated with radiation. With improved understanding of radiobiology and late sequelae, there has gradually been more judicial use of radiation as well decreased number of patients treated with radiation for benign conditions.

Although the use of ionizing radiation in malignant conditions has been well established, its application in benign conditions has not been fully accepted and has been inadequately recognized by health care providers outside of radiation therapy. Most frequently, radiation therapy in these benign conditions is used along with other treatment modalities, such as surgery, in instances where the condition causes significant disability or could even lead to death. Radiation therapy can be helpful for inflammatory/proliferative disorders. For example, patients undergoing major orthopedic surgeries may benefit from adjuvant low-dose radiation therapy to help prevent heterotopic bone formation, and radiation therapy can help prevent progression and need for surgery in Dupuytren disease. Low to intermediate doses of radiation have been shown to provide effective improvement in conditions, such as Graves ophthalmopathy and keloid recurrence. Eye pterygium can be treated with brachytherapy using a strontium applicator. Arteriovenous malformations (AVMs) can be obliterated successfully with precise stereotactic radiosurgery (SRS). This article discusses the current use of radiation therapy on some of the more common benign conditions but excludes certain benign tumors, such as meningiomas and pituitary adenomas, that are frequently discussed in major textbooks or are very rare.

RADIOBIOLOGICAL BASIS

The therapeutic effect of radiation therapy is a result of energy interacting with matter and causing ionization or excitation. Ionization, which is the ejection of a charged particle from an atom, is important clinically due its resultant direct and indirect effects on DNA. Direct effects cause damage when the charged particles interacts with DNA, whereas indirect effects lead to the production of intermediary products that then cause damage to the DNA. For example, charged particles react with water to create highly reactive free radicals. The free radicals form a hydroxyl radical that then interacts with DNA to cause lethal cellular damage, like a DNA double-strand break. Because mammalian cells are 80% water, indirect effects of radiation drive the majority of the resultant DNA damage.[2] Oxygen facilitates the production of free radicals. As well-oxygenated tumor cells are killed and hypoxic tumor cells gain a better vascular supply, reoxygenation of previously hypoxic cells makes subsequent doses of radiation more efficacious. Fractionation of radiation allows for the exploitation of reoxygenation. It also takes of advantage of the reassortment of cells from more radioresistant phases of the cell cycle to more radiosensitive phases, specifically Gap 2 (G2 [subphase of interphase in the cell cycle])/mitosis. As the sensitive cells are eliminated, the surviving cells progress through the cell cycle to radiosensitive phases. Therefore, when the next dose of radiation is administered, the cells render themselves more sensitive to radiation.[3] A cell's ability to delay the progression to the G2 phase may correspond to its resistance to irradiation. Regardless, some cells appear intrinsically more radiosensitive to radiation therapy than others. Whether radiation directly or indirectly causes damage to the cell, sublethal damage can be repaired by cells if given enough time. Cancer cells, however, often have aberrant DNA repair mechanisms, so they are less able to repair DNA damage and subsequently die when they attempt to undergo mitosis prior to repairing damage. For cancers cells that survive, there is an accelerated regrowth of cells seen after irradiation that is called repopulation. The timing and length of radiation therapy must take into account the 5 radiobiologic principles that define the interaction of radiation with mammalian tissue during conventionally fractionated radiation: reoxygenation, reassortment, repair, repopulation, and radiosensitivity.[4] The goal is to achieve optimal disease control while allowing for sufficient sparing of normal tissue.

RADIATION TOXICITY AND TISSUE TOLERANCE

Radiation therapy can produce acute and late side effects, which depend on the volume of tissue receiving dose above a tissue-specific threshold. The risk of side effects in the treatment of benign diseases is generally uncommon because the dose of radiation used often is lower than that used in the treatment of malignancies. Furthermore, with modern radiation therapy techniques, radiation treatment plans are optimized with dose-volume constraints to minimize the risk of side effects in nontarget tissues. These constraints are based on the radiation tolerance of each organ system, which depend on the organization of the organ (such as in series or parallel) and intrinsic cellular properties of the tissue (**Table 1** lists example tissue constraints). The variable radiation tolerance of different tissues demonstrates that the risk of toxicity from radiation therapy depends on the site being treated and the nearby structures. For example, skin toxicities, such as acute dermatitis and late fibrosis, are of concern when treating an extremity target, whereas bowel toxicities, such as acute nausea and vomiting and late risk of bowel necrosis, are of concern when treating an abdominal target. Normal tissue tolerance and the risk of toxicities stratified by dose and volume of tissue treated are published with the results of radiation therapy clinical trials.[5-7]

ARTERIOVENOUS MALFORMATIONS

AVMs are complex congenital lesions of the cerebral vasculature in which blood flows directly from feeding arteries to draining veins without passing through a capillary

Table 1
Example dose constraints

Tissue	Toxicities	Common Constraints (Reference Trial)
Brain stem	Necrosis	Volume receiving 60 Gy <0.03 mL (RTOG 0825)
Heart	Pericarditis	V30 Gy <50% of organ (RTOG 1308)
Lung	Pneumonitis	V20 Gy <25% (RTOG 1010)
Optic chiasm	Blindness	V56 Gy <0.03 mL (RTOG 0825)
Parotid	Xerostomia	Mean dose to organ <26 Gy (RTOG 1016)
Rectum	Proctitis/necrosis	V75 Gy <15% (RTOG 0815)
Stomach	Ulceration/perforation	Maximum dose to organ <54 Gy (RTOG 0848)

Note, these constraints are for radiation delivered in 1.8 Gy to 2 Gy per fraction. Normal tissues are more sensitive to higher doses of radiation per fraction (20 Gy in 1 fraction does not equal 20 Gy in 5 fractions of 4 Gy each).
Abbreviation: RTOG, Radiation Therapy Oncology Group; V, volume receiving.

system. The annual risk of AVM hemorrhage is approximately 3%.[8] During the first year after hemorrhage, the risk of another hemorrhage increases to 6% to 15%.[8] AVMs may be observed or treated with surgical resection, embolization, or SRS. For AVMs that are less suitable to surgical intervention, such as those with deep venous drainage or in high-risk areas of the brain, or for patients who are not surgical candidates, SRS is an effective treatment strategy to ablate the AVM and reduce the risk of hemorrhage.[9] SRS may be delivered using cobalt beams (as with Gamma Knife), protons, or linear accelerators.

Radiosurgery works by injuring vascular walls within the AVM, thereby causing sclerosis of the lesion.[10] Response to SRS typically takes 2 years to 4 years.[8] The goal of treatment is complete obliteration of the lesion. Obliteration is associated with an 85% risk reduction of hemorrhage.[8] After SRS, but before obliteration, there is a 54% reduction in bleeding risk.[11] SRS is generally recommended for lesions less than 3.5 cm in diameter,[5] but staged radiosurgery, in which different parts of the lesion are treated in separate sessions, can be used for larger lesions.[12] The ideal management strategy for AVMs is an ongoing topic of debate, especially after recent randomized data suggested that medical management may be preferable for unruptured AVMs.[13] **Fig. 1** shows a typical AVM case treated with linear accelerator–based SRS. **Table 2** presents published outcomes using radiation therapy to treat AVMs.

DESMOID TUMOR

Desmoid tumor (also known as aggressive fibromatosis) is a locally aggressive benign growth arising from connective tissue in the muscular aponeurotic structures. The name, desmoid, is derived from the Greek word, *desmos*, meaning relating to bonds, connections, or ligaments, and was originally used in the nineteenth century to describe a growth with tendon-like consistency. The estimated incidence of occurrence is 2 million to 4 per million people, with slightly more incidence in women.[20] Although desmoid tumors are benign without the potential for metastatic spread, they have a high rate of local recurrence with surgical excision, especially in the presence of positive margin status.[21] Desmoid tumors can occur in most body sites, but they are differentiated into extra-abdominal (70%), abdominal wall (20%), and intra-abdominal (10%), with APC mutations associated with intra-abdominal and abdominal wall locations.[22] **Fig. 2** demonstrates a recurrent desmoid tumor along the right elbow as well as a clinical setup for the treatment. Although most desmoid tumors arise

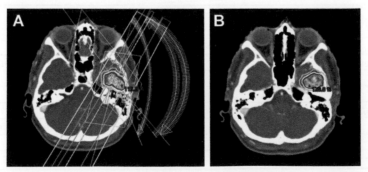

Fig. 1. AVM in the Left temporal lobe and a volumetric modulated arc therapy treatment plan using a linear accelerator (Linac). (*A*) Three noncoplanar arcs were used to treat the lesion. (*B*) Isodose lines, from out to in, 60%, 90%, and 100%. The prescription dose was 17.5 Gy in 1 fraction.

Table 2
Summary of selected treatment results for arteriovenous malformations

Author, Year	Total No. Patients	Technique	Dose	Results (%)
Hanakita et al,[14] 2016	292	GKS	20 Gy	73 obliteration at 6 y 53 bleeding risk reduction after RS 85 bleeding risk reduction after obliteration
Ding et al,[15] 2015	66 elderly, ≥60 y	GKS	21.7 Gy (mean)	77 obliteration at 10 y 1.1 hemorrhage risk after RS
Yen et al,[16] 2014	31	GKS	15–26 Gy	61 obliteration (at median 51 mo) 6.5 hemorrhage
Starke et al,[9] 2013	1012	GKS	21.2 Gy (mean)	69 obliteration at mean 8 y 8.7 hemorrhage
Sirin et al,[12] 2008	28 with large AVMs	GKS (staged volume)	16 Gy (median)	AVM volume range 10.2–57.7 cm³ 39 total or near-total obliteration (only half followed >36 mo) 14 hemorrhage
Maruyama et al,[11] 2005	500	GKS	20 Gy	91 obliteration at 6 y 6.6 complication rate 5.8 hemorrhage after RS
Vernimmen et al, 2005[17]	64	Protons	10–22 GyE	67 obliteration rate (vol <14 cm³) 43 obliteration rate (vol ≥14 cm³)
Nicolato et al,[13] 2005	63 children, <16 y	GKS	16–26 Gy	77 obliteration rate at 4 y 2 with complications No hemorrhage reported
Zabel et al,[18] 2005	110	Linac SRS	18 Gy	67 obliteration at 4 y 0 complications 8 hemorrhage after RS
Bollet et al,[19] 2004	118	Linac SRS	10–25 Gy	77 obliteration rate 6.7 complications 6 hemorrhage

Abbreviations: GKS, Gamma Knife radiosurgery; RS, radiosurgery.

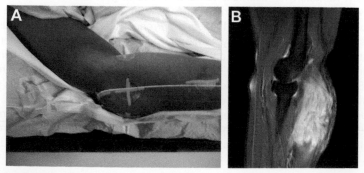

Fig. 2. Extra-abdominal desmoid tumor of the right elbow. (*A*) The clinical setup of the right elbow for the AP/PA treatment of the right elbow. (*B*) T1 Sagittal postcontrast MRI demonstrating the desmoid tumor along the right elbow. AP, anterior-posterior; MRI, magnetic resonance imaging; PA, posterior-anterior.

sporadically, approximately 7.5% to 16% arise from familial adenomatous polyposis.[23] Diagnosis of desmoid tumor is achieved through biopsy, with histologic identification of elongated clonal spindle-shaped cells in fibrous stroma.

Desmoid tumors can regress spontaneously, and, as such, close observation may be used for asymptomatic tumors, especially locations associated with significant morbidity after resection.[24,25] Per current National Comprehensive Cancer Network (NCCN) guidelines, surgery is a first-line treatment of desmoid tumors that are symptomatic or impairing or threatening in function as well as for tumors that have progressed after proceeding with observation. When proceeding with surgery, obtaining negative margins should be attempted and would require re-resection for positive margins due to the increased rates of local recurrence associated with positive margins.[26,27] There is also evidence, however, that status of surgical margins is not predictive of recurrence.[28,29] When negative margins are obtained, no further therapy is needed.

Radiation therapy is an effective definitive treatment of patients with unresectable desmoid tumors, and radiation alone, to doses of 50 Gy to 56 Gy using conventional fractionation of 1.8 Gy to 2.0 Gy per fraction, is associated with local control rates of 75% to 83%.[30–32] Keus and colleagues[31] performed a multicenter phase II study for moderate-dose radiotherapy for inoperable desmoid tumors, delivering 56 Gy using 28 fractions of 2 Gy per fraction and demonstrated 3-year local control rate of 81.5% as well as demonstrating a slow response, with some cases demonstrating continued response after 3 years. Radiation therapy also is used in the postoperative for resections with microscopic (R1) and macroscopic (R2) margins. The utility of radiation in R1 resections has been more debated, with NCCN giving a category 2B recommendation for adjuvant radiation in that setting. The retrospective study from MD Anderson Cancer Center demonstrated a benefit for resection combined with radiation versus surgery alone for postoperative cases,[27] whereas an Italian experience[33] and a cohort from Memorial Sloan Kettering Cancer Center[28] did not demonstrate a significant association between positive margins and local recurrence. There was a recent meta-analysis, however, looking at 16 studies and a combined 1295 patients demonstrated improved recurrence rates with adjuvant radiation for patients with primary tumors and recurrent tumors who had incomplete surgical resection.[34] There also was evidence of a higher risk of local recurrence for patients who had microscopic positive resection margins after receiving surgery alone, with a relative risk of 1.78.

A limited number of studies from Princess Margaret Hospital may indicate a role for neoadjuvant radiation for desmoid tumors. In the largest study, 58 patients were treated with preoperative radiation using 50 Gy in 25 fractions, and with median follow-up of 69 months, there were 11 local recurrences (19%), with major wound complications in 2 patients (3.4%).[35] Systemic therapy also remains a component of the treatment cascade, with effects of antiestrogen agents contributing growth inhibitory effects and often may be used in combination with nonsteroidal anti-inflammatory drugs (NSAIDs).[36,37] Per NCCN guidelines, systemic therapy can be used as frontline treatment or can be used in instances of gross residual disease or recurrence. In addition to noncytotoxic options of antiestrogen agents and NSAIDs, targeted therapy with imatinib (Bcr-Abl tyrosine kinase inhibition) and cytotoxic chemotherapy remain options for treatment. **Table 3** summarizes some of the selected treatment results.

DUPUYTREN CONTRACTURE

Dupuytren contracture is a noncancerous condition where the fingers can become permanently bent in a flexed position, typically occurring in individuals over 50 years

Table 3
Summary of selected treatment results of desmoid tumor

Authors, Year	No. Lesions	Dose	Recurrence	Comments
Janssen et al,[34] 2017	1295	35–66 Gy although some doses were not reported	Positive margins Primary tumor Surgery alone: LC 60% Surgery + RT: LC 77% Recurrent tumor Surgery alone: LC 22% Surgery + RT: LC 59%	Meta-analysis that demonstrates reduced risk of recurrence with adjuvant radiation for positive margins.
Keus et al,[31] 2013	44 (17 were recurrent)	56 Gy in 28 fractions	3-y LC 81.5%	Single modality radiation demonstrated good control in primary and recurrent setting.
Zlotecki et al,[32] 2002	65	50–56 Gy	5-y LRC 83%	There was a decreased probability of control with multiple prior recurrences.
Ballo et al,[30] 1998	75	60 Gy (range 46–66 Gy)	After GTR: 5-y LC 82% Gross disease: 5-y LC 69%	There were increased rates of complications >56 Gy. Doses >50 Gy were associated with higher control rates.
O'Dea et al,[35] 2003	58	Neoadjuvant 50 Gy in 25 fractions	At median 69 mo, LC was 81%	Demonstrates efficacy of preoperative radiation for desmoid tumors

Abbreviations: GTR, gross total resection; LC, local control; LRC, locoregional control; RT, radiation therapy.

of age. The underlying cause is unknown, but there is thought to be an abnormal formation of connective tissue in this condition. Patients present with nodules and cord-like structures in the palm of their hands, stretching from their palms to fingers. The contraction of these tendons can cause permanent flexion of the fingers, most

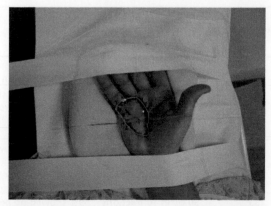

Fig. 3. This patient with Dupuytren contracture is receiving radiation treatment to the affected hand.

commonly affecting the fourth and fifth digits. Symptoms can include pain, burning, or itching in the affected area.[38–42]

Dupuytren contracture can be treated with surgery, injections, or radiation. The choice of treatment largely depends on the degree the affected finger(s) is bent toward the palm. A staging system is used to characterize the degree of flexion, and this is called the Dupuytren staging system. For patients with a contracture between 0° and 10°, radiation is the primary treatment modality (**Fig. 3**). In addition, if there are only nodules and cords present in the palm without contracture, radiation can be used. Patients that have contractures greater than 10° are usually offered surgery, collagenase injections, or needle aponeurotomy. Radiation is not offered to patients with severe Dupuytren contracture, because these patients have a greater chance of worsening disease if treated with radiation alone.[38–42]

A total dose of 30 Gy in 10 fractions is the typical treatment; 5 treatments are given consecutively every day and then a 6-week to 8-week period follows to allow the targeted area to respond and the surrounding tissue time to heal. After that 6-week to 8-week period, the last 5 treatments are completed. Patients also may receive a total dose of 21 Gy in 7 fractions.[39,42–44] This regimen has comparable long-term control over the disease to the standard total dose of 30 Gy divided in 10 fractions but has more acute side effects, such as redness and skin irritation. Patients and health care providers may decide on the 21-Gy regimen if the longer course is not possible in accommodating a patient's schedule. Treatment fields consist of proximal/distal margin of 1 cm to 2 cm and lateral margin of 1 cm. Orthovoltage treatment consists of 120-kv to 150-kv photons with bolus and electron treatment consists of 6 MeV to 9 MeV with bolus, with preference of electrons to photons given superior target coverage.[45]

The most common short-term side effect is erythema and long-term side effect is hand atrophy. No secondary malignancies have been identified, although follow-up for most studies has been limited to 5 years.[2,46] Although there have been some studies in analyzing radiotherapy in Dupuytren contractures, these have been mostly retrospective in nature and do not always differentiate the stage of contracture. Further randomized controlled studies are required to confirm the efficacy of radiation in treating early-stage Dupuytren contracture and to understand the possible long-term effects. **Table 4** presents some of the selected treatment results.

Table 4
Summary of selected treatment results of Dupuytren contracture

Study	No. Patients	Dose	Results
Keilholz et al,[40] 1996	96	30 Gy in 10 fractions	77% with no progression and 23% with progression
Adamietz et al,[38] 2001	99	30 Gy in 10 fractions	Stage N 84% and stage N/I 67% of cases with no progression. Stage I 65% and stage II 83% showed progression.
Seegenschmiedt et al,[41] 2001	129	Group A: 30 Gy in 10 fractions Group B: 21 Gy in 7 fractions	Group A: 93% showed no progression. Group B: 91% showed no progression.
Betz et al,[42] 2010	135	30 Gy in 10 fractions	69% showed no progression.
Zirbs et al,[44] 2015	206	32 Gy in 4 fractions	80% showed no progression.

GRAVES OPHTHALMOPATHY

Graves ophthalmopathy is an inflammatory condition of the orbital tissues and the extraocular muscles. It is thought to be autoimmune in nature and frequently occurs in women aged 40 years old to 44 years old and 60 years old to 64 years old.[47] It is most commonly associated with hyperthyroidism, because 20% to 25% of patients with Graves hyperthyroidism have Graves ophthalmopathy,[48] but it also can occur in euthyroid or hypothyroid patients.

Histologic features include interstitial edema, widespread lymphocytic infiltration, and varying degrees of muscle damage. Inflammatory reaction leads to venous engorgement, inadequate drainage of interstitial fluid, periorbital edema, proptosis, and ultimately compression of the optic nerve.[49] This compression may cause irreversible neuronal death and diminished nerve function that can manifest as decreased visual acuity and pupillary dysfunction as well as constriction of the visual fields. The most common clinical presentation of Graves ophthalmopathy usually involves the constellation of proptosis, periorbital edema, upper eyelid retraction, and excessive tearing.[50]

Management of this disease process can be medical, surgical (orbital decompression, eye muscle, or lid surgery), or radiologic or involve a combined modality approach.[51] High-dose systemic glucocorticoids are the first line of treatment. Favorable results have been reported in 60% of patients.[52] Orbital decompression may help in some cases that are resistant to steroid treatment, particularly in the presence of marked proptosis and optic neuropathy.[53] Although 1 study showed no benefit of radiation therapy,[54] many other investigators have found radiation therapy, usually in combination with steroids, as an alternative and efficacious anti-inflammatory therapy, with response rates of 50% to 88%.[55–58] A meta-analysis showed that a combination of radiation therapy with corticosteroids was better than either therapy alone.[59] If combination therapy is utilized, intravenous corticosteroids seem better tolerated and more effective than oral corticosteroids.[58] Other therapies, such as immunosuppressive drugs, intravenous immunoglobulins, and plasmapheresis, have resulted in less than significant outcomes.[60] When severe ophthalmopathy is present, permanent control of thyroid hyperfunction by radioiodine or thyroidectomy is sometimes recommended.[61]

Radiation therapy should be reserved for those who are symptomatic, who have not responded to a course of high-dose systemic steroids, or for whom steroids are contraindicated (those who have optic neuropathy or corneal ulceration).[62] Because of the risk of worsening retinopathy, diabetes mellitus can be a relative contraindication for radiation.[63] **Table 5** summarizes some of the results of radiation therapy treatments.

The most common dose of radiation is 20 Gy, which is administered using opposed lateral fields with posterior angulation. **Fig. 4** illustrates a common opposed lateral field design with a half-beam block posterior to the lens and the corresponding isodose color wash. Radiation treatment requires several weeks to take effect and may transiently cause increased inflammation. Thus, patients are sometimes maintained on steroids during the first few weeks of treatment.

Potential side effects include cataract formation, radiation retinopathy, and radiation optic neuropathy, which often manifests between 6 months and 3 years after ophthalmic radiation but may occur as late as 7 years after treatment.[66,67] The risk of cataract formation does not appear to be higher than the risk in the general population when radiation is delivered with modern linear accelerators.[68] In addition, the use of intensity-modulated radiation therapy may further reduce the risk of cataract

Table 5
Summary of selected treatment results of Graves ophthalmopathy

Author, Year	Number of Patients	Treatment	Results	Comments
Kulig et al,[64] 2004	101	20 Gy/2 wk + steroids	Donaldson ophthalmopathy index decreased significantly. Right eye: from 6.35 to 1.2; left eye: from 6.1 to 1.15.	Combined therapy is effective. Persistent diplopia in 16/101 patients
Prummel et al,[55] 2004	88 (RT vs sham RT)	20 Gy/2 wk	52% vs 27% responded	Less need for follow-up in RT group
Alpert et al,[63] 2003	47 (30 with optic neuropathy)	20 Gy/10 fx	75% improved. (retropulsion improved in 83%)	Early intervention (<6 mo) better
Pitz et al,[57] 2002	104 (29 RT, 75 RT + steroids)	10–20 Gy	75% pain improved 25% motility improved	No additional benefit seen with steroids No adverse side effects up to 16 y
Mourits et al,[56] 2000	60 (RT vs sham RT)	20 Gy/10 fx	Qualitative improvement (diplopia): 60% vs 31% Proptosis, lid swelling not better	25% RT patients spared from additional strabismus surgery
Beckendorf et al,[65] 1999	199	20 Gy/2 wk	26% excellent response 50% partial response 19% stable 5% progression	Patients treated within 7 mo after having ophthalmopathy had better responses.
Marcocci et al,[58] 2001	82 (RT + IV GC (41) vs RT + oral GC (41)	20 Gy/10 fx	87.8% response with RT + IV GC vs 63.4% in RT + oral GC	IV GC resulted in fewer side effects than oral GC (56.1% vs 85.4%)

Abbreviations: fx, fraction(s); GC, glucocorticoids; IV, glucocorticoids; RT, radiation therapy.

formation, with a cataract formation rate of 1.72% presented in a single-institution retrospective study.[69] These side effects generally do not occur if treatment is appropriately fractionated and carefully planned.

GYNECOMASTIA

Gynecomastia is a benign proliferation of glandular male breast tissue usually caused by an imbalance between estrogen and testosterone. The most common pathologic cause of gynecomastia is the use of antiandrogen therapy (AT) for treatment of prostate cancer. Gynecomastia can occur in 60% to 70% of patients receiving AT for prostate cancer.[70] Hormone-induced gynecomastia is usually bilateral and often

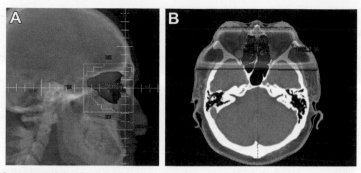

Fig. 4. (A) A typical half-beam block approach posterior to the lens to help with lens sparing. (B) The corresponding isodose color wash for treatment of Graves ophthalmopathy using opposed lateral fields.

accompanied by painful swelling. These side effects can lead to patients discontinuing AT in up to 16.4% of cases.[71] This issue is increasingly relevant, given an increasing life expectancy in patients.

There are several treatment options for hormone-induced gynecomastia, including low-dose radiotherapy. This is an effective method for both the prevention and treatment of gynecomastia.[72,73] Radiation is more effective if given prophylactically before the administration of antiandrogens, but it also has been used with some success for patients with existing gynecomastia. The largest randomized trial comparing radiation therapy for prevention of gynecomastia versus existing gynecomastia was conducted in 2003. For the prevention arm, gynecomastia rates decreased from 71% to 28%. For treating existing gynecomastia, 33% of patients had visible improvement and 39% experienced improvement in pain.[74] **Fig. 5** shows a patient with symptomatic gynecomastia after 6 months of hormonal therapy for prostate cancer. His symptoms were relieved with low-dose radiotherapy. **Table 6** summarizes several studies, including the aforementioned largest randomized trial, for evaluating radiotherapy for gynecomastia. Although this section focuses on radiotherapy in treating gynecomastia, it is important to recognize other treatment alternatives for gynecomastia. Tamoxifen has demonstrated its efficacy in treating hormone-induced gynecomastia via a small randomized trial.[76]

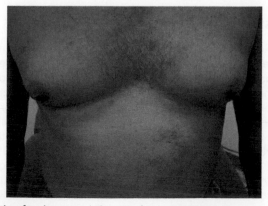

Fig. 5. Gynecomastia after hormonal therapy for prostate cancer.

Table 6
Summary of selected treatment results of gynecomastia

Study	No. Patients	Dose	Results
Ozen et al,[75] 2010	125 (prophylactic RT vs no RT)	12 Gy/1 fx	15.8% had gynecomastia in prophylactic RT arm, and 50.8% had gynecomastia in the nonprophylactic arm ($P<.001$). Breast pain rate 36.4% and 49.2% in prophylactic and non-RT arms, respectively
Perdona et al,[76] 2005	151 (AT only vs AT + tamoxifen vs AT + RT)	12 Gy/1 fx	69% developed gynecomastia in AT only arm, 1% in tamoxifen arm, and 34% in RT arm
Van Poppel et al,[77] 2005	65 with existing gynecomastia	12 Gy/2 fx	Gynecomasatia improved or resolved 33%; breast pain improved or resolved 39%
Tyrrell et al,[78] 2004	106 (prophylactic RT vs no RT)	10 Gy/1 fx	Gynecomastia rate: 52% vs 85% ($P>.001$)
Widmark et al,[74] 2003	253 (prophylactic RT vs no RT)	12–15 Gy/1fx	Gynecomastia rate: 28% vs 71% ($P>.001$)

Abbreviations: fx, fraction(s); RT, radiation therapy.

Tamoxifen has shown more effective in treating gynecomastia compared with radiotherapy, but tamoxifen must be taken concurrently with AT, whereas radiation may take up to only a few sessions.[79,80] Additionally, aromatase inhibitors or mastectomy with liposuction also can be used.[81,82]

Dosing typically is anywhere from 12 Gy in 2 fractions to 20 Gy in 5 fractions for existing gynecomastia.[77,83] For prophylaxis, 10 Gy to 15 Gy in 1 to 3 fractions has been published in the literature.[5–9] Radiation portal fields should cover the entire breast bud. Generally, electrons are used due to shallow depth–dose characteristics. Electron energy should be chosen depending on the thickness of the chest wall, typically 6 MeV to 12 MeV. Side effects tend to be minimal when treating gynecomastia. The most common side effect is mild skin erythema. Secondary malignancies, in particular breast cancer, from radiation therapy for gynecomastia is low.[84]

HETEROTOPIC OSSIFICATION

Heterotopic ossification (HO), ossification of soft tissues around the hip, is a potential complication after total hip arthroplasty, hip trauma, acetabular fracture, or central nervous injury. Primitive mesenchymal cells surrounding soft tissues can be transformed into osteoblastic tissue, which then forms mature bones. The most common location of HP is around the femoral neck or adjacent to the greater trochanter. Other less common locations include jaw, elbow, spine, and other joints after trauma. HO occurs in approximately 43% of the patients who underwent hip arthroplasty, with the incidence greater than 80% in those who have a history of HO, either ipsilateral or contralateral.[85] Among patients with a history of hypertrophic osteoarthritis, ankylosing spondylitis, diffuse idiopathic skeletal hyperostosis, and Paget disease, the incidence of HO can be more than 60%.[86]

The most common presenting symptom is hip stiffness, not hip pain. A majority of the patients with radiographically low-grade or early HO are asymptomatic. Those with severe HO may develop signs of inflammation, such as fever, joint erythema, swelling, warmth, and tenderness. Further work-up is needed to rule out infection. Plain films usually are sufficient for diagnosis. Ossification can be visualized on plain films within 4 weeks postoperatively. Bone scan typically shows increased uptake in the soft tissue next to the hip but it is not specific. The most widely adopted HO classification system is the Brooker system. It grades HO based on an anteroposterior radiograph of the pelvis and hip.[87] Bones that appear to be bridging, however, may be located either anterior or posterior to the hip, which may not cause significant loss of range of motion.

Table 7
Summary of selected radiation treatment results of heterotopic ossification prophylaxis

Study	Design	N	Results	Conclusion
Lo et al,[93] 1988	Retrospective postoperative 7 Gy in 1 fx	24	No grade 3–4 HO	Single fraction of 7 Gy appears effective.
Pellegrini et al,[94] 1992	PRT of postoperative 8 Gy (1 fx) vs postoperative 10 Gy (5 fx)	62	Grade 1–4 HO: Single fraction 21% Fractionated 21%	Single fraction appears equally effective as fractionated RT.
Gregoritch et al,[86] 1994	PRT of 7–8 Gy (1 fx) preoperative vs postoperative	124	Grade 1–4 HO: preoperative 26%; postoperative 28%	Preoperative may be similar to postoperative in HO prevention.
Healy et al,[95] 1995	Retrospective study of postoperative 7 Gy (1 fx) and postoperative 5.5 Gy (1 fx)	107	Grade 1–4 HO: 7 Gy 10%; 5.5 Gy 63% ($P = .03$)	5.5 Gy (1 fx) is insufficient.
Seegenschmiedt et al,[96] 1997	PRT of preoperative 7 Gy (1 fx) vs postoperative 17.5 (5 fx)	161	Grade 1–4 HO: preoperative 24%; postoperative 5% ($P = .05$)	Preoperative inferior to postoperative for HO prevention
Padgett et al,[97] 2003	PRT of postoperative 5 Gy (2 fx) vs 10 Gy (5 fx)	59	Grade 1–4 HO: 5 Gy 69%; 10 Gy 43% ($P = .09$)	5 Gy (2 fx) may be inferior to 10 Gy (5 fx) for HO prevention.
Burd et al,[98] 2003	PRT of RT (8 Gy in 1 fx) vs indomethacin 6 wk	166	Grade 3–4 HO: RT 7%; indomethacin 14%; ($P = .22$)	NSAIDs not statistically inferior to RT for HO prevention but may be due to small sample size
Pakos and Ioannidis,[90] 2004	Meta-analysis 7 PRTs of RT vs NSAIDs	1143	Grade 3–4 HO: OR 0.42 (95% CI, 0.18–0.97) favoring RT	RT more effective than NSAIDs for HO prevention. 1.2% absolute risk difference

Abbreviations: fx, fraction(s); PRT, prospective randomized trial; OR, odds ratio; RT, radiation therapy.

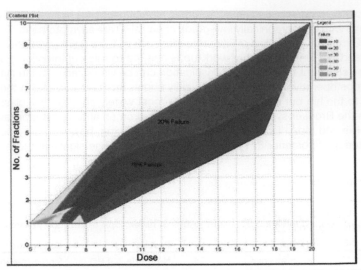

Fig. 6. Graphic retrospective analysis of 32 studies. Red (*center*) represents a failure rate of less than 10%. The lowest dose and number of fractions to achieve failure rate of less than 10% seems to be 7 Gy in 1 fraction. (*From* Luh JY, Cavanaugh SX, Eng TY, et al. A graphic retrospective analysis of 32 studies investigating optimal dose and fractionation schedules in the prevention of heterotopic ossification after hip arthroplasty. Int J Radiat Oncol Biol Phys 2004;60(1S):S547; with permission.)

The general treatment regimen for HO is surgical excision with HO prophylaxis, which may include NSAIDs, or external beam radiation therapy (EBRT) because recurrence rate after surgical excision alone is high. Effective prophylaxis of HO generally should be given to patients at high risk of HO. Indomethacin is the most common NSAID used for HO prophylaxis. The recommended dose of indomethacin is 75 mg/d to 100 mg/d and should be continued for 7 days to 14 days postoperatively. Matta and Siebenrock[88] showed indomethacin was not effective in preventing ectopic bone formation. Other NSAIDs also have been used. Bleeding and gastrointestinal side effects are potential disadvantages of using NSAIDs.

EBRT is another effective option for HO prophylaxis. A prospective randomized study showed both EBRT and indomethacin are effective in postoperative HO prevention.[89] A 2004 meta-analysis of 7 randomized studies comparing EBRT with NSAIDs demonstrated that EBRT is more effective.[90] Various radiation doses have been used. A 2010 retrospective study by Pakos and colleagues[91] showed great efficacy of combined EBRT and indomethacin in preventing HO after total hip arthroplasty. A fractionated total dose of 10 Gy does not seem to offer additional benefit compared with a single dose of 7 Gy. Several randomized studies demonstrated that the failure

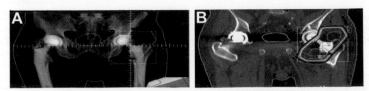

Fig. 7. (*A*) A small treatment field encompassing the soft tissue surrounding the hip joint and hardware but avoiding the bowels and genitals. (*B*) Isodose plan.

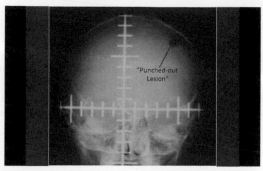

Fig. 8. A typical punched-out skull lesion in a 10-year-old boy who had histiocytosis.

rates are similar among those who received EBRT preoperatively (within 4 hours) or postoperatively (within 72 hours).[86,92] Delivering radiation preoperatively helps reduce patients' discomfort but scheduling is challenging, especially if surgery is delayed.

Table 8
Summary of selected treatment results of histiocytosis

Authors, Year	No. Patients	Follow-up	Treatment	Outcome	Comments
Laird et al,[115] 2018	39	Med 45 mo	7.5–50.4 Gy/ varied fx sizes	LC 89% (100% in bone lesions)	Bone lesions well controlled with low doses of RT
Kotecha et al,[119] 2014	69	Med 6 y	2.5–45 Gy using 0.66–6 Gy per fraction	LC 91.4%	Increased long-term morbidity in pediatric patients
Jahraus et al,[116] 2004	24	Med 28 mo	3–20 Gy/varied fx sizes	1.8–2.0 Gy/fx, score 1.29; if <1.8 Gy/fx, score 2.1 ($P = .013$)	Recommended fx <1.8 Gy
Rosenzweig et al,[120] 1997	14 diabetes insipidus	7.3 y	6–14.4 Gy/3–9 fx med 7.5 Gy	14% CR	Early disease responded
Minehan et al,[121] 1992	47 diabetes insipidus	Med 14.7 y	10–11 Gy mean (hypothalamic-pituitary RT vs no RT)	RT: 22% CR, 14% PR No RT: 0% CR/PR	Actuarial survival at 40 y was 65%
el-Sayed and Brewin,[111] 1992	15	1–20 y	Low doses RT	14/15 bone CR; 2/2 (DI) responded	
Selch and Parker,[112] 1990	22 (40 bony, 16 soft tissue sites)	1–13 y	6–26 Gy Med 9 Gy (bone) Med 15 (soft tissue)	All LC 82% Bone 88% Soft tissue 69%	Pediatric LC 100%

Score system: 1, CR; 2, greater than 50% PR; 3, less than 50% PR; 4, NR.
Abbreviations: CR, complete response; DI, diabetes insipidus; fx, fraction; LC, local control; med, median; NR, no response; PR, partial response; RT, radiation therapy.

Table 7 summarizes some of the selected treatment results. **Fig. 6** shows a graphic analysis of radiation doses and failure rates of HO prevention. **Fig. 7** illustrates a typical radiation treatment field used in HO.

Secondary malignancy induced by single-fraction radiation therapy is extremely rare. The University of Mississippi reports a 51 year-old patient who developed high grade undifferentiated sarcoma of the proximal thigh 16 months after prophylactic RT.[99] There is a relative contraindication for radiation in patients who have a posterior hip dislocation with a femoral head fracture because there is a theoretic risk of contributing to avascular necrosis or nonunion.

HISTIOCYTOSIS

Langerhans cell histiocytosis (LCH), previously known as histiocytosis X, is a rare disorder that consists of a cohort of idiopathic mononuclear cell regulation derangements[100] that present as infiltrative collections of monocytic cells with telltale cytoplasmic inclusions (Birbeck granules). LCH received its name from the due to the resemblance of the morphology and immunophenotype to Langerhans cells. LCH cells were discovered to be myeloid dendritic cells distinct from Langerhans dendritic cells of skin using gene expression array.[101] LCH is a monoclonal disorder characterized by the by the accumulation of CD207+ dendritic cells with BRAF V600E mutation in stem cell and dendritic cells demonstrating support for LCH being a myeloid neoplasia.[102]

LCH may present in multiple organ sites with a wide number of presentations,[103] many of which possess eponymous historical designations (for example, the classic exophthalmos, punched-out cranial lesions, and diabetes insipidus of Hand-Schüller-Christian disease or the pediatric hepatosplenomegaly, anemia, and hemorrhagic diathesis of Letterer-Siwe syndrome).[104] LCH has a predilection for bone involvement but may also include many other sites, including skin, lymph nodes, bone marrow, liver, and lungs.[105] **Fig. 8** shows a 10-year-old boy who has a typical punched-out skull lesion. He was treated with low-dose radiation therapy and had a complete response.

Multiple treatments exist for the treatment of LCH, including steroids, systemic therapy, and surgery.[106–110] The role of radiation in LCH has not been well defined[111,112] because treatment strategies have been changing over time. Bone pain and vertebral lesions remain an area that may benefit from radiation[113]; however, there is a decreased need for radiation, with cure rates of 70% to 90% with frontline surgical intervention.[114] When surgery is contraindicated, or for palliation of multifocal, persistent, or osseous disease, low-dose conventional fractionation of 6 Gy to 10 Gy may be utilized with good results.[113,115–118] Multiple series report local control greater than 80% with radiotherapy and local control in more than 90% of localized bone lesions.[112,115,117,119] **Table 8** summarizes some of the results of radiation therapy in LCH.

ACKNOWLEDGMENTS

This article was supported in part by the Departments of Radiation Oncology at Winship Cancer Institute of Emory University and University of Texas Health Science Center at San Antonio.

REFERENCES

1. Kogelnik HD. The history and evolution of radiotherapy and radiation oncology in Austria. Int J Radiat Oncol Biol Phys 1996;35:219–26.
2. Hall EJ, Giaccia AJ. Radiobiology for the radiologist. Philadelphia: Wolters Kluwer; 2019.
3. Withers RH. Four R's of radiotherapy. Advances in Radiation Biology 1975;5: 241–71.
4. Steel GG, McMillan TJ, Peacock JH. The 5Rs of radiobiology. Int J Radiat Biol 1989;56:1045–8.
5. Cox JD, Stetz J, Pajak TF. Toxicity criteria of the Radiation Therapy Oncology Group (RTOG) and the European Organization for Research and Treatment of Cancer (EORTC). Int J Radiat Oncol Biol Phys 1995;31:1341–6.
6. Emami B, Lyman J, Brown A, et al. Tolerance of normal tissue to therapeutic irradiation. Int J Radiat Oncol Biol Phys 1991;21:109–22.
7. Marks LB, Yorke ED, Jackson A, et al. Use of normal tissue complication probability models in the clinic. Int J Radiat Oncol Biol Phys 2010;76:S10–9.
8. Narayanan M, Atwal GS, Nakaji P. Multimodality management of cerebral arteriovenous malformations. Handb Clin Neurol 2017;143:85–96.
9. Starke RM, Yen CP, Ding D, et al. A practical grading scale for predicting outcome after radiosurgery for arteriovenous malformations: analysis of 1012 treated patients. J Neurosurg 2013;119:981–7.
10. Ajiboye N, Chalouhi N, Starke RM, et al. Cerebral arteriovenous malformations: evaluation and management. ScientificWorldJournal 2014;2014:649036.
11. Maruyama K, Kawahara N, Shin M, et al. The risk of hemorrhage after radiosurgery for cerebral arteriovenous malformations. N Engl J Med 2005;352: 146–53.
12. Sirin S, Kondziolka D, Niranjan A, et al. Prospective staged volume radiosurgery for large arteriovenous malformations: indications and outcomes in otherwise untreatable patients. Neurosurgery 2008;62(Suppl 2):744–54.
13. Nicolato A, Foroni R, Seghedoni A, et al. Leksell gamma knife radiosurgery for cerebral arteriovenous malformations in pediatric patients. Childs Nerv Syst 2005;21:301–7 [discussion: 308].
14. Hanakita S, Shin M, Koga T, et al. Risk reduction of cerebral stroke after stereotactic radiosurgery for small unruptured brain arteriovenous malformations. Stroke 2016;47:1247–52.
15. Ding D, Xu Z, Yen CP, et al. Radiosurgery for cerebral arteriovenous malformations in elderly patients: effect of advanced age on outcomes after intervention. World Neurosurg 2015;84:795–804.
16. Yen CP, Ding D, Cheng CH, et al. Gamma Knife surgery for incidental cerebral arteriovenous malformations. J Neurosurg 2014;121:1015–21.
17. Vernimmen FJ, Slabbert JP, Wilson JA, et al. Stereotactic proton beam therapy for intracranial arteriovenous malformations. Int J Radiat Oncol Biol Phys 2005; 62:44–52.
18. Zabel A, Milker-Zabel S, Huber P, et al. Treatment outcome after linac-based radiosurgery in cerebral arteriovenous malformations: retrospective analysis of factors affecting obliteration. Radiother Oncol 2005;77:105–10.
19. Bollet MA, Anxionnat R, Buchheit I, et al. Efficacy and morbidity of arc-therapy radiosurgery for cerebral arteriovenous malformations: a comparison with the natural history. Int J Radiat Oncol Biol Phys 2004;58:1353–63.

20. Escobar C, Munker R, Thomas JO, et al. Update on desmoid tumors. Ann Oncol 2012;23:562–9.
21. Goy BW, Lee SP, Eilber F, et al. The role of adjuvant radiotherapy in the treatment of resectable desmoid tumors. Int J Radiat Oncol Biol Phys 1997;39: 659–65.
22. Nieuwenhuis MH, Casparie M, Mathus-Vliegen LM, et al. A nation-wide study comparing sporadic and familial adenomatous polyposis-related desmoid-type fibromatoses. Int J Cancer 2011;129:256–61.
23. Koskenvuo L, Peltomaki P, Renkonen-Sinisalo L, et al. Desmoid tumor patients carry an elevated risk of familial adenomatous polyposis. J Surg Oncol 2016; 113:209–12.
24. Salas S, Dufresne A, Bui B, et al. Prognostic factors influencing progression-free survival determined from a series of sporadic desmoid tumors: a wait-and-see policy according to tumor presentation. J Clin Oncol 2011;29: 3553–8.
25. Bonvalot S, Ternes N, Fiore M, et al. Spontaneous regression of primary abdominal wall desmoid tumors: more common than previously thought. Ann Surg Oncol 2013;20:4096–102.
26. Abbas AE, Deschamps C, Cassivi SD, et al. Chest-wall desmoid tumors: results of surgical intervention. Ann Thorac Surg 2004;78:1219–23 [discussion: 1219–23].
27. Ballo MT, Zagars GK, Pollack A, et al. Desmoid tumor: prognostic factors and outcome after surgery, radiation therapy, or combined surgery and radiation therapy. J Clin Oncol 1999;17:158–67.
28. Merchant NB, Lewis JJ, Woodruff JM, et al. Extremity and trunk desmoid tumors: a multifactorial analysis of outcome. Cancer 1999;86:2045–52.
29. Crago AM, Denton B, Salas S, et al. A prognostic nomogram for prediction of recurrence in desmoid fibromatosis. Ann Surg 2013;258:347–53.
30. Ballo MT, Zagars GK, Pollack A. Radiation therapy in the management of desmoid tumors. Int J Radiat Oncol Biol Phys 1998;42:1007–14.
31. Keus RB, Nout RA, Blay JY, et al. Results of a phase II pilot study of moderate dose radiotherapy for inoperable desmoid-type fibromatosis–an EORTC STBSG and ROG study (EORTC 62991-22998). Ann Oncol 2013;24:2672–6.
32. Zlotecki RA, Scarborough MT, Morris CG, et al. External beam radiotherapy for primary and adjuvant management of aggressive fibromatosis. Int J Radiat Oncol Biol Phys 2002;54:177–81.
33. Gronchi A, Casali PG, Mariani L, et al. Quality of surgery and outcome in extra-abdominal aggressive fibromatosis: a series of patients surgically treated at a single institution. J Clin Oncol 2003;21:1390–7.
34. Janssen ML, van Broekhoven DL, Cates JM, et al. Meta-analysis of the influence of surgical margin and adjuvant radiotherapy on local recurrence after resection of sporadic desmoid-type fibromatosis. Br J Surg 2017;104:347–57.
35. O'Dea FJ, Wunder J, Bell RS, et al. Preoperative radiotherapy is effective in the treatment of fibromatosis. Clin Orthop Relat Res 2003;(415):19–24.
36. Brooks MD, Ebbs SR, Colletta AA, et al. Desmoid tumours treated with triphenyl-ethylenes. Eur J Cancer 1992;28A:1014–8.
37. Francis WP, Zippel D, Mack LA, et al. Desmoids: a revelation in biology and treatment. Ann Surg Oncol 2009;16:1650–4.
38. Adamietz B, Keilholz L, Grunert J, et al. Radiotherapy of early stage Dupuytren disease. Long-term results after a median follow-up period of 10 years. Strahlenther Onkol 2001;177:604–10 [in German].

39. Kadhum M, Smock E, Khan A, et al. Radiotherapy in Dupuytren's disease: a systematic review of the evidence. J Hand Surg Eur 2017;42:689–92.

40. Keilholz L, Seegenschmiedt MH, Sauer R. Radiotherapy for prevention of disease progression in early-stage Dupuytren's contracture: initial and long-term results. Int J Radiat Oncol Biol Phys 1996;36:891–7.

41. Seegenschmiedt MH, Olschewski T, Guntrum F. Radiotherapy optimization in early-stage Dupuytren's contracture: first results of a randomized clinical study. Int J Radiat Oncol Biol Phys 2001;49:785–98.

42. Betz N, Ott OJ, Adamietz B, et al. Radiotherapy in early-stage Dupuytren's contracture. Long-term results after 13 years. Strahlenther Onkol 2010;186: 82–90.

43. Schuster J, Saraiya S, Tennyson N, et al. Patient-reported outcomes after electron radiation treatment for early-stage palmar and plantar fibromatosis. Pract Radiat Oncol 2015;5:e651–8.

44. Zirbs M, Anzeneder T, Bruckbauer H, et al. Radiotherapy with soft X-rays in Dupuytren's disease - successful, well-tolerated and satisfying. J Eur Acad Dermatol Venereol 2015;29:904–11.

45. Meredith R, Carlisle J, Dover L, et al. Dosimetric comparison of radiation methods for palmar fibrosis. J Clin Radiat Oncol 2017;2:1–3.

46. Trott KR, Kamprad F. Estimation of cancer risks from radiotherapy of benign diseases. Strahlenther Onkol 2006;182:431–6.

47. Bartalena L, Marcocci C, Pinchera A. Graves' ophthalmopathy: a preventable disease? Eur J Endocrinol 2002;146:457–61.

48. Tanda ML, Piantanida E, Liparulo L, et al. Prevalence and natural history of Graves' orbitopathy in a large series of patients with newly diagnosed graves' hyperthyroidism seen at a single center. J Clin Endocrinol Metab 2013;98: 1443–9.

49. Bahn RS. Clinical review 157: Pathophysiology of Graves' ophthalmopathy: the cycle of disease. J Clin Endocrinol Metab 2003;88:1939–46.

50. Bahn RS. Graves' ophthalmopathy. N Engl J Med 2010;362:726–38.

51. Wakelkamp IM, Baldeschi L, Saeed P, et al. Surgical or medical decompression as a first-line treatment of optic neuropathy in Graves' ophthalmopathy? A randomized controlled trial. Clin Endocrinol (Oxf) 2005;63:323–8.

52. Jaulerry C. [The role of radiotherapy in Graves' ophthalmopathy]. J Fr Ophtalmol 2004;27:825–7.

53. Bartalena L, Marcocci C, Pinchera A. Treating severe Graves' ophthalmopathy. Baillieres Clin Endocrinol Metab 1997;11:521–36.

54. Gorman CA. Radiotherapy for Graves' ophthalmopathy: results at one year. Thyroid 2002;12:251–5.

55. Prummel MF, Terwee CB, Gerding MN, et al. A randomized controlled trial of orbital radiotherapy versus sham irradiation in patients with mild Graves' ophthalmopathy. J Clin Endocrinol Metab 2004;89:15–20.

56. Mourits MP, van Kempen-Harteveld ML, Garcia MB, et al. Radiotherapy for Graves' orbitopathy: randomised placebo-controlled study. Lancet 2000;355: 1505–9.

57. Pitz S, Kahaly G, Rosler HP, et al. Retrobulbar irradiation for Graves' ophthalmopathy – long-term results. Klin Monbl Augenheilkd 2002;219:876–82 [in German].

58. Marcocci C, Bartalena L, Tanda ML, et al. Comparison of the effectiveness and tolerability of intravenous or oral glucocorticoids associated with orbital radiotherapy in the management of severe Graves' ophthalmopathy: results of a

prospective, single-blind, randomized study. J Clin Endocrinol Metab 2001;86: 3562–7.

59. Stiebel-Kalish H, Robenshtok E, Hasanreisoglu M, et al. Treatment modalities for Graves' ophthalmopathy: systematic review and metaanalysis. J Clin Endocrinol Metab 2009;94:2708–16.

60. Cockerham KP, Kennerdell JS. Does radiotherapy have a role in the management of thyroid orbitopathy? View 1. Br J Ophthalmol 2002;86:102–4.

61. Bartalena L, Tanda ML, Piantanida E, et al. Relationship between management of hyperthyroidism and course of the ophthalmopathy. J Endocrinol Invest 2004; 27:288–94.

62. Bartalena L, Marcocci C, Gorman CA, et al. Orbital radiotherapy for Graves' ophthalmopathy: useful or useless? Safe or dangerous? J Endocrinol Invest 2003;26:5–16.

63. Alpert TE, Alpert SG, Bersani TA, et al. Radiotherapy for moderate-to-severe Graves' ophthalmopathy: improved outcomes with early treatment. Cancer J 2003;9:472–5.

64. Kulig G, Kazmierczyk-Puchalska A, Krzyzanowska-Swiniarska B, et al. Effectiveness of treatment for thyroid orbitopathy in patients hospitalized at the Endocrinology Department of Pomeranian Medical University. Przegl Lek 2004;61: 852–4 [in Polish].

65. Beckendorf V, Maalouf T, George JL, et al. Place of radiotherapy in the treatment of Graves' orbitopathy. Int J Radiat Oncol Biol Phys 1999;43:805–15.

66. Wakelkamp IM, Tan H, Saeed P, et al. Orbital irradiation for Graves' ophthalmopathy: Is it safe? A long-term follow-up study. Ophthalmology 2004;111:1557–62.

67. Miller ML, Goldberg SH, Bullock JD. Radiation retinopathy after standard radiotherapy for thyroid-related ophthalmopathy. Am J Ophthalmol 1991;112:600–1.

68. Marcocci C, Bartalena L, Rocchi R, et al. Long-term safety of orbital radiotherapy for Graves' ophthalmopathy. J Clin Endocrinol Metab 2003;88:3561–6.

69. Li YJ, Luo Y, He WM, et al. Clinical outcomes of graves' ophthalmopathy treated with intensity modulated radiation therapy. Radiat Oncol 2017;12:171.

70. See WA, Wirth MP, McLeod DG, et al. Bicalutamide as immediate therapy either alone or as adjuvant to standard care of patients with localized or locally advanced prostate cancer: first analysis of the early prostate cancer program. J Urol 2002;168:429–35.

71. Heidenreich A, Bastian PJ, Bellmunt J, et al. EAU guidelines on prostate cancer. Part II: Treatment of advanced, relapsing, and castration-resistant prostate cancer. Eur Urol 2014;65:467–79.

72. Dicker AP. The safety and tolerability of low-dose irradiation for the management of gynaecomastia caused by antiandrogen monotherapy. Lancet Oncol 2003; 4:30–6.

73. Tyrrell CJ. Gynaecomastia: aetiology and treatment options. Prostate Cancer Prostatic Dis 1999;2:167–71.

74. Widmark A, Fossa SD, Lundmo P, et al. Does prophylactic breast irradiation prevent antiandrogen-induced gynecomastia? Evaluation of 253 patients in the randomized Scandinavian trial SPCG-7/SFUO-3. Urology 2003;61:145–51.

75. Ozen H, Akyol F, Toktas G, et al. Is prophylactic breast radiotherapy necessary in all patients with prostate cancer and gynecomastia and/or breast pain? J Urol 2010;184:519–24.

76. Perdona S, Autorino R, De Placido S, et al. Efficacy of tamoxifen and radiotherapy for prevention and treatment of gynaecomastia and breast pain caused

by bicalutamide in prostate cancer: a randomised controlled trial. Lancet Oncol 2005;6:295–300.

77. Van Poppel H, Tyrrell CJ, Haustermans K, et al. Efficacy and tolerability of radiotherapy as treatment for bicalutamide-induced gynaecomastia and breast pain in prostate cancer. Eur Urol 2005;47:587–92.

78. Tyrrell CJ, Payne H, Tammela TL, et al. Prophylactic breast irradiation with a single dose of electron beam radiotherapy (10 Gy) significantly reduces the incidence of bicalutamide-induced gynecomastia. Int J Radiat Oncol Biol Phys 2004;60:476–83.

79. Viani GA, Bernardes da Silva LG, Stefano EJ. Prevention of gynecomastia and breast pain caused by androgen deprivation therapy in prostate cancer: tamoxifen or radiotherapy? Int J Radiat Oncol Biol Phys 2012;83:e519–24.

80. Fagerlund A, Cormio L, Palangi L, et al. Gynecomastia in Patients with Prostate Cancer: A Systematic Review. PLoS One 2015;10:e0136094.

81. Prezioso D, Piccirillo G, Galasso R, et al. Gynecomastia due to hormone therapy for advanced prostate cancer: a report of ten surgically treated cases and a review of treatment options. Tumori 2004;90:410–5.

82. de Ronde W, de Jong FH. Aromatase inhibitors in men: effects and therapeutic options. Reprod Biol Endocrinol 2011;9:93.

83. Chou JL, Easley JD, Feldmeier JJ, et al. Effective radiotherapy in palliating mammalgia associated with gynecomastia after DES therapy. Int J Radiat Oncol Biol Phys 1988;15:749–51.

84. Aksnessaether BY, Solberg A, Klepp OH, et al. Does prophylactic radiation therapy to avoid gynecomastia in patients with prostate cancer increase the risk of breast cancer? Int J Radiat Oncol Biol Phys 2018;101:211–6.

85. Neal B, Gray H, MacMahon S, et al. Incidence of heterotopic bone formation after major hip surgery. ANZ J Surg 2002;72:808–21.

86. Gregoritch SJ, Chadha M, Pelligrini VD, et al. Randomized trial comparing preoperative versus postoperative irradiation for prevention of heterotopic ossification following prosthetic total hip replacement: preliminary results. Int J Radiat Oncol Biol Phys 1994;30:55–62.

87. Brooker AF, Bowerman JW, Robinson RA, et al. Ectopic ossification following total hip replacement. Incidence and a method of classification. J Bone Joint Surg Am 1973;55:1629–32.

88. Matta JM, Siebenrock KA. Does indomethacin reduce heterotopic bone formation after operations for acetabular fractures? A prospective randomised study. J Bone Joint Surg Br 1997;79:959–63.

89. Kienapfel H, Koller M, Wust A, et al. Prevention of heterotopic bone formation after total hip arthroplasty: a prospective randomised study comparing postoperative radiation therapy with indomethacin medication. Arch Orthop Trauma Surg 1999;119:296–302.

90. Pakos EE, Ioannidis JP. Radiotherapy vs. nonsteroidal anti-inflammatory drugs for the prevention of heterotopic ossification after major hip procedures: a meta-analysis of randomized trials. Int J Radiat Oncol Biol Phys 2004;60:888–95.

91. Pakos EE, Tsekeris PG, Paschos NK, et al. The role of radiation dose in a combined therapeutic protocol for the prevention of heterotopic ossification after total hip replacement. J BUON 2010;15:74–8.

92. Seegenschmiedt MH, Makoski HB, Micke O, German Cooperative Group on Radiotherapy for Benign Diseases. Radiation prophylaxis for heterotopic

ossification about the hip joint–a multicenter study. Int J Radiat Oncol Biol Phys 2001;51:756–65.

93. Lo TC, Healy WL, Covall DJ, et al. Heterotopic bone formation after hip surgery: prevention with single-dose postoperative hip irradiation. Radiology 1988;168: 851–4.

94. Pellegrini VD Jr, Konski AA, Gastel JA, et al. Prevention of heterotopic ossification with irradiation after total hip arthroplasty. Radiation therapy with a single dose of eight hundred centigray administered to a limited field. J Bone Joint Surg Am 1992;74:186–200.

95. Healy WL, Lo TC, DeSimone AA, et al. Single-dose irradiation for the prevention of heterotopic ossification after total hip arthroplasty. A comparison of doses of five hundred and fifty and seven hundred centigray. J Bone Joint Surg Am 1995; 77:590–5.

96. Seegenschmiedt MH, Keilholz L, Martus P, et al. Prevention of heterotopic ossification about the hip: final results of two randomized trials in 410 patients using either preoperative or postoperative radiation therapy. Int J Radiat Oncol Biol Phys 1997;39:161–71.

97. Padgett DE, Holley KG, Cummings M, et al. The efficacy of 500 CentiGray radiation in the prevention of heterotopic ossification after total hip arthroplasty: a prospective, randomized, pilot study. J Arthroplasty 2003;18:677–86.

98. Burd TA, Hughes MS, Anglen JO. Heterotopic ossification prophylaxis with indomethacin increases the risk of long-bone nonunion. J Bone Joint Surg Br 2003; 85:700–5.

99. Mourad WF, Packianathan S, Shourbaji RA, et al. Radiation-induced sarcoma following radiation prophylaxis of heterotopic ossification. Pract Radiat Oncol 2012;2:151–4.

100. Osband ME. Histiocytosis X. Langerhans' cell histiocytosis. Hematol Oncol Clin North Am 1987;1:737–51.

101. Allen CE, Li L, Peters TL, et al. Cell-specific gene expression in Langerhans cell histiocytosis lesions reveals a distinct profile compared with epidermal Langerhans cells. J Immunol 2010;184:4557–67.

102. Berres ML, Lim KP, Peters T, et al. BRAF-V600E expression in precursor versus differentiated dendritic cells defines clinically distinct LCH risk groups. J Exp Med 2014;211:669–83.

103. Buckwalter JA, Brandser E, Robinson RA. The variable presentation and natural history of Langerhans cell histiocytosis. Iowa Orthop J 1999;19:99–105.

104. Arceci RJ. The histiocytoses: the fall of the tower of babel. Eur J Cancer 1999; 35:747–67 [discussion 767–9].

105. Grois N, Potschger U, Prosch H, et al. Risk factors for diabetes insipidus in langerhans cell histiocytosis. Pediatr Blood Cancer 2006;46:228–33.

106. Yasko AW, Fanning CV, Ayala AG, et al. Percutaneous techniques for the diagnosis and treatment of localized Langerhans-cell histiocytosis (eosinophilic granuloma of bone). J Bone Joint Surg Am 1998;80:219–28.

107. Gadner H, Grois N, Potschger U, et al. Improved outcome in multisystem Langerhans cell histiocytosis is associated with therapy intensification. Blood 2008; 111:2556–62.

108. Gadner H, Minkov M, Grois N, et al. Therapy prolongation improves outcome in multisystem Langerhans cell histiocytosis. Blood 2013;121:5006–14.

109. Gadner H, Grois N, Arico M, et al. A randomized trial of treatment for multisystem Langerhans' cell histiocytosis. J Pediatr 2001;138:728–34.

110. Atalar B, Miller RC, Dincbas FO, et al. Adult langerhans cell histiocytosis of bones : a rare cancer network study. Acta Orthop Belg 2010;76:663–8.
111. el-Sayed S, Brewin TB. Histiocytosis X: does radiotherapy still have a role? Clin Oncol (R Coll Radiol) 1992;4:27–31.
112. Selch MT, Parker RG. Radiation therapy in the management of Langerhans cell histiocytosis. Med Pediatr Oncol 1990;18:97–102.
113. Bertram C, Madert J, Eggers C. Eosinophilic granuloma of the cervical spine. Spine (Phila Pa 1976) 2002;27:1408–13.
114. Berry DH, Gresik M, Maybee D, et al. Histiocytosis X in bone only. Med Pediatr Oncol 1990;18:292–4.
115. Laird J, Ma J, Chau K, et al. Outcome after radiation therapy for langerhans cell histiocytosis is dependent on site of involvement. Int J Radiat Oncol Biol Phys 2018;100:670–8.
116. Jahraus CD, Russo S, Penagaricano J, et al. Radiotherapy dose fractionation in pediatric Langerhans cell histiocytosis. South Med J 2004;97:1268–9.
117. Greenberger JS. Radiation therapy in children: continued need to assess risk versus gain. Int J Radiat Oncol Biol Phys 1992;23:675–6.
118. Richter MP, D'Angio GJ. The role of radiation therapy in the management of children with histiocytosis X. Am J Pediatr Hematol Oncol 1981;3:161–3.
119. Kotecha R, Venkatramani R, Jubran RF, et al. Clinical outcomes of radiation therapy in the management of Langerhans cell histiocytosis. Am J Clin Oncol 2014;37:592–6.
120. Rosenzweig KE, Arceci RJ, Tarbell NJ. Diabetes insipidus secondary to Langerhans' cell histiocytosis: is radiation therapy indicated? Med Pediatr Oncol 1997;29:36–40.
121. Minehan KJ, Chen MG, Zimmerman D, et al. Radiation therapy for diabetes insipidus caused by Langerhans cell histiocytosis. Int J Radiat Oncol Biol Phys 1992;23:519–24.

Radiation Therapy for Benign Disease
Keloids, Macular Degeneration, Orbital Pseudotumor, Pterygium, Peyronie Disease, Trigeminal Neuralgia

Tony Y. Eng, MD[a],*, Mustafa Abugideiri, MD[a],
Tiffany W. Chen, MD[b], Nicholas Madden, MD[a],
Tiffany Morgan, MD[a], Daniel Tanenbaum, MD[a],
Narine Wandrey, MD[b], Sarah Westergaard, MD[a], Karen Xu, MD[a]

KEYWORDS

- Radiation therapy • Benign disease • Keloids • Macular degeneration
- Orbital pseudotumor • Pterygium • Peyronie disease • Trigeminal neuralgia

KEY POINTS

- Although the use of ionizing radiation on malignant conditions has been well established, its application on benign conditions has not been fully accepted and has been inadequately recognized by health care providers outside of radiation therapy.
- Radiation therapy has been shown to be effective as one of the treatment modalities for several benign conditions.
- Most patients experience no or very few symptomatic side effects and achieve good long-term control and improved quality of life.
- Clinicians must still carefully balance all of the potential risks against the benefits before proceeding with radiation therapy, especially in younger patients and children.

This is an update of an article that first appeared in the *Hematology/Oncology Clinics of North America*, Volume 20, Issue 2, April 2006.
Disclosure: The authors have nothing to disclose.
[a] Radiation Oncology Department, Winship Cancer Institute of Emory University, 1365 Clifton Road Northeast, Building C, Atlanta, GA 30322, USA; [b] Department of Radiation Oncology, University of Texas Health Science Center at San Antonio, 7979 Wurzbach Road, San Antonio, TX 78229, USA
* Corresponding author.
E-mail address: t.y.eng@emory.edu

KELOIDS

Keloids are benign dermal disorders that consist of raised scars formed from excessive tissue proliferation and excess collagen in the skin, mostly resulting from pathologic wound healing after injuries to the deep dermis, including surgery, trauma, and burn injuries.[1] Some other inciting events include body piercings, acne, insect bites, and vaccinations. However, some keloids form spontaneously and usually in areas with high skin tension, such as presternal, back, and posterior neck regions. Although sometimes painful and pruritic, keloids are usually asymptomatic and mainly of cosmetic concern.[2–4]

The exact pathophysiologic mechanisms causing keloid formation are unknown. Unlike hypertrophic scars, keloids extend beyond the boundary of the original site of injury. Fibroblasts in keloids seem to have different properties compared with normal skin of hypertrophic scars, because they show greater capacity to proliferate and produce high levels of primarily type I collagen, elastin, fibronectin, and proteoglycan.[5–7] In contrast, hypertrophic scars only show a modest increase in collagen production and respond normally to growth factors.[8] Several studies have shown an association between transforming growth factor-β and increased collagen or fibronectin synthesis by keloid fibroblasts.[8–10] It is hypothesized that radiation acts on fibroblasts to prevent their repopulation after excision, modulates humoral or cellular factors that would otherwise recruit or stimulate fibroblasts, or inhibits angiogenesis.[11,12]

Keloids are common, occurring in 5% to 15% of wounds and affecting both sexes equally.[13] They mainly affect people 10 to 30 years old[14] and are more commonly seen in those with family history of keloids.[15] Marneros and colleagues[16] studied 14 pedigrees and determined that keloids were an autosomal dominant entity with incomplete penetrance and variable expression. Keloids are more prominent in those with darker skin phototypes, such as black and Hispanic populations, in which the incidence is 4.5% to 16%.[17,18] **Fig. 1** shows a common keloid occurring after ear piercing in a female African American.

Although there have been many articles and studies done on management of keloids, there is no universally accepted treatment protocol for them. Choice of treatment modality often depends on factors such as size, depth, and location of the

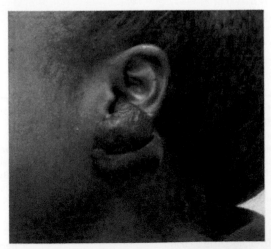

Fig. 1. A keloid develops slowly after ear piercing in a female African American.

lesion as well as the patient's age and prior response to treatment.[19] Radiation is usually indicated for recurrent keloids or keloids suspected to be at high risk of recurrence because of marginal resections, wider spread, or unfavorable locations.[20] Recurrence rates after surgical debulking or resection range from 45% to 100%[21] and are lowest in earlobe keloids.[22] With adjuvant radiation therapy, there is a 60% to 90% success rate in preventing new scar formation and achieving good cosmetic outcomes.[13,23,24] Other treatment modalities that keloids respond to include pressure therapy, cryotherapy, intralesional injections of corticosteroid, interferon and fluorouracil, pulsed-dye laser treatment, and topical silicone and other dressings.

Radiation therapy can be applied in the form of low-energy x-rays (150–200 kV), low-energy electrons (4–10 MeV), or brachytherapy.[25] Radiation can most effectively prevent keloid recurrence when it is started within 24 hours after surgical excision.[1,26] Borok and colleagues[27] reported a 2.4% recurrence rate within 50 years on 393 keloids in 250 patients after excision. In a 2011 meta-analysis, Flickinger[22] determined from a review of 2515 resected keloids that earlobe location, biologically effective dose, and treatment with electron beam or Co-60 versus other techniques, including x-rays and Sr-90, were correlated with decreased keloid recurrence by multivariate stepwise logistic regression analysis. In addition, postoperative keloid radiotherapy requires moderately high doses with a limited number of fractions and high doses per fraction to obtain optimum results, given that the dose-response function for keloids has a low α/β ratio. Using electron beam radiation, 18.3 to 19.2 Gy achieves 95% control of earlobe keloids, whereas 23.4 to 24.8 Gy achieves 95% control of other sites. Electron beam or Co-60 were thought to achieve lower rates of recurrence of resected keloids because of their less rapid dose decline with depth. Multiple studies have shown that a biologic equivalent dose 2 Gy (BED_2) greater than 35 Gy (ie, 13 Gy/1 fraction, 16 Gy/2 fractions, 18 Gy/3 fractions) yields favorable local control across all keloid sites.[22,23] The most commonly seen side effects of radiation therapy are hyperpigmentation, pruritus, and erythema.[24] **Table 1** summarizes the results from several radiation therapy studies on keloids.

Most studies on the radiation treatment of keloids are either retrospective studies or meta-analyses. A meta-analysis by Mankowski and colleagues[28] analyzed 72 studies of 9048 keloids and showed that, among brachytherapy, electron, and x-ray treatment modalities, postoperative brachytherapy yielded the lowest recurrence rate of 15%. High-dose brachytherapy is an alternative for patients who are resistant to adjuvant external beam radiation therapy and has been shown to result in a recurrence rate of 4.7% to 21%.[29–32] Jiang and colleagues[32] did a prospective trial of 29 patients with 37 recurrent keloids, in which all patients received 18 Gy in 3 fractions within 36 hours of local excision, with a subsequent 8.1% recurrence rate after a median follow-up of 49.7 months and complete resolution of pretherapeutic symptoms without recurrence.

MACULAR DEGENERATION

Macular degeneration is a common disease of the eye, characterized by deterioration of the central area of the retina known as the macula and resulting in blurry, distorted, or lost central vision. Age-related macular degeneration (AMD) is a major cause of visual impairment in the United States for people more than 65 years of age and is the leading cause of legal blindness in Western countries.[38] Approximately 30 million people worldwide are blind because of this disease.[39] The 2 common forms of macular degeneration are dry and wet. Dry AMD is the most common form, accounting for 90% of all AMD. The classic lesion in the dry form is geographic atrophy, which causes

Table 1
Summary of selected treatment results of keloids

Study	No. Patients	Cohort	No. Lesions	Dose	Response Rate (%)	Notes/Findings
Jiang et al,[32] 2018	29	HDR brachytherapy	37	18 Gy/3 fx	91.9	All patients started with recurrent keloids
Kim et al,[33] 2015	28	WLE + RT	39	12 Gy/3 fx (group 1) or 15 Gy/3 fx (group 2)	50 (group 1), 50 (group 2)	Recurrence was indirectly assessed by observing for reelevation of keloids
Shen et al,[34] 2015	568	WLE + RT	834	18 Gy/2 fx	90.41	Electron beam of 6 or 7 MeV was used
Emad et al,[35] 2010	26	WLE + RT (group A), cryotherapy + intralesional steroid (group B)	76	12 Gy/3 fx (group A)	70.4 (group A), 68.8 (group B)	Treatment using surgery plus immediate radiotherapy was more efficacious and safer than cryotherapy and adjuvant steroid injection
Malaker et al,[36] 2004	64	RT alone	86	37.5 Gy/5 fx	97	Unresectable keloids; 63% satisfied with outcome
Lo et al,[37] 1990	199	WLE + RT	354	2–20 Gy/1 fx	87 ($\geq$9 Gy); 43 (<9 Gy)	Difference nonsignificant statistically
Borok et al,[27] 1988	250	WLE + RT	393	4–16 Gy/varied fx	98	Excellent cosmetic results in 92% of pts; recommend 12 y in 3 fx

Abbreviations: fx, fractions; HDR, high dose rate; RT, radiation therapy; WLE, wide local excision.

severe central visual loss (**Fig. 2**). In most cases, this loss is self-limited and causes no dramatic visual deterioration. No treatment can reverse the progression of this type of AMD. Approximately 20% of patients who have dry AMD progress to wet AMD over a 5-year period.[40] Wet macular degeneration is less common but is more severe than the dry form. It accounts for 10% of all AMD but results in 90% of all blindness from the disease. Wet macular degeneration is characterized by choroidal neovascularization macular degeneration, which is the development of abnormal vessels beneath the retinal pigment of the retina. These vessels can bleed and eventually cause macular scarring, resulting in profound loss of central vision. The pathophysiology of macular degeneration is not completely understood. Some of the causal factors that have been proposed include primary retinal pigment epithelium, Bruch membrane senescence, genetic susceptibility, primary ocular perfusion abnormalities, and oxidative injury.[41] Several therapeutic strategies are available to treat macular degeneration, but the progression of disease often cannot be reversed. Laser treatment has shown some potential benefit and may halt or decrease vision loss. Often, a scar is left and may produce a permanent loss of vision secondary to damage of the overlying retina.

Subretinal surgery may be an option but does not always give optimal results.[42] In photodynamic therapy, a light-activated drug, verteporfin, is given intravenously and a laser is used to close the abnormal vessels while leaving the retina intact.[43] Intravitreal anti–vascular endothelial growth factor (VEGF) drugs are the mainstay of treatment, with multiple approved drugs, including bevacizumab, ranibizumab, and aflibercept. They function by inhibiting angiogenesis and permeability.[44]

The treatment with ionizing radiation is to prevent the proliferation of endothelial cells necessary for neovascularization as well as inhibiting inflammation and fibrosis. It induces the regression of vascular tissue and inhibits growth of new blood vessels. Some advantages in treating AMD with low-dose radiotherapy include the absence of iatrogenic mechanical or laser damage, absence of systemic side effects, and absence of local side effects caused by ocular injection. An additional advantage for patients who have primarily large, occult choroidal neovascularization is that radiation can be used for this type of macular degeneration. One of the major potential side effects is radiation retinopathy, which is dose dependent.[45] Some of the common techniques include 6-MV to 9-MV photons with a lateral-port half-beam technique, episcleral brachytherapy with strontium-90 plaques, and more recently proton

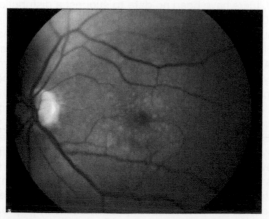

Fig. 2. Macular degeneration with atrophic-appearing macula.

therapy, kilovoltage stereotactic radiotherapy (SRT), and epimacular brachytherapy (EMBT).

External beam SRT allows more accurate delivery of dose than a half-beam technique with external beam radiotherapy would, with potential benefits of allowing for dose decline and dose escalation. Multiple commercial systems are available. SRT was evaluated in a randomized trial of 16-Gy or 24-Gy SRT using the IRay system or sham radiation therapy in patients previously treated with anti-VEGF injections. Patients treated with radiation had a significant reduction in intravitreal injections over 2 years, and only 1% of eyes had microvascular changes related to radiation that possibly affected vision.[46] Long-term follow-up showed 30.3% of cases treated developed retinal microvascular abnormalities, although this contributed to vision loss in only 5 out of 37 cases.[47]

EMBT uses an intraocular probe containing a radioactive source that emits β radiation. A randomized trial did not support use of EMBT with anti-VEGF versus VEGF alone in a randomized trial.[48] A recent trial treated patients with a combination of proton therapy and anti-VEGF with ranibizumab, the first study using this combination therapy. Proton therapy has an advantage of limited distal dose because of the properties of the Bragg peak. There was no change in visual acuity at 24 months, but, for newly diagnosed patients, there was some improvement in visual acuity; fewer injections of ranibizumab were noted than with the standard protocol and no cases of radiation retinopathy were reported at 3 years.[49]

Although several clinical studies have shown some benefit with radiation therapy, conclusive data have not been established despite multiple trials, many of which were completed before anti-VEGF therapy became standard-of-care treatment. **Table 2** presents some of the recent radiation treatment results.

ORBITAL PSEUDOTUMOR

Orbital pseudotumor, also called idiopathic orbital inflammation, is an inflammatory process of unknown cause that sometimes results in a palpable mass resembling a tumor. It can affect the orbit in its entirety or parts of the orbit, such as the extraocular muscles, lacrimal gland, fat, and sclera. In addition to a palpable mass, orbital pseudotumor may present as pain, edema, proptosis, chemosis, ophthalmoplegia, and diplopia.[57] It can manifest acutely or chronically, and it presents bilaterally around 25% of the time. Distant metastases are rare, but local recurrence is common. To date, there have been no data to suggest a distribution based on age, gender, or race. Orbital pseudotumor is generally a diagnosis of exclusion. Other causes to rule out include neoplasms, infection, Graves ophthalmology, ocular lymphoma, sarcoidosis, orbital myositis, scleritis, Sjögren disease, and Wegener granulomatosis. An appropriate work-up includes a physical examination, medical history, laboratory work, and imaging.[58] Usually, there are nonspecific markers of inflammation found on serologic studies. Computed tomography (CT) scans may show soft tissue swelling and inflammation, but contrast-enhanced MRI with fat saturation is recommended. Some clinicians argue a biopsy is not required for diagnosis, but it is often obtained in order to rule out other causes. Histopathology shows infiltrative inflammatory cells that can be further classified as lymphoid (necessitating flow cytometry to rule out lymphoma), granulomatous, or sclerosing.[59] Besides a biopsy, a diagnosis can be confirmed by an improvement of symptoms on a trial of systemic corticosteroids, which then are slowly tapered. Although most patients experience an improvement, only approximately 50% of patients have a complete resolution of symptoms. Radiation therapy can be

Table 2
Summary of selected treatment results of macular degeneration

Study	No. Patients/Eyes	Treatment	Results	Notes
Park et al,[49] 2012	6	24 CGE proton therapy/2 fx 24 h apart with 4 monthly injections ranibizumab	No change VA at 24 mo; no radiation retinopathy at 3 y	Fewer injections of ranibizumab than would be standard
Jackson et al,[46] 2015	230	16 Gy vs 24 Gy SRT vs sham RT; all received concurrent ranibizumab	SRT reduces intravitreal injections at 2 y; 30.3% of cases developed microvascular abnormalities at 3 y; no improvement VA with SRT	—
Jackson et al,[48] 2016	363	Ranibizumab monotherapy vs 24 Gy EMBT + ranibizumab	No difference in PRN ranibizumab injections, mean VA change −4.8 vs −0.9 letters favoring EMBT, proportion of patients losing fewer than 15 letters 84% EMBT vs 92%	One patient with RT-induced retinal vascular abnormality; safety good but only 12 mo follow-up
Jaakkola et al,[50] 2005	86/88	15 Gy 12.6 Gy (Sr90)	VA loss >3 lines: Control 84% RT 80%	No long-term benefits (at 3.5 mo)
Marcus et al,[51] 2004	88 (randomized RT vs no RT)	20 Gy/fx	At 6 mo, 26% vs 43% 3-line VA loss At 12 mo, 42% vs 49% 3-line VA loss	RT had a short-term benefit in preserving visual acuity
Prettenhofer et al,[52] 2004	80	14.4 Gy 25.2 Gy	VA deteriorated in 85% (14.4 Gy) and 65% (25.2 Gy) of patients	After 4 y, irradiated eyes were similar to the natural course of the disease
Hart et al,[53] 2002	203 (randomized to RT vs no RT)	12 Gy/6 fx	RT better than control group but not statistical significance	Negative trial
Valmaggia et al,[54] 2002	161 (prospective double-blinded study)	1 Gy/4 fx vs 8 Gy/4 fx vs 16 Gy/4 fx	No difference among treatment groups. Classic CNV, initial VA >20/100 benefited more from higher doses	Higher doses resulted in stabilization of the VA without any difference in efficacy
Schittkowski et al,[55] 2001	118/126	20 Gy in 2 wk	VA decreased but most had decreased metamorphopsia and increased color and contrast perception with RT	8 patients reported epiphora, and 4 patients complained of transient sicca syndrome
Kobayashi & Kobayashi,[56] 2000	101 (randomized RT vs no RT)	20 Gy in 2 wk	Smaller choroidal neovascular membrane or better baseline VA benefited. Mean VA 20/168 vs 20/327	RT seems to have a beneficial effect in selected patients

Abbreviations: CGE, cobalt gray equivalent; CNV, choroidal neovascularization; PRN, as needed; VA, visual acuity.

considered when there is a lack of response to steroids, a recurrence after steroids, or an inability to tolerate steroids. Treatment is delivered using en face electron therapy, opposed lateral field three-dimensional conformal radiation therapy, or intensity modulated radiation therapy (IMRT). **Fig. 3** shows a right orbital pseudotumor treated with IMRT. Radiation doses range from 2000 to 3000 cGy given at 180 to 200 cGy per fraction. **Table 3** provides a summary of radiation therapy results.[60–67] Using proper radiation techniques, such as lens shielding, these studies show a good local control rate with minimal morbidity. patients who are older at the time of diagnosis and who have a complete response to radiation therapy were significantly less likely to experience a recurrence of symptoms. Outside of radiation therapy, other treatment modalities include immunosuppressive agents (cyclosporine, tacrolimus), cytotoxic agents (azathioprine, cyclophosphamide, methotrexate), biologic agents (rituximab, infliximab), and surgery for lesions that are well localized or lesions that are refractory to other treatment modalities.[57,68] However, although an orbital pseudotumor may start as a benign process, it may progress and compress critical orbital structures, such as the optic nerve, leading to optic nerve atrophy and vision loss.

PTERYGIUM

A pterygium is a triangular wedge, usually of medial nasal conjunctiva, that extends onto the cornea. It is sometimes confused with pinguecula, which is a similar disorder that arises from but remains confined to the conjunctiva. The name pterygium describes the shape of the tissue, which resembles a wing. Although considered a benign proliferation of subconjunctival fibroblasts, pterygia can block the visual axis, directly reducing visual acuity, and induce astigmatism. It also is of concern to patients because of the abnormal appearance of the eye and often is associated with redness and irritation, which can make wearing contact lenses uncomfortable. Pterygia occur most commonly in tropical regions where there is a high rate of sun exposure.[69] Lower rates of pterygium are associated with using sunglasses, using prescription glasses, and smoking cigarettes.[70] Diagnosis is made clinically by

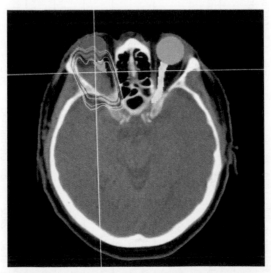

Fig. 3. A right orbital pseudotumor treated with IMRT.

Table 3
Summary of selected treatment results of orbital pseudotumor

Study	No. Patients (Orbits)	Radiation Therapy Treatment	Outcomes	Comments
Mokhtech et al,[67] 2018	20 (24)	20 Gy (4.8–40 Gy) at 2 Gy (0.8–2 Gy)/fx	40% CR, 35% PR, 20% SD, 5% DP	Most common toxicities; cataracts (10%) and dry eye (10%)
Prabhu et al,[66] 2013	20 (26)	Median 27 Gy (25.2–30.6 Gy)	35% PR, 5% CR with reduction in steroids, 45% CR with cessation of steroids	Older age and complete clinical response to RT reduced symptom recurrence
Matthiesen et al,[65] 2011	16 (20)	Mean 20 Gy (14–30 Gy)	25% CR with reduction in steroids, 56.3% CR with cessation of steroids, 18.7% required same steroid dose	3 patients received orbital retreatment. No increased morbidity noted on follow-up
Keleti et al,[64] 1992	28 benign, 20 lymphoma, 17 indeterminate	20–30 Gy/10–15 fx	RT efficacious in all groups. 84% DFS at 42 mo med FU; benign group did better	Cataracts developed in 46% of the patients treated with anterior-posterior fields
Lanciano et al,[63] 1990	23 (26)	20 Gy/10 fx	Overall CR 66%; soft tissue swelling 87% CR; proptosis 82% CR; extraocular dysfunction 78%; pain 75% CR; durable LC 77% (median FU 41 mo)	70% recurrence during steroid taper, 17% no response to steroids, 13% no steroids treatment before RT
Mittal et al,[62] 1986	20 benign, 12 lymphoma, 10 indeterminate	Mean 25 Gy	100% ultimate control rate	Very high local control, minimal morbidity
Austin-Seymour et al,[61] 1985	20 (20)	Mean 23.6 Gy (20–30 Gy)	75% complete resolution	Most steroid-refractory disease; no complications
Sergott et al,[60] 1981	19 (21)	10–20 Gy	Improvement 74% (decreased proptosis, lid edema, and conjunctival injection; improved ocular motility and VA	79% recurrence during steroid taper before RT. RT responders remained recurrence free × 25 mo FU with no further steroids

Abbreviations: CR, complete response; DFS, disease-free survival; DP, disease progression; FU, follow-up; LC, local control; PR, partial response; SD, stable disease.

recognizing the classic appearance of a wedge-shaped growth onto the cornea. **Fig. 4** shows a typical medial (nasal) pterygium that is extending onto the cornea. There is no commonly accepted scale for grading the severity of pterygia. Although surgery has been the primary therapy for this condition, recurrence rates are high, at 20% to 67%.[71] Medications can be used for symptomatic relief but do not stop progression. Postoperative radiation using a strontium-90/yttrium-90 beta-emitting contact applicator has been shown to reduce recurrence rates significantly, to 20% or less,[71,72] and in a randomized trial has shown to be significantly more effective than observation, with recurrence rates of 68% versus 0% with radiation therapy at a median follow-up of 14 months.[73]

Because pterygium is often considered a trivial problem, most datasets are small, and more evidence-based data are needed. The largest study analyzing the use of postoperative radiation in the treatment of pterygium was performed by Van den Brenk,[74] who found that using prophylactic postoperative beta radiation treatment with a strontium-90 applicator resulted in recurrences of only 1.4% of 1300 pterygia in 1064 patients (**Table 4**). Treatment consisted of 8 to 10 Gy given immediately after surgery followed by 2 more treatments at 7-day intervals. Local control is best when the radiation is given immediately after surgery,[75] with most published protocols requiring treatment within 3 days.[76–78] A retrospective study comparing high-dose (n = 28; 40 Gy in 2 fractions 1 week apart) and low-dose (n = 67; 20 Gy in a single fraction) strontium-90 treatment of pterygium suggested a benefit to higher doses. All recurrences (11) occurred in the low-dose group, with older age a marginal negative predictor of recurrence in the low-dose group, with no severe complications, including scleromalacia, occurring in either dose group with a median follow-up of 10 years.[79]

Kal and colleagues[80] performed a meta-analysis and found that recurrence rates for pterygia were less than or equal to 10% with a BED greater than or equal to 30. However, 2 randomized trials comparing dosing regimens in pterygium did not show improved control with higher doses. The first randomized patients to 30 Gy in 3 fractions over 15 days or 40 Gy in 4 fractions in 22 days, with no significant difference in 2-year local control (85% vs 75%) and no serious acute or late complications in either arm.[78] The second randomized patients to 35 Gy in 7 fractions (3 d/wk) or 20 Gy in 10 fractions (5 d/wk) using strontium-90 applicators. There was no significant difference in crude recurrence rates (7.1% vs 6.7%) or pterygium control (92.3% vs 93.9%; $P = .616$). Excellent or good cosmetic effect was favored in the lower-dose group (92% vs 70%; $P = .034$), and scleromalacia was more common in the high-dose group (5.6% vs 0%; $P = .17$).[77]

Other dosing schedules are also effective, as shown in **Table 4**. The primary use of radiation therapy as a nonsurgical treatment of pterygium also has been successful in

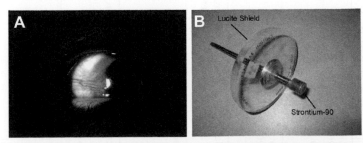

Fig. 4. Pterygium of the left eye. (*A*) The medial conjunctival tissue extends laterally onto the cornea, affecting the patient's vision. (*B*) The strontium eye applicator.

Table 4
Summary of selected treatment results of pterygium

Study	No. Lesions	Dose	Recurrence (%)	Comments
Viani et al,[77] 2012	216	5 Gy × 7 vs 2 Gy × 10 (randomized)	3-y LC 93.8% (35 Gy) vs 92.3% (20 Gy), $P = .616$	Significant benefit in lower group for cosmetic effect ($P = .034$), photophobia ($P = .02$), irritation ($P = .001$), scleromalacia ($P = .017$)
Nakamatsu et al,[78] 2011	74	30 Gy × 3 (15 d) vs 40 Gy × 4 (22 d) (randomized)	2-y LC 85% (30 Gy) vs 75% (40 Gy); no significant difference	No serious acute/late toxicity in either arm. Supports lower dose
Yamada et al,[79] 2011	95	40 Gy (n = 28) vs 20 Gy (n = 67) (retrospective)	Crude rates 0 vs 16.4	Suggests benefit for higher doses, including for larger size pterygia and in younger patients
Schultze et al,[87] 1996	64	5 Gy × 6	12.5 (median FU 5.5 y)	0% recurrence for primary lesions treated within 3 d after surgery
Paryani et al,[88] 1994	825	10 Gy × 6	1.7 (median FU 8 y)	No complications with higher doses
Dusenbery et al,[76] 1992	36 (recurrent lesions)	24 Gy (median) in 2–4 fractions	8	36% complications, higher if previously irradiated
Monselise et al,[89] 1984	135	6 Gy × 3	7.4	Relatively low doses
Alaniz-Camino,[72] 1982	485	7–8 Gy × 4	4.3	—
Van Den Brenk,[74] 1968	1300	8–10 Gy × 3	1.7	Largest series reported

reducing the size of pterygia.[81,82] Acute self-limited side effects of radiation include ocular irritation, scleral atrophy, and neovascularization. No late complications or side effects have been reported with fractionated therapy. Major complications, such as severe scleromalacia and corneal ulceration, have been seen in 4% to 5% of patients receiving single fractions of 20 to 22 Gy given postoperatively,[83] but rates can be lower or even absent in lower-dose treatments.[77,78] Significant complications have been reported in patients who received reirradiation.[76] Alternative methods for preventing recurrence include intraoperative or postoperative mitomycin C, postoperative thiotepa solution, postoperative 5-fluorouracil, and conjunctival autografting.[84–86] Successful prevention of pterygium involves educating the public to wear sunglasses, particularly those who spend significant time outdoors.

PEYRONIE DISEASE

Named after the personal physician of King Louis XVI of France, Francois Gigot de la Peyronie, who in 1743 described "rosary beads" of scar tissue extending the full length of the dorsal penis, Peyronie disease (PD) occurs in 3% to 5% of men between the ages of 40 and 70 years.[90,91] However, the true prevalence of PD may be underestimated because some men may are reluctant to report because of embarrassment and some attribute the condition to aging.

Also known as induratio penis plastica, PD is a localized connective tissue disorder characterized by severe curvature of the erected penis.[92] Scarring and formation of plaques that do not stretch with erection are thought to occur as a result of penile injury, trauma, or other nonspecific inflammation of the tunica albuginea.[90,91] Patients may initially present with painful erections, curvature, distortion and shortening of the penis, and psychological issues caused by associated physiologic or functional impotence.[93,94] Some degree of erectile dysfunction, either as a direct result of or in association with PD, has been observed in as many as 40% of affected men.[93]

Diagnosis is usually apparent from patient history and penile examination. A well-defined plaque or induration can be palpated on physical examination, especially in classic PD. Several imaging modalities have been applied to diagnose PD, including ultrasonography, plain radiography, CT, and MRI. Ultrasonography has the highest sensitivity for plaques in the tunica albuginea compared with other methods.[95]

Disease stabilization may take up to 6 months and occurs in approximately half of the cases. Reassurance alone is appropriate for patients who have minimal pain or deformity. PD has an overall spontaneous regression rate of 13%.[96] Penile pain occurs primarily during erection and usually resolves with 12 to 24 months of initial onset. Mulhall and colleagues[97] showed about 90% of 246 men who did not receive medical or surgical intervention reported complete resolution of pain at a mean follow-up of 18 months. At this moment, there are no placebo-controlled randomized trials that evaluate conservative therapy to reduce inflammation and pain in early-stage PD. Therefore, treatment of PD is symptom directed and it can include pentoxifylline, vitamin E, ibuprofen, and colchicine.[91,96] In addition to oral therapies, intralesional drug therapy is another potential option. Collagenase clostridium histolyticum is the only intralesional treatment approved by US Food and Drug Administration (FDA) for PD.[98] Other potential options include interferon alfa-2b, verapamil, and corticosteroids. Topical therapy is not recommended for the treatment of PD outside of clinical trials. Surgery to straighten the penis is indicated if the curvature interferes with sexual intercourse, and penile prosthesis is the treatment of choice for PD with erectile dysfunction.[91] Penile traction therapy has shown some efficacy in small case studies.[99,100] Iontophoresis, electromotive drug administration, has also been used but it needs further studies.[101] Extracorporeal shockwave therapy is currently under investigation.

Low-dose radiation therapy has been used to relieve pain and to improve plaque resolution.[93,102,103] External beam radiation, electron, and brachytherapy techniques using isotopic molds have been reported, with doses ranging from 250 to 2000 cGy.[92,96,104] **Table 5** presents some of the results of radiation therapy. The patient must be counseled, and special care must be given to gonadal protection and shielding. The potential for either spontaneous regression or progression must be considered. **Fig. 5** shows a patient who has PD being treated with electrons. The wax-coated shields protect the scrotum and the base of penis.

Table 5
Summary of selected treatment results of Peyronie disease

Study	No. of Patients	RT Treatment	Outcome	Comments
Pietsch et al,[102] 2018	83	32 Gy in 8 fx superficial x-ray	78% patients reported some response. 47% had symptom regression. Only 7% reported PD progression. Penile curvature was improved in 49% of patients	71% reported substantial pain relief. Transient erythema in 38.6% and 9.6% reported transient or chronic dryness. No severe side effects
Niewald et al,[103] 2006	154	30 or 36 Gy at 2 Gy per fx Co-60 gamma rays or 4-MV/6-MV photon beams	Improvement of deviation in 47%, reduction of number of foci in 32%, reduction of size of foci in 49%, and less induration in 52%. 50% reported pain relief	28 patients with mild acute dermatitis and only 4 patients with mild urethritis. No long-term side effects
Incrocci et al,[93] 2000	179	13.5 Gy/9 fx x-rays or 12 Gy/6 fx electrons	Pain relief 83% Deformity improved 23% Sexually active 72% Erectile dysfunction 48% Dissatisfied 49%	82% responded to questionnaire regarding sexual function. 29% had post-RT penile surgery
Koren et al,[92] 1996	265	Iridium-192 moulage	Success 66.4% fibromatous foci: CR 9% PR>50%: 29.7% PR<50%: 27.7% Pain relief: 61.4%	Pain relief and regression of deviation correlated with improved erectile function. 41 pretreated with potassium p-aminobenzoate, vitamins, topical corticosteroids, or RT
Rodrigues et al,[90] 1995	38	9 Gy/5 fx x-rays. Reirradiation for minimal response: 9 Gy/5 fx (16 patients)	Pain relief 66% (CR 12%, PR 54%). Improved curvature 40% Sexual function 47% Plaque: CR 24%, PR 8% Reirradiated group: pain relief 25% Improved curvature 28% Sexual function 28%	No RT morbidity Vitamin E effects not clear
Viljoen et al,[94] 1993	98	25 Gy (10 × 2.5 2.5 Gy), x-rays	Pain relief: 84% Angulation improved: 38.6% Sexual function: 87.2%	Progression in 18% Decline in sexual activity seemed age related

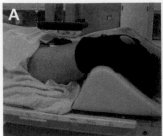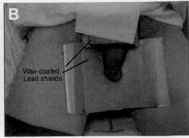

Fig. 5. Radiation treatment setup for Peyronie disease. (*A*) The patient is treated in a supine frog-legged position. (*B*) With proper lead shields, only the penis is exposed to radiation. (*Courtesy of* J. Mira, MD, San Antonio, TX.)

TRIGEMINAL NEURALGIA

Trigeminal neuralgia (TN) is characterized by recurrent brief episodes of unilateral electric shock–like pains, abrupt in onset and termination, in the distribution of 1 or more divisions of the trigeminal nerve (V1, ophthalmic; V2, maxillary; V3, mandibular), typically triggered by innocuous stimuli. TN is uncommon, with an annual incidence of 4 to 13 per 100,000 people.[105] It affects women more than men. Most cases of TN are caused by compression of the trigeminal nerve root by an aberrant loop of an artery or vein, usually in the root entry zone.[106] According to the International Classification of Headache Disorders, Third Edition (ICHD-3), TN is divided into classic TN, secondary TN, and idiopathic TN.[107] Classic TN includes cases caused by vascular compression. Secondary TN is caused by an underlying disease such as multiple sclerosis or a tumor along the trigeminal nerve. TN without clear cause is categorized as idiopathic.

TN is usually unilateral but it is bilateral occasionally. V2 and V3 subdivisions are more commonly involved than V1. Autonomic symptoms may include lacrimation, conjunctival injection, and rhinorrhea.[108] The diagnostic criteria for TN are listed in the ICHD-3.[107] It is recommended that all patients with suspected TN get brain MRI with and without contrast to look for an underlying cause such as brain lesion, demyelinating disease, or vascular compression. The preferred imaging modality is high-resolution MRI with thin cuts through the region of the trigeminal ganglion and heavy T2 weighting, a constructive interference in steady-state fusion study.[108] If a patient cannot get MRI, a CT cisternogram can be obtained. Sometimes TN can be confused with postherpetic neuralgia. Isolated involvement of the V1 subdivision is less than 5% in TN but very common in postherpetic neuralgia.[109] Dental causes of pain sometimes can be misdiagnosed as TN. Dental pain is usually continuous, intraoral pain that is dull or throbbing.

Carbamazepine is the first-line initial treatment of TN. Several randomized trials have shown its effectiveness (200–2400 mg daily).[110–112] Some studies suggest oxcarbazepine, clonazepam, gabapentin, baclofen, and lamotrigine can also be beneficial. Botulinum toxin injections may be beneficial for patients who do not respond to first-line medical therapies.[113] For patients with medically refractory TN, surgical options include microvascular decompression, rhizotomy with radiofrequency thermocoagulation, mechanical balloon compression, glycerol injection, and peripheral neurectomy and nerve block.[114,115]

Stereotactic radiosurgery (SRS) is a minimally invasive option for TN. It is preferred for patients with medically refractory TN who are not good surgical candidates. It aims at the proximal trigeminal nerve root. A typical dose of 70 to 90 Gy in a single fraction is prescribed to the 100% isodose line via a 4-mm cone. Stereotactic frame and high-

Table 6
Summary of selected treatment results of trigeminal neuralgia

Study	No. of Patients	Type of TN	RT Treatment	Outcome	Side Effects
Regis et al,[121] 2016	497	Classic	GKS, 70–90 Gy	91.75% pain free in a median time of 10 d (range 1–180 d). Probabilities of remaining pain free without medication at 3, 5, 7, and 10 y were 71.8%, 64.9%, 59.7%, and 45.3%	Hypesthesia rate at 5 y was 20.4%, but remained stable until 14 y. Very bothersome facial hypesthesia was reported in only 3 patients
Lucas et al,[118] 2014	446	Mixed	GKS, 80–97 Gy	Pain relief of BNI 1–3 at 1, 3, and 5 y in 86.1%, 74.3%, and 51.3% of type 1 patients; 79.3%, 46.2%, and 29.3% of type 2 patients; and 62.7%, 50.2%, and 25% of atypical facial pain patients	Only 13% of patients with atypical facial pain achieved BNI 1 response; 42% of patients developed post-GKS radiation surgery trigeminal dysfunction
Young et al,[122] 2013	315	Mixed	GKS, 90 Gy	170 patients (71.4%) were pain free and 213 (89.5%) had at least 50% pain relief	Eighty patients (32.9%) developed numbness after GKS, and 74.5% of patients with numbness had complete pain relief
Marshall et al,[123] 2012	448	Mixed	GKS, 80–97 Gy	By 3 mo after GKS, 86% of patients achieved BNI 1–3 pain scores, with 43% of patients achieving a BNI 1 pain score	26% patients reported facial numbness; 28% reported a post-GKS procedure for relapsed pain, and median time to next procedure was 4.4 y
Kondziolka et al,[124] 2010	503	Idiopathic	GKS, 80 Gy	Significant pain relief was achieved in 73% at 1 y, 65% at 2 y, and 41% at 5 y 43% of 450 patients reported recurrent pain 3–144 mo after initial relief (median 50 mo)	10.5% (53) developed new subjective facial paresthesia; these symptoms resolved in 17 patients
Smith et al,[125] 2011	179	Mixed	LINAC, 70–90 Gy	134 (79.3%) experienced significant relief at a mean of 28.8 mo (range, 5–142 mo). Average time to relief was 1.92 mo (range, 0–6 mo)	Numbness, averaging 2.49 on a subjective scale of 1–5, was experienced by 49.7% of the patients
Herman et al,[119] 2004	18	Recurrent	GKS, median dose of 75 Gy for first SRS and 70 Gy for second SRS	Among those with recurrent pain after initial SRS, 14 patients (93%) achieved excellent or good pain outcomes after repeat SRS	Two patients (11%) reported new or increased facial numbness after retreatment
Hasegawa et al,[120] 2002	31	Recurrent	GKS, median dose of 75 Gy for first SRS and 64 Gy for second SRS	After second SRS, 5 patients had an excellent response, 8 had a good response, 10 had a fair response, and 4 had a poor response. 48% achieved complete pain relief	2 patients (7.4%) experienced new sensory symptoms after first SRS, and 3 (12.7%) experienced new sensory symptoms after second SRS

Abbreviation: GKS, Gamma Knife radiosurgery.

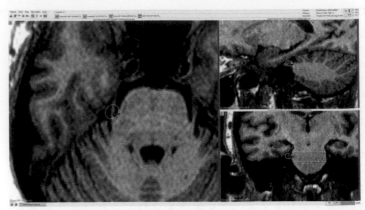

Fig. 6. High-resolution MRI with the target trigeminal nerve clearly identified for Gamma Knife radiosurgery treatment planning.

resolution MRI brain are generally required for treatment planning. The high-dose radiation causes axonal degeneration and necrosis. The major complication is facial numbness/paresthesia (<10%).[116] Both Gamma Knife SRS and linear accelerator (LINAC) SRS have been used. The typical response rate is 60% to 70%. The only prospective controlled trial that included 100 patients with at least 12-month follow-up showed that 83% patients were pain free at last visit. Six patients reported facial paresthesia and 4 patients reported hypesthesia.[117] There are more than 60 retrospective studies that showed the effectiveness of SRS for TN. Lucas and colleagues[118] described an Internet-based nomogram that predicts durability of pain relief based on pretreatment and posttreatment factors following SRS. Barrow Neurologic Institute (BNI) pain scale was used. Some studies suggest that repeat SRS after recurrent TN can still be beneficial with a reasonable safety profile.[119,120] **Fig. 6** shows an example of target delineation on MRI brain. **Table 6** provides a summary of the major studies.

SUMMARY

Although the evidence for radiation therapy efficacy on benign disease is largely retrospective, it has been shown to be quite effective as one of the treatment modalities for several benign conditions. In many cases, patients benefit from adjuvant radiation therapy in a multidisciplinary approach. By following the general radiation safety principles and established guidelines, the risk of major radiation therapy toxicity is low because only lower doses and smaller fields of radiation are normally used than those used to treat cancer. Most patients experience no or very few symptomatic side effects and achieve good long-term control and improved quality of life. However, clinicians must still carefully balance all of the potential risks against the benefits before proceeding with radiation therapy, especially in younger patients and children, who are expected to live long and may be at a higher risk of potential secondary malignancies and other late sequelae.

ACKNOWLEDGMENTS

This article was supported in part by the Departments of Radiation Oncology at Winship Cancer Institute of Emory University and University of Texas Health Science Center at San Antonio.

REFERENCES

1. Rodel F, Fournier C, Wiedemann J, et al. Basics of radiation biology when treating hyperproliferative benign diseases. Front Immunol 2017;8:519.
2. Berman B, Flores F. The treatment of hypertrophic scars and keloids. Eur J Dermatol 1998;8:591–5.
3. Niessen FB, Spauwen PH, Schalkwijk J, et al. On the nature of hypertrophic scars and keloids: a review. Plast Reconstr Surg 1999;104:1435–58.
4. English RS, Shenefelt PD. Keloids and hypertrophic scars. Dermatol Surg 1999; 25:631–8.
5. Abergel RP, Pizzurro D, Meeker CA, et al. Biochemical composition of the connective tissue in keloids and analysis of collagen metabolism in keloid fibroblast cultures. J Invest Dermatol 1985;84:384–90.
6. Bettinger DA, Yager DR, Diegelmann RF, et al. The effect of TGF-beta on keloid fibroblast proliferation and collagen synthesis. Plast Reconstr Surg 1996;98: 827–33.
7. Calderon M, Lawrence WT, Banes AJ. Increased proliferation in keloid fibroblasts wounded in vitro. J Surg Res 1996;61:343–7.
8. Younai S, Nichter LS, Wellisz T, et al. Modulation of collagen synthesis by transforming growth factor-beta in keloid and hypertrophic scar fibroblasts. Ann Plast Surg 1994;33:148–51.
9. Babu M, Diegelmann R, Oliver N. Fibronectin is overproduced by keloid fibroblasts during abnormal wound healing. Mol Cell Biol 1989;9:1642–50.
10. Smith P, Mosiello G, Deluca L, et al. TGF-beta2 activates proliferative scar fibroblasts. J Surg Res 1999;82:319–23.
11. Keeling BH, Whitsitt J, Liu A, et al. Keloid removal by shave excision with adjuvant external beam radiation therapy. Dermatol Surg 2015;41:989–92.
12. van Leeuwen MC, Stokmans SC, Bulstra AE, et al. Surgical excision with adjuvant irradiation for treatment of keloid scars: a systematic review. Plast Reconstr Surg Glob Open 2015;3:e440.
13. Guix B, Andres A, Salort P. Keloids and hypertrophic scars. Berlin: Springer; 2008.
14. McKeown SR, Hatfield P, Prestwich RJ, et al. Radiotherapy for benign disease; assessing the risk of radiation-induced cancer following exposure to intermediate dose radiation. Br J Radiol 2015;88:20150405.
15. Brown JJ, Bayat A. Genetic susceptibility to raised dermal scarring. Br J Dermatol 2009;161:8–18.
16. Marneros AG, Norris JE, Olsen BR, et al. Clinical genetics of familial keloids. Arch Dermatol 2001;137:1429–34.
17. Rockwell WB, Cohen IK, Ehrlich HP. Keloids and hypertrophic scars: a comprehensive review. Plast Reconstr Surg 1989;84:827–37.
18. Abrams BJ, Benedetto AV, Humeniuk HM. Exuberant keloidal formation. J Am Osteopath Assoc 1993;93:863–5.
19. Poochareon VN, Berman B. New therapies for the management of keloids. J Craniofac Surg 2003;14:654–7.
20. Zainib M, Amin NP. Radiation therapy in the treatment of keloids. Treasure Island (FL): StatPearls; 2019.
21. Mustoe TA, Cooter RD, Gold MH, et al. International clinical recommendations on scar management. Plast Reconstr Surg 2002;110:560–71.
22. Flickinger JC. A radiobiological analysis of multicenter data for postoperative keloid radiotherapy. Int J Radiat Oncol Biol Phys 2011;79:1164–70.

23. Kal HB, Veen RE. Biologically effective doses of postoperative radiotherapy in the prevention of keloids. Dose-effect relationship. Strahlenther Onkol 2005; 181:717–23.

24. Kutzner J, Schneider L, Seegenschmiedt MH. Radiotherapy of keloids. Patterns of care study – results. Strahlenther Onkol 2003;179:54–8 [in German].

25. Arnault JP, Peiffert D, Latarche C, et al. Keloids treated with postoperative Iridium 192* brachytherapy: a retrospective study. J Eur Acad Dermatol Venereol 2009;23:807–13.

26. Ollstein RN, Siegel HW, Gillooley JF, et al. Treatment of keloids by combined surgical excision and immediate postoperative X-ray therapy. Ann Plast Surg 1981; 7:281–5.

27. Borok TL, Bray M, Sinclair I, et al. Role of ionizing irradiation for 393 keloids. Int J Radiat Oncol Biol Phys 1988;15:865–70.

28. Mankowski P, Kanevsky J, Tomlinson J, et al. Optimizing radiotherapy for keloids: a meta-analysis systematic review comparing recurrence rates between different radiation modalities. Ann Plast Surg 2017;78:403–11.

29. Bertiere MN, Jousset C, Marin JL, et al. Value of interstitial irradiation of keloid scars by Iridium 192. Apropos of 46 cases. Ann Chir Plast Esthet 1990;35: 27–30 [in French].

30. Escarmant P, Zimmermann S, Amar A, et al. The treatment of 783 keloid scars by iridium 192 interstitial irradiation after surgical excision. Int J Radiat Oncol Biol Phys 1993;26:245–51.

31. Garg MK, Weiss P, Sharma AK, et al. Adjuvant high dose rate brachytherapy (Ir-192) in the management of keloids which have recurred after surgical excision and external radiation. Radiother Oncol 2004;73:233–6.

32. Jiang P, Geenen M, Siebert FA, et al. Efficacy and the toxicity of the interstitial high-dose-rate brachytherapy in the management of recurrent keloids: 5-year outcomes. Brachytherapy 2018;17:597–600.

33. Kim K, Son D, Kim J. Radiation therapy following total keloidectomy: a retrospective study over 11 years. Arch Plast Surg 2015;42:588–95.

34. Shen J, Lian X, Sun Y, et al. Hypofractionated electron-beam radiation therapy for keloids: retrospective study of 568 cases with 834 lesions. J Radiat Res 2015;56:811–7.

35. Emad M, Omidvari S, Dastgheib L, et al. Surgical excision and immediate postoperative radiotherapy versus cryotherapy and intralesional steroids in the management of keloids: a prospective clinical trial. Med Princ Pract 2010;19:402–5.

36. Malaker K, Vijayraghavan K, Hodson I, et al. Retrospective analysis of treatment of unresectable keloids with primary radiation over 25 years. Clin Oncol (R Coll Radiol) 2004;16:290–8.

37. Lo TC, Seckel BR, Salzman FA, et al. Single-dose electron beam irradiation in treatment and prevention of keloids and hypertrophic scars. Radiother Oncol 1990;19:267–72.

38. Byrne S, Beatty S. Current concepts and recent advances in the management of age-related macular degeneration. Ir J Med Sci 2003;172:185–90.

39. Verma L, Das T, Binder S, et al. New approaches in the management of choroidal neovascular membrane in age-related macular degeneration. Indian J Ophthalmol 2000;48:263–78.

40. Noble KG, Carr RE. Acquired macular degeneration. I. Nonexudative (dry) macular degeneration. Ophthalmology 1985;92:591–2.

41. Young RW. Pathophysiology of age-related macular degeneration. Surv Ophthalmol 1987;31:291–306.
42. Votruba M, Gregor Z. Neovascular age-related macular degeneration: present and future treatment options. Eye (Lond) 2001;15:424–9.
43. Comer GM, Ciulla TA, Criswell MH, et al. Current and future treatment options for nonexudative and exudative age-related macular degeneration. Drugs Aging 2004;21:967–92.
44. van Wijngaarden P, Coster DJ, Williams KA. Inhibitors of ocular neovascularization: promises and potential problems. JAMA 2005;293:1509–13.
45. Flaxel CJ. Use of radiation in the treatment of age-related macular degeneration. Ophthalmol Clin North Am 2002;15:437–44, v.
46. Jackson TL, Chakravarthy U, Slakter JS, et al. Stereotactic radiotherapy for neovascular age-related macular degeneration: year 2 results of the INTREPID study. Ophthalmology 2015;122:138–45.
47. Freiberg FJ, Michels S, Muldrew A, et al. Microvascular abnormalities secondary to radiation therapy in neovascular age-related macular degeneration: findings from the INTREPID clinical trial. Br J Ophthalmol 2019;103:469–74.
48. Jackson TL, Desai R, Simpson A, et al. Epimacular brachytherapy for previously treated neovascular age-related macular degeneration (MERLOT): a phase 3 randomized controlled trial. Ophthalmology 2016;123:1287–96.
49. Park SS, Daftari I, Phillips T, et al. Three-year follow-up of a pilot study of ranibizumab combined with proton beam irradiation as treatment for exudative age-related macular degeneration. Retina 2012;32:956–66.
50. Jaakkola A, Heikkonen J, Tommila P, et al. Strontium plaque brachytherapy for exudative age-related macular degeneration: three-year results of a randomized study. Ophthalmology 2005;112:567–73.
51. Marcus DM, Sheils WC, Young JO, et al. Radiotherapy for recurrent choroidal neovascularisation complicating age related macular degeneration. Br J Ophthalmol 2004;88:114–9.
52. Prettenhofer U, Haas A, Mayer R, et al. Long-term results after external radiotherapy in age-related macular degeneration. A prospective study. Strahlenther Onkol 2004;180:91–5.
53. Hart PM, Chakravarthy U, Mackenzie G, et al. Visual outcomes in the subfoveal radiotherapy study: a randomized controlled trial of teletherapy for age-related macular degeneration. Arch Ophthalmol 2002;120:1029–38.
54. Valmaggia C, Ries G, Ballinari P. Radiotherapy for subfoveal choroidal neovascularization in age-related macular degeneration: a randomized clinical trial. Am J Ophthalmol 2002;133:521–9.
55. Schittkowski M, Schneider H, Gruschow K, et al. 3 years experience with low dosage fractionated percutaneous teletherapy in subfoveal neovascularization. Clinical results. Strahlenther Onkol 2001;177:345–53 [in German].
56. Kobayashi H, Kobayashi K. Age-related macular degeneration: long-term results of radiotherapy for subfoveal neovascular membranes. Am J Ophthalmol 2000;130:617–35.
57. Chaudhry IA, Shamsi FA, Arat YO, et al. Orbital pseudotumor: distinct diagnostic features and management. Middle East Afr J Ophthalmol 2008;15:17–27.
58. Jacobs D, Galetta S. Diagnosis and management of orbital pseudotumor. Curr Opin Ophthalmol 2002;13:347–51.
59. Fujii H, Fujisada H, Kondo T, et al. Orbital pseudotumor: histopathological classification and treatment. Ophthalmologica 1985;190:230–42.

60. Sergott RC, Glaser JS, Charyulu K. Radiotherapy for idiopathic inflammatory orbital pseudotumor. Indications and results. Arch Ophthalmol 1981;99: 853–6.
61. Austin-Seymour MM, Donaldson SS, Egbert PR, et al. Radiotherapy of lymphoid diseases of the orbit. Int J Radiat Oncol Biol Phys 1985;11:371–9.
62. Mittal BB, Deutsch M, Kennerdell J, et al. Paraocular lymphoid tumors. Radiology 1986;159:793–6.
63. Lanciano R, Fowble B, Sergott RC, et al. The results of radiotherapy for orbital pseudotumor. Int J Radiat Oncol Biol Phys 1990;18:407–11.
64. Keleti D, Flickinger JC, Hobson SR, et al. Radiotherapy of lymphoproliferative diseases of the orbit. Surveillance of 65 cases. Am J Clin Oncol 1992;15:422–7.
65. Matthiesen C, Bogardus C Jr, Thompson JS, et al. The efficacy of radiotherapy in the treatment of orbital pseudotumor. Int J Radiat Oncol Biol Phys 2011;79: 1496–502.
66. Prabhu RS, Kandula S, Liebman L, et al. Association of clinical response and long-term outcome among patients with biopsied orbital pseudotumor receiving modern radiation therapy. Int J Radiat Oncol Biol Phys 2013;85:643–9.
67. Mokhtech M, Nurkic S, Morris CG, et al. Radiotherapy for orbital pseudotumor: the University of Florida experience. Cancer Invest 2018;36:330–7.
68. Char DH, Miller T. Orbital pseudotumor. Fine-needle aspiration biopsy and response to therapy. Ophthalmology 1993;100:1702–10.
69. Threlfall TJ, English DR. Sun exposure and pterygium of the eye: a dose-response curve. Am J Ophthalmol 1999;128:280–7.
70. Luthra R, Nemesure BB, Wu SY, et al. Frequency and risk factors for pterygium in the Barbados eye study. Arch Ophthalmol 2001;119:1827–32.
71. de Keizer RJ, Swart-van den Berg M, Baartse WJ. Results of pterygium excision with Sr 90 irradiation, lamellar keratoplasty and conjunctival flaps. Doc Ophthalmol 1987;67:33–44.
72. Alaniz-Camino F. The use of postoperative beta radiation in the treatment of pterygia. Ophthalmic Surg 1982;13:1022–5.
73. de Keizer RJ. Pterygium excision with or without postoperative irradiation, a double-blind study. Doc Ophthalmol 1982;52:309–15.
74. Van den Brenk HAS. Results of prophylactic post-operative irradiation in 1300 cases of pterygium. Am J Roentgenol 1968;103:723.
75. Aswad MI, Baum J. Optimal time for postoperative irradiation of pterygia. Ophthalmology 1987;94:1450–1.
76. Dusenbery KE, Alul IH, Holland EJ, et al. Beta irradiation of recurrent ptergia: results and complications. Int J Radiat Oncol Biol Phys 1992;24:315–20.
77. Viani GA, De Fendi LI, Fonseca EC, et al. Low or high fractionation dose beta-radiotherapy for pterygium? A randomized clinical trial. Int J Radiat Oncol Biol Phys 2012;82:e181–5.
78. Nakamatsu K, Nishimura Y, Kanamori S, et al. Randomized clinical trial of postoperative strontium-90 radiation therapy for pterygia: treatment using 30 Gy/3 fractions vs. 40 Gy/4 fractions. Strahlenther Onkol 2011;187:401–5.
79. Yamada T, Mochizuki H, Ue T, et al. Comparative study of different beta-radiation doses for preventing pterygium recurrence. Int J Radiat Oncol Biol Phys 2011;81:1394–8.
80. Kal HB, Veen RE, Jurgenliemk-Schulz IM. Dose-effect relationships for recurrence of keloid and pterygium after surgery and radiotherapy. Int J Radiat Oncol Biol Phys 2009;74:245–51.

81. Pajic B, Greiner RH. Long term results of non-surgical, exclusive strontium-/yttrium-90 beta-irradiation of pterygia. Radiother Oncol 2005;74:25–9.

82. Monteiro-Grillo I, Gaspar L, Monteiro-Grillo M, et al. Postoperative irradiation of primary or recurrent pterygium: results and sequelae. Int J Radiat Oncol Biol Phys 2000;48:865–9.

83. MacKenzie FD, Hirst LW, Kynaston B, et al. Recurrence rate and complications after beta irradiation for pterygia. Ophthalmology 1991;98:1776–80 [discussion: 1781].

84. Chen PP, Ariyasu RG, Kaza V, et al. A randomized trial comparing mitomycin C and conjunctival autograft after excision of primary pterygium. Am J Ophthalmol 1995;120:151–60.

85. Bekibele CO, Baiyeroju AM, Ajayi BG. 5-fluorouracil vs. beta-irradiation in the prevention of pterygium recurrence. Int J Clin Pract 2004;58:920–3.

86. Asregadoo ER. Surgery, thio-tepa, and corticosteroid in the treatment of pterygium. Am J Ophthalmol 1972;74:960–3.

87. Schultze J, Hinrichs M, Kimmig B. Results of adjuvant radiation therapy after surgical excision of pterygium. Ger J Ophthalmol 1996;5:207–10.

88. Paryani SB, Scott WP, Wells JW Jr, et al. Management of pterygium with surgery and radiation therapy. The North Florida Pterygium Study Group. Int J Radiat Oncol Biol Phys 1994;28:101–3.

89. Monselise M, Schwartz M, Politi F, et al. Pterygium and beta irradiation. Acta Ophthalmol (Copenh) 1984;62:315–9.

90. Rodrigues CI, Njo KH, Karim AB. Results of radiotherapy and vitamin E in the treatment of Peyronie's disease. Int J Radiat Oncol Biol Phys 1995;31:571–6.

91. Tunuguntla HS. Management of Peyronie's disease–a review. World J Urol 2001; 19:244–50.

92. Koren H, Alth G, Schenk GM, et al. Induratio penis plastica: effectivity of low-dose radiotherapy at different clinical stages. Urol Res 1996;24:245–8.

93. Incrocci L, Wijnmaalen A, Slob AK, et al. Low-dose radiotherapy in 179 patients with Peyronie's disease: treatment outcome and current sexual functioning. Int J Radiat Oncol Biol Phys 2000;47:1353–6.

94. Viljoen IM, Goedhals L, Doman MJ. Peyronie's disease–a perspective on the disease and the long-term results of radiotherapy. S Afr Med J 1993;83:19–20.

95. Andresen R, Wegner HE, Miller K, et al. Imaging modalities in Peyronie's disease. An intrapersonal comparison of ultrasound sonography, X-ray in mammography technique, computerized tomography, and nuclear magnetic resonance in 20 patients. Eur Urol 1998;34:128–34 [discussion: 135].

96. Furlow WL, Swenson HE Jr, Lee RE. Peyronie's disease: a study of its natural history and treatment with orthovoltage radiotherapy. J Urol 1975;114:69–71.

97. Mulhall JP, Hall M, Broderick GA, et al. Radiation therapy in Peyronie's disease. J Sex Med 2012;9:1435–41.

98. Gelbard M, Goldstein I, Hellstrom WJ, et al. Clinical efficacy, safety and tolerability of collagenase clostridium histolyticum for the treatment of peyronie disease in 2 large double-blind, randomized, placebo controlled phase 3 studies. J Urol 2013;190:199–207.

99. Levine LA, Newell M, Taylor FL. Penile traction therapy for treatment of Peyronie's disease: a single-center pilot study. J Sex Med 2008;5:1468–73.

100. Levine LA, Rybak J. Traction therapy for men with shortened penis prior to penile prosthesis implantation: a pilot study. J Sex Med 2011;8:2112–7.

101. Di Stasi SM, Giannantoni A, Stephen RL, et al. A prospective, randomized study using transdermal electromotive administration of verapamil and dexamethasone for Peyronie's disease. J Urol 2004;171:1605–8.
102. Pietsch G, Anzeneder T, Bruckbauer H, et al. Superficial radiation therapy in peyronie's disease: an effective and well-tolerated therapy. Adv Radiat Oncol 2018;3:548–51.
103. Niewald M, Wenzlawowicz KV, Fleckenstein J, et al. Results of radiotherapy for Peyronie's disease. Int J Radiat Oncol Biol Phys 2006;64:258–62.
104. Mira JG, Chahbazian CM, del Regato JA. The value of radiotherapy for Peyronie's disease: presentation of 56 new case studies and review of the literature. Int J Radiat Oncol Biol Phys 1980;6:161–6.
105. Katusic S, Williams DB, Beard CM, et al. Epidemiology and clinical features of idiopathic trigeminal neuralgia and glossopharyngeal neuralgia: similarities and differences, Rochester, Minnesota, 1945-1984. Neuroepidemiology 1991;10:276–81.
106. Love S, Coakham HB. Trigeminal neuralgia: pathology and pathogenesis. Brain 2001;124:2347–60.
107. Headache Classification Committee of the International Headache Society (IHS) the international classification of headache disorders, 3rd edition. Cephalalgia 2018;38:1–211.
108. Antonini G, Di Pasquale A, Cruccu G, et al. Magnetic resonance imaging contribution for diagnosing symptomatic neurovascular contact in classical trigeminal neuralgia: a blinded case-control study and meta-analysis. Pain 2014;155:1464–71.
109. Maarbjerg S, Gozalov A, Olesen J, et al. Trigeminal neuralgia–a prospective systematic study of clinical characteristics in 158 patients. Headache 2014;54:1574–82.
110. Rockliff BW, Davis EH. Controlled sequential trials of carbamazepine in trigeminal neuralgia. Arch Neurol 1966;15:129–36.
111. Nicol CF. A four year double-blind study of tegretol in facial pain. Headache 1969;9:54–7.
112. Campbell FG, Graham JG, Zilkha KJ. Clinical trial of carbazepine (tegretol) in trigeminal neuralgia. J Neurol Neurosurg Psychiatry 1966;29:265–7.
113. Guardiani E, Sadoughi B, Blitzer A, et al. A new treatment paradigm for trigeminal neuralgia using Botulinum toxin type A. Laryngoscope 2014;124:413–7.
114. Jannetta PJ. Microsurgical management of trigeminal neuralgia. Arch Neurol 1985;42:800.
115. Kanpolat Y, Ugur HC. Systematic review of ablative neurosurgical techniques for the treatment of trigeminal neuralgia. Neurosurgery 2005;57:E601.
116. Nurmikko TJ, Eldridge PR. Trigeminal neuralgia–pathophysiology, diagnosis and current treatment. Br J Anaesth 2001;87:117–32.
117. Regis J, Metellus P, Hayashi M, et al. Prospective controlled trial of gamma knife surgery for essential trigeminal neuralgia. J Neurosurg 2006;104:913–24.
118. Lucas JT Jr, Nida AM, Isom S, et al. Predictive nomogram for the durability of pain relief from gamma knife radiation surgery in the treatment of trigeminal neuralgia. Int J Radiat Oncol Biol Phys 2014;89:120–6.
119. Herman JM, Petit JH, Amin P, et al. Repeat gamma knife radiosurgery for refractory or recurrent trigeminal neuralgia: treatment outcomes and quality-of-life assessment. Int J Radiat Oncol Biol Phys 2004;59:112–6.
120. Hasegawa T, Kondziolka D, Spiro R, et al. Repeat radiosurgery for refractory trigeminal neuralgia. Neurosurgery 2002;50:494–500 [discussion: 500–2].

121. Regis J, Tuleasca C, Resseguier N, et al. Long-term safety and efficacy of Gamma Knife surgery in classical trigeminal neuralgia: a 497-patient historical cohort study. J Neurosurg 2016;124:1079–87.
122. Young B, Shivazad A, Kryscio RJ, et al. Long-term outcome of high-dose gamma knife surgery in treatment of trigeminal neuralgia. J Neurosurg 2013; 119:1166–75.
123. Marshall K, Chan MD, McCoy TP, et al. Predictive variables for the successful treatment of trigeminal neuralgia with gamma knife radiosurgery. Neurosurgery 2012;70:566–72 [discussion: 572–3].
124. Kondziolka D, Zorro O, Lobato-Polo J, et al. Gamma Knife stereotactic radiosurgery for idiopathic trigeminal neuralgia. J Neurosurg 2010;112:758–65.
125. Smith ZA, Gorgulho AA, Bezrukiy N, et al. Dedicated linear accelerator radiosurgery for trigeminal neuralgia: a single-center experience in 179 patients with varied dose prescriptions and treatment plans. Int J Radiat Oncol Biol Phys 2011; 81:225–31.

Palliative Radiotherapy
Inpatients, Outpatients, and the Changing Role of Supportive Care in Radiation Oncology

William Tristram Arscott, MD[a], Jaclyn Emmett, MSN, CNRP[b],
Alireza Fotouhi Ghiam, MD, MSc[c], Joshua A. Jones, MD, MA[d],*

KEYWORDS

- Palliative radiotherapy • Palliative care • Supportive oncology • Radiation oncology

KEY POINTS

- Palliative radiotherapy is a safe, effective treatment of many symptoms of advanced cancer.
- Wait times and poor care collaboration have led to the growth of dedicated palliative radiotherapy services in Canada, the United States, and around the world.
- Dedicated palliative radiotherapy programs have shown improved outcomes for patients in the inpatient and outpatient settings, including increased use of hypofractionated radiotherapy regimens, decreased hospital length of stay, and better collaboration with palliative care and hospice.
- The role of advanced radiotherapy techniques in palliative radiotherapy is still being explored, but may be more important as new data emerge.

INTRODUCTION

Shortly after radiotherapy was first used in the treatment of cancer in the late 1800s, a distinction was created between radical or curative radiotherapy and palliative radiotherapy with markedly divergent goals. In contrast with radical radiotherapy, in which the treatment goal is cure of cancer, palliative radiotherapy focuses on the application of radiotherapy to improve symptoms, with the goal of maximizing quality of life.[1] Palliative radiotherapy prescriptions have generally followed a less-is-more principle, in that short but effective regimens are chosen to maximize the ratio of palliative benefit to potential treatment toxicity, often using regimens containing 10 or fewer fractions, or even a single treatment. Palliative radiotherapy is appropriate both for treatment of primary

[a] Compass Oncology, 265 North Broadway Street, Portland, OR 97227, USA; [b] Inpatient Oncology, Department of Hematology/Oncology, Massachusetts General Hospital, 55 Fruit Street, Boston, MA 02114, USA; [c] Department of Radiation Oncology, British Columbia Cancer Agency (BCCA), University of British Columbia, 2410 Lee Avenue, Victoria, British Columbia V8R 6V5, Canada; [d] Palliative Radiotherapy Service, Department of Radiation Oncology, University of Pennsylvania Health System, Philadelphia, PA, USA
* Corresponding author. Department of Radiation Oncology, Perelman Center for Advanced Medicine, 3400 Civic Center Boulevard, TRC 2 West, Philadelphia, PA 19104.
E-mail address: Joshua.Jones@pennmedicine.upenn.edu

Hematol Oncol Clin N Am 34 (2020) 253–277
https://doi.org/10.1016/j.hoc.2019.09.009
0889-8588/20/© 2019 Elsevier Inc. All rights reserved.

cancers[2] as well as in the treatment of bone metastases,[3] brain metastases,[4] advanced disease in the lung,[5] and bleeding in various contexts.[6] Because of wait times in some health systems, dedicated palliative radiotherapy programs were created to help expedite consultation, simulation, and treatment of patients referred for palliative radiotherapy.[7] Clinics such as these show that patients referred for palliative radiotherapy often have symptoms that extend beyond radiotherapy indications,[8] leading to questions about how optimally to support patients referred for palliative radiotherapy. Many institutions have studied similar clinics in different contexts, with the aim of improving convenience, efficacy, and collaboration with other teams in caring for patients with advanced cancer who are referred for palliative radiotherapy.[9–12]

The modern era of cancer treatment includes personalized medicine, targeted therapies, and immunotherapies as well as complex radiotherapy treatment planning with three-dimensional (3D) conformal radiotherapy, intensity-modulated radiotherapy (IMRT), and stereotactic radiotherapy treatments available. In this era, questions have arisen about the utility of such advanced radiation techniques in palliative radiotherapy.[13] Algorithms are being developed to differentiate when simple palliative radiotherapy treatments are appropriate and when more advanced techniques are necessary. Treatment decisions may be divided into 2 distinct categories: 1 in which patients present with signs concerning for potential complications, and those already with symptoms that need to be addressed.[14] With the former, weight is placed on disease control to prevent complications, in which higher doses and longer treatment courses can be justified. In the latter, rapid relief of symptoms is crucial, thus using higher doses per fraction and fewer overall treatments.

Palliative radiotherapy assessments need to include an understanding of the patient's disease burden, performance status, prognosis, alternative treatments, potential side effects from treatment, and patient and family goals/values/priorities to come to a treatment decision regarding radiotherapy.[15] Moreover, an overall treatment plan should incorporate a multidisciplinary team, with consideration of how radiotherapy will be beneficial in the context of the patient as a whole and potential other treatment options. Once a decision has been made to proceed with a course of palliative radiotherapy, clear expectations for the effect of radiation treatments should be established. In addition, a plan must be made for addressing the additional components of caring for patients with advanced illness, using resources within the radiation oncology department or in the institution as a whole.

This article provides an update on the impact that dedicated palliative radiotherapy programs have had on the use of palliative radiotherapy, patient outcomes, and broader health system outcomes.

PRINCIPLES OF PALLIATIVE RADIOTHERAPY

Radiotherapy has long been established as an effective treatment of a multitude of symptoms of advanced cancer.[2,16,17] Potential indications for radiotherapy for patients with stage IV solid malignancies are described in **Box 1**. These indications include radiotherapy for pain from primary tumors or sites of metastatic disease, including bone, skin, and visceral metastases; neurologic deficits from primary and metastatic tumors to the brain, spinal cord, vertebral bodies (including spinal cord compression and cauda equina syndrome), and leptomeningeal metastases; bleeding from primary or metastatic cancer to the lung, head and neck, gastrointestinal (GI) tract, genitourinary tract, and gynecologic malignancies; respiratory symptoms from tumors of the head and neck and lung; obstructive symptoms; and after other palliative interventions have failed.

Box 1
Indications for palliative radiotherapy

Pain from:
- Bone metastases, including epidural spinal cord compression
- Bulky/painful nodal metastases
- Bulky primary or metastatic soft tissue site (including skin)

Neurologic symptoms from:
- Brain metastases
- Leptomeningeal carcinomatosis (or other malignant spread to leptomeninges)
- Spinal cord/nerve root compression
- Cauda equina syndrome
- Orbital/optic nerve metastases

Bleeding from:
- Oozing from any uncontrolled primary or metastatic disease site, including skin, head and neck, gastrointestinal (GI), genitourinary (GU), and gynecologic cancers
- Note: radiotherapy is generally not appropriate for control of arterial bleeding, and embolization or surgery should be considered in that context

Respiratory symptoms, including cough, dyspnea, and hemoptysis, from:
- Advanced primary or metastatic cancer in the lung, head and neck, or esophagus

Obstructive symptoms from compression of:
- Superior vena cava (SVC) causing SVC syndrome
- Airway obstruction
- Esophageal obstruction causing dysphagia
- Distal GI or GU obstructive symptoms
- Less well described for obstructive symptoms of the mid-GI tract, including bowel obstruction

Impending symptoms from:
- Impending pathologic fracture, asymptomatic cord compression, and so forth
- Note: this is less well described in the palliative radiotherapy literature and merits consideration of higher biological effective doses if the goal is durable palliation in a patient who begins asymptomatic; it also merits more detailed discussion for patients with short anticipated survival given balance between risk of side effects and potential benefits

Following other palliative intervention or other intervention that has not controlled symptoms:
- Surgery to bone, vertebral augmentation, stenting (ie, airway, SVC, GI tract), decompression of brain metastases, or spinal cord compression

Adapted from Jones JA, Simone CB. Palliative radiotherapy for advanced malignancies in a changing oncologic landscape: guiding principles and practice implementation. Ann Palliat Med 2014;3(3):193; with permission.

Several questions are critical to understand the goals of palliative radiotherapy. **Fig. 1** indicates some of the critical factors that are important in understanding potential options for palliative radiotherapy. Although formal algorithms exist for some disease sites (eg, brain metastases[18–20] and spine metastases[21,22]), these questions may help patients and clinicians to better reach decisions about the type and indications for palliative radiotherapy, regardless of clinical metastasis site.

Although shortened radiotherapy regimens (especially single fraction) with lower doses are appropriate for most patients referred for palliative radiotherapy, durable control may be important. For patients with a solitary metastasis and good performance status, the data for radical therapy is emerging, whether it be with ablative doses of radiotherapy, radiofrequency ablation/chemoablation, or surgery.[23–27] Recent data have also shown that patients with a low burden of metastatic disease (<3–5 metastatic sites) have a survival benefit following use of radiotherapy to

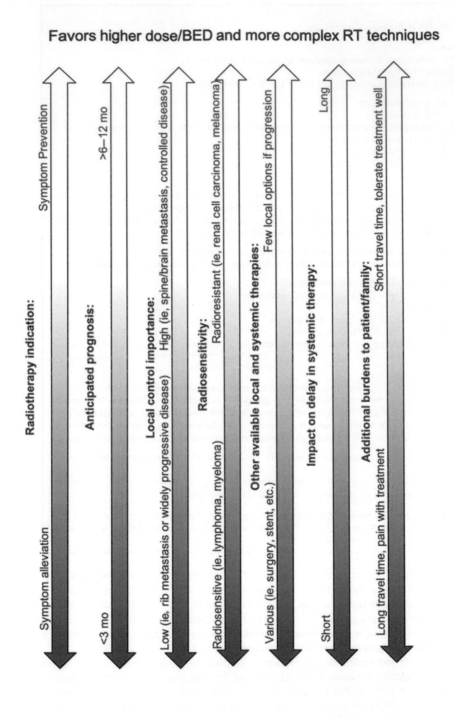

Fig. 1. Factors that affect radiotherapy in patients with stage IV malignancies. Enrollment in clinical trials should be considered for patients who are candidates for higher doses, including ablative therapies, or with more complex techniques. BED, Biological Equivalent Dose; RT, radiotherapy.

Table 1
Indications and sample palliative radiotherapy regimens by site and prognosis

Site	Common Symptoms	Poor Prognosis	Average Prognosis
Primary CNS malignancy	• Headache, nausea/vomiting • Focal neurologic deficits • Personality changes • Seizures	• 30–40 Gy in 10–15 fx • Supportive care alone	• 59–60 Gy in 30–35 fx
Brain metastases	• Headache, nausea/vomiting • Focal neurologic deficits	• Supportive care alone • Whole-brain radiotherapy, 20 Gy in 5 fx	• Based on size and number of brain metastases: • Whole-brain radiotherapy ± hippocampal avoidance IMRT • Stereotactic radiosurgery • Surgical resection
Head and neck	• Dysphagia/pain • Malnutrition • Speech changes • Bleeding • Airway issues: cough/dyspnea	• 14 Gy in 4 fx (BID)/mo to 42 Gy • 8 Gy in 1–3 fx • Supportive care alone	• 70 Gy in 35 fx • Altered fractionation • CRT
Breast	• Pain • Ulceration/bleeding • Brachial plexopathy	• 20–30 Gy in 4–5 fx • 8–10 Gy in 1 fx • Supportive care alone	• 30 Gy in 10 fx • 50 Gy in 20 fx • 42–66 Gy in 16–33 fx
Lung	• Pain (chest wall/plexopathy) • Cough/dyspnea • Hemoptysis • SVC syndrome	• 17 Gy in 2 fx in 2 wk • 8–10 Gy in 1 fx • Supportive care alone	• BED of 30 Gy in 10 fx or equivalent • Endobronchial brachytherapy for obstruction
GI (esophagus, stomach, colorectal cancers)	• Obstruction/compression of lumen • Dysphagia/odynophagia • Bleeding • Pain	• 30 Gy in 10 fx • 8–24 Gy in 1–3 fx • Supportive care alone	• 50 Gy in 25 fx • 50 Gy in 20 fx • 30–35 Gy in 10–14 fx • Brachytherapy
GU (bladder cancer, prostate cancer)	• Pelvic pain • Dysuria, frequency/urgency • Obstruction • Bleeding	• 14.8 Gy in 4 fx (BID) per month to 44.4 Gy • 8–2 1 Gy in 1–3 fx • Supportive care alone	• 30 Gy in 10 fx • 50–60 Gy in 20–30 fx • Brachytherapy
GYN	• Pelvic pain • Obstruction (ureteral, bladder, colon) • Dyspareunia • Bleeding	• 14.8 Gy in 4 fx (BID) per month to 44.4 Gy • 8–10 Gy in 1 fx • Supportive care alone	• 30 Gy in 10 fx • 50 Gy in 20 fx • Brachytherapy
Lymphoma	• Pain, obstruction, nerve root compression	• 4–8 Gy in 2 fx	• 20–40 Gy in 10–20 fx

(continued on next page)

Table 1 (continued)			
Site	Common Symptoms	Poor Prognosis	Average Prognosis
Oligometastases	• May be asymptomatic	• Consider no ablative therapy	• Stereotactic ablative radiotherapy by site or longer course radiotherapy
Uncomplicated bone metastasis	• Nociceptive pain • Neuropathic pain	• 8 Gy in 1 fx • Supportive care alone	• 8 Gy in 1 fx • 20 Gy in 5 fx • 24 Gy in 6 fx • 30 Gy in 10 fx • Stereotactic ablative radiotherapy if oligometastatic
Spinal cord compression	• Pain • Neurologic deficits including weakness, paralysis, numbness, bowel and bladder incontinence	• 8 Gy in 1 fx • Supportive care alone	• 20 Gy in 5 fx • 30 Gy in 10 fx • Separation surgery and stereotactic ablative radiotherapy (SABR alone only if clinical trial)

Abbreviations: BED, Biological Equivalent Dose; BID, twice a day; CRT, chemoradiation therapy; CNS, central nervous system; fx, fractions; GYN, gynecologic; stereotactic ablative body radiotherapy; SVC, superior vena cava.

Adapted from Lutz ST, Jones J, Chow E. Role of Radiation Therapy in Palliative Care of the Patient with Cancer. J Clin Oncol 2014;32(26):2915; with permission.

consolidate sites of active disease.[26,27] However, care must be used in applying these data, because there is still a risk of severe toxicity (in Palma and colleagues,[26] grade 5 toxicity was 4.5%). In more widely metastatic disease, care must be taken to choose dose and fractionation regimens that are likely to provide the intended benefit (ie, palliation of symptoms or preserving function) and not expose the patient to added toxicity (whether physical toxicity or from the burden of treatment time on the patient/family). Anatomic sites where disease progression is not salvageable (either by radiation or surgery), would result in potential functional loss (particularly neurologic), or could put the patient in a critical condition (hemorrhage or fistula formation) warrant careful consideration of the radiotherapy plan chosen. In these instances ensuring durable local control may warrant a higher dose and/or proceeding with a longer treatment regimen. However, the decision must account for the patient's performance status; the added risk of side effects from higher doses of radiation to improve local control may not be worthwhile in patients with a more limited life expectancy.

Table 1 provides a summary of dose and fractionation schemes, as well as suggested indications.

Palliative radiotherapy is an important component of cancer treatment for many patients with metastatic disease. It can alleviate symptoms, provide local control, and improve patients' quality of life. There is a vast array of indications for palliative radiotherapy.[28] Herein and previously,[17] the authors have reviewed the commonly used indications of palliative radiotherapy across the spectrum of patients with advanced and metastatic cancer. As shown in **Table 2**, a wide range of radiotherapy dose-fractionation schedules are available. Because, in many cases, there is insufficient evidence to recommend a particular dose-fractionation schedule rather than any other, the choice of the radiotherapy regimen is frequently based on the physician's clinical

Table 2
Prognostic models among patients referred for palliative radiotherapy

	Risk Factor	Points and Median LE
TEACHH Score		
Type of primary tumor	Breast, prostate	0
	Lung, other	1
ECOG performance status	0–1	0
	2–4	1
Age	≤ 60 y	0
	> 60 y	1
Number of prior palliative chemotherapy lines	≤ 2	0
	> 2	1
Hepatic metastases	Absent	0
	Present	1
Hospitalizations in prior 3 mo	No	0
	Yes	1
Sum points	0–1	20 mo
	2–4	5 mo
	5–6	1 mo
Chow Score		
Primary cancer	Breast	0
	Other	1
Site of metastases	Bone only	0
	Other	1
KPS	> 60	0
	≤ 60	1
Sum points	0–1	55–64 mo[a]
	2	19–28 mo[a]
	3	9–10 mo[a]
Oswestry Risk Index		
Primary tumor	Slow growth: breast, thyroid, prostate, myeloma, hemangioma, endothelioma, non-Hodgkın lymphoma	1
	Moderate growth: kidney, uterus, tonsils, epipharynx, synovial cell sarcoma, metastatic thymoma	2
	Rapid growth: stomach, colon, liver, melanoma, teratoma, sigmoid colon, pancreas, rectum, unknown origin	3
	Very rapid growth: lung	4
General condition (KPS)	Good: KPS 80%–100%	0
	Moderate: KPS 50%–70%	1
	Poor: KPS 10%–40%	2
Sum points	1	23 mo
	2–3	6 mo
	4–5	4 mo
	6	2 mo
	7	1 mo

Abbreviations: ECOG, European Collaborative Oncology Group; KPS, Karnofsky performance scale; LE, life expectancy.

[a] The median overall survival (OS) varied between the training, temporal validation, and external validation sets.

From Dosani M, Tyldesley S, Bakos B, et al. The TEACHH model to predict life expectancy in patients presenting for palliative spine radiotherapy: external validation and comparison with alternate models. Support Care Cancer. 2018;26(7):2219; with permission.

Table 3
Prospective studies using stereotactic body radiotherapy for patients with metastatic cancer

Study	Type of Study	Sample Size	Population	Treatment Arms	Dose/ Fractionation	Modality	Response Rate	Tumor Control	Survival Outcomes	Toxicity	Comments
Brain Metastases											
Sahgal et al	Meta-analysis of 3 RCTs	364	Patients with 1–4 metastases	SRS vs SRS + WBRT	—	SRS and conventional WBRT	—	Rates of distant brain failure similar in the 2 arms for patients ≤50 y of age; distant failure reduced with WBRT for patients >50 y of age Patients with single metastasis had lower risk of distant brain failure than patients who had 2–4 metastases. LC favored WBRT in all ages	Survival significantly favored SRS alone in patients ≤50 y of age. No significant differences observed in older patients. Patients with a single metastasis had significantly better survival than those who had 2–4 metastases	—	—
Yamamoto et al	Prospective observational	1194	Patients with 5–10 brain metastases with KPS ≥70	Single-fx SRS	22 Gy if <4 cm³, 20 Gy if 4–10 cm³	SRS	—	—	Median OS 13.9 mo with 1 tumor, 10.3 mo with 2–4 tumors, 10.3 mo with 5–10 tumors; OS for 2–4 tumors not noninferior to 5–10 tumors	AE in 8% total, 1 or more grade 3–4 events seen in 2% of patients with 1 tumor, 2% with 2–4 tumors, 3% with 5–10 tumors; no significant difference in proportion between patients with 2–4 tumors vs 5–10 tumors; 4 patient deaths (2 with 1 tumors, 1 with 5–10 tumors)	—

		N							
Chang et al	Prospective RCT	53	Patients with 1–3 newly diagnosed brain metastases	SRS vs SRS and WBRT	18 Gy for tumors ≤20 mm, 15 Gy for those 21–30 mm, and 12 Gy for those 31–40 mm in maximum diameter. Dose was prescribed to the 50%–90% isodose line	SRS and conventional WBRT	—	—	Freedom from CNS recurrence at 1 y: 73% in combined vs 27% SRS	Death at 4 mo: 13% SRS vs 29% SRS + WBRT	Probability of decline in learning/memory function at 4 mo 52% in SRS + WBRT vs 24% SRS alone; 1 G3 AE in SRS + WBRT vs 1 G3 AE in SRS, 2 G4 AE in SRS alone (radiation necrosis)
Shaw et al	Prospective phase 1	156	Adults with recurrent previously irradiated solitary primary and metastatic cerebral/cerebellar tumors ≤40 mm in maximum diameter (nonbrainstem)	SRS	18 Gy for tumors ≤20 mm, 15 Gy for those 21–30 mm, and 12 Gy for those 31–40 mm in maximum diameter. Dose was prescribed to the 50–90% isodose line	SRS	—	48% with tumor progression within SRS target volume (primary brain tumors with 2.85 relative risk and tumors treated on linac with 2.84 relative risk compared with GK)	—	Actuarial incidence of radionecrosis was 5%, 8%, 9%, and 11% at 6, 12, 18, and 24 mo following radiosurgery, respectively; 4 (3%) G5 toxicities	MTD was 24 Gy, 16 Gy, and 15 Gy for tumors ≤20 mm, 21–30 mm, and 31–40 mm in maximum diameter, respectively. Tumors 21–40 mm were 7.3–16 times more likely to develop grade 3–5 neurotoxicity compared with tumors <20 mm

(continued on next page)

Table 3
(continued)

Study	Type of Study	Sample Size	Population	Treatment Arms	Dose/ Fractionation	Modality	Response Rate	Tumor Control	Survival Outcomes	Toxicity	Comments
Lung Malignancy											
Bezjak et al	Prospective phase I/II	120	Medically inoperable patients with centrally located biopsy-proven, NSCLC ≤5 cm, node negative	SBRT	10–12 Gy/fx for 5 fx over 1.5–2 wk	SBRT	—	89.4% and 87.9% LC for 11.5 and 12.0 Gy/fx at 2 y	67.9% and 72.7% OS for 113 and 12.0 Gy/fx at 2 y, 52.2% and 54.5% PFS or 11.5 and 12.0 Gy/fx at 2 y	MTD 12.0 Gy/fx with DLT 7.2%	MTD was defined as the SBRT dose at which the probability of DLT was closest to 20% without exceeding it
Nonspine Bone Metastases											
Nguyen et al	Prospective, randomized, phase II noninferiority tria1	160	Adults with mostly nonspine bone lesions	SBRT or standard MFRT	Single-fx SBRT, 12 Gy for ≥4-cm lesions or 16 Gy for <4-cm lesions; MFT, 30 Gy in 10 fx	SBRT and conventional MFRT	SBRT had more pain responders than the MFRT group (complete response + partial response) at 2 wk (62% vs36%) (P = .01), 3 mo (72% vs 49%) (P = .03), and 9 mo (77% vs 46%) (P = .03)	Local PFS100% vs 90.5% at 1 y and 100% vs 75.6% at 2 y in SBRT vs MFRT, respectively	No difference in mOS (6.7 mo) or OS in ITT analysis	No differences were found in treatment-related toxic effects or quality-of-life scores after SBRT vs MFRT	Reirradiation rates nonsignificantly (P = .1) lower in SBRT group (0%) vs MFRT (2.2% and 5.3% at 1 and 2 y)
Spine Metastases											

Study	Design	N	Population	Comparison	Dose	Arm	Pain outcome		AE	Comments
Sprave et al	Prospective phase II	55	Patients with confirmed previously untreated spinal metastases	SBRT vs 3DCRT	24 Gy in 1 fx (SBRT) vs 30 Gy in 10 fx (3DCRT)	SBRT	No differences in VAS pain score at 3 mo, but pain values decreased faster with SBRT within 3 mo. Significantly lower pain at 6 mo with SBRT. No differences in OMED consumption at 3 and 6 mo. Trend toward improved pain response in SBRT arm at 3 mo, and significantly so after 6 mo	—	No G3 or higher AE in SBRT arm	—
Ryu et al	Prospective phase II	44	Patients with 1–3 spine metastases with NRPS score ≥5	SRS	16 Gy in 1 fx	SRS	—	—	No cases of G4 or G5 AEs	Phase II design showed the feasibility and accurate use of SRS to treat spinal metastases. Phase III component of RTOG 0631 to follow to compare pain relief and QOL between SRS and EBRT

(continued on next page)

Table 3
(continued)

Study	Type of Study	Sample Size	Population	Treatment Arms	Dose/ Fractionation	Modality	Response Rate	Tumor Control	Survival Outcomes	Toxicity	Comments
Garg et al	Prospective phase I/II	59	Patients reirradiated with SBRT after conventional RT	SBRT	27 Gy in 3 fx or 30 Gy in 5 fx	SBRT	—	76% radiographic 1-y LC	76% 1-y OS	2 patients with grade 3 lumbar plexopathy. No ambulatory dysfunction or grade 4 neurologic toxicity. Freedom from neurologic deterioration 92% at 1 y and 81% at 3 y	13 of 16 patients who progressed had tumors within 5 mm of the spinal cord; 6 of 13 developed SCC
Spinal Cord Compression											
Ryu et al	Prospective feasibility study	10	Patients with 1–2 contiguous vertebral metastases with or without SCC	EBRT followed by SRS	25 Gy in 10fx EBRT followed by SRS boost 6–8 Gy in 1 fx	EBRT and SRS	Complete relief in 5 of 9 patients, remaining 4 of 9 able to reduce pain medication; time to pain relief 2–4 wk, 2 patients with 0 out of 5 strength before treatment, 1 with complete motor recovery the other with partial recovery	—	—	No acute toxicity clinically detected during mean follow-up to 6 mo	—

		N	Population	Modality	Dose		Local Control	Overall Survival	Toxicity	Notes
Ghia et al	Prospective phase I	32	inoperable patients with MESCC	SRS	18–24 Gy in 1 fx depending on histology	—	1-y LC 89%	mOS 28.6 mo	No cases of RM with median f/u 17 mo	Incremental spinal cord constraint relaxation up to dose maximum of 16 Gy was performed
Liver Metastases										
Rusthoven et al	Prospective multi-institutional phase I/II trial	47	Patients with 1–3 hepatic lesions diameter <6 cm	SBRT	60 Gy in 3 fx in phase II arm	—	Local progression only in 3 lesions at median of 7.5 mo, 95% in-field LC at 1 y, 92% in-field LC at 2 y (100% if maximum diameter <3 cm)	mOS 205 mo	1 patient with G3 or higher AE	47 patients with 63 lesions, median f/u 16 mo, median maximal tumor diameter 2.7 cm
Hong et al	Prospective phase II trial	89	Patients with 1–4 liver metastases and Child-Pugh A	Proton SBRT	30–50 Gy equivalent in 5 fx, median dcse 40 GyE	—	1-y and 3-y LC 71.9% and 61.2%, respectively. Tumors ≥ 6 cm with similar 1 y LC 73.9%	mOS 18.1 mo	No G3–G5 toxicity	Median tumor size 2.5 cm. Median f/u 30.1 mo, KRAS mutation strongly predicted poor LC

(continued on next page)

Table 3
(continued)

Study	Type of Study	Sample Size	Population	Treatment Arms	Dose/ Fractionation	Modality	Response Rate	Tumor Control	Survival Outcomes	Toxicity	Comments
Oligometastatic Disease											
Palma et al	Randomized, phase II trial	99	Patients with controlled primary tumor and 1–5 metastatic lesions (93%–94% with 1–3 metastases)	SOC palliative treatment vs SOC and SBRT	Palliative, 8 Gy in 1 fx to 30 Gy in 10fx; SBRT, 30–60 Gy in 3–8 fx or single fx of 16–24 Gy for brain and vertebrae	3DCRT and SBRT	—	—	mOS 41 mo vs 28 mo control, mPFS 12.0 vs 6.0 in SBRT and SOC, respectively	AE grade >2 in 9% of control group vs 29% of SBRT group. TRD 4.554 in SBRT group vs 0% in control group	Randomized phase II screening design with a 2-sided alpha of 0.20
Gomez et al	Randomized, phase II trial	49	Patients with NSCLC and 3 or fewer metastatic lesions without progression after first-line systemic therapy	LCT (CRT/RT or resection) ± maintenance therapy vs maintenance therapy alone or observation (no LCT)	Wide variation (see study supplement)	SBRT, SRS, hypofractio-nated radiation (15 fx), or concurrent CRT	—	Local progression 52% with LCT vs 70.8% in no LCT	mPFS 11.9 mo vs 3.9 mo, 1 y PFS 48% vs 20% (consolidative vs maintenance)	5 patients in LCT with AE G <3,3 patients in no LCT with AE G <3, no G4 events or deaths in either arm	—

Abbreviations: 3DCRT, 3D conformal radiotherapy; AE, Adverse Event; EBRT, external beam radiotherapy; DLT, Dose Limiting Toxicity; f/u, follow-up; G3, grade 3; G4, grade 4; GK, gamma knife; GyE, gray equivalent; ITT, intention to treat; LC, local control; LCT, local consolidative therapy; linac, linear accelerator; MESCC, metastatic epidural spinal cord compression; MFRT, multifraction radiotherapy; mOS, median overall survival; mPFS, median progression-free survival; MTD, maximum tolerated dose; NSCLC, non–small cell lung cancer; NRPS, numerical rating pain scale; OMED, oral morphine equivalent dose; OS, overall survival; PFS, progression-free survival; QOL, quality of life; RCT, randomized controlled trial; RM, radiation myelopathy; RT, radiotherapy; RTOG, Radiation Therapy Oncology Group; SCC, spinal cord compression; SOC, standard of care; TRD, treatment-related deaths; VAS, visual analog scale; WBRT, whole-brain radiotherapy.

Adapted from Butala AA, Lo SS, Jones JA. Advanced radiotherapy for metastatic disease—a major stride or a futile effort? Ann Palliat Med 2019;8(3):337-351; with permission.

judgment and experience and must account for other factors, including the patient's physical and psychosocial status. A detailed discussion on the various radiotherapy dose-fractionation schedules in different clinical indications is outside the scope of this article.

High-dose palliative radiotherapy using advanced radiotherapy techniques, including IMRT, stereotactic body radiotherapy (SBRT) and stereotactic radiosurgery (SRS), are increasingly being offered to patients to gain durable local control with acceptable toxicities.[29] SBRT is becoming a more attractive radiotherapy option, particularly with radioresistant disorders (eg, renal cell carcinoma, sarcoma, and melanoma) and in patients with oligometastatic disease.[27] Data from a recent phase 2 study of 160 patients with bone metastases randomized to single-fraction SBRT versus 30 Gy in 10 fractions with conventional techniques show pain response rates at 3 months of 72% versus 49% and at 9 months of 77% versus 46%.[29] Although these data have not been replicated elsewhere, they raise the possibility that, in the future, more patients may benefit from complex radiotherapy techniques to help attain symptom control. **Table 3** summarizes the studies that compared conventional radiotherapy and SBRT in treating patients with metastatic disease.

DEDICATED PALLIATIVE RADIOTHERAPY SERVICES

The Rapid Response Radiotherapy Program was initially created at Sunnybrook Hospital in Toronto, Canada, to help with wait times for patients referred for palliative radiotherapy.[7] This program has become a model for programs in Canada and around the world, facilitating evidence-based radiotherapy delivered in a timely fashion and studying relevant outcomes of palliative radiotherapy including symptom relief, overall symptom clusters, patient and provider satisfaction with the clinic, as well as prognostic models for patients referred for palliative radiotherapy.[9] Moreover, the program has become a model for other inpatient and outpatient palliative radiotherapy programs, including the Dana-Farber/Brigham and Women's Supportive and Palliative Radiation Oncology (SPRO) program,[10] the Mount Sinai New York Hospital's Palliative Radiation Oncology Consultation service,[30] the InPROV service at Vanderbilt,[31] and the Palliative Radiation Oncology (PRADO) service at Oregon Health Sciences University.[32] Other groups have looked to move into more specialized areas, including establishing collaborations with palliative care for patients with brain metastases at the University of North Carolina[33] and Alberta, Canada,[18] as well as the STAT-RT[12] clinic at the University of Virginia.

The first clinical inpatient palliative radiotherapy program in the United States was developed between the Dana-Farber and Brigham and Women's Cancer Center's Departments of Radiation Oncology and Palliative Medicine.[10,34] This service, founded in 2011 and known as SPRO, provides a 24-hour clinical team of physicians and nurse practitioners to support the urgent and complex clinical care needs of patients with advanced cancers. Key clinical activities include comprehensive evaluation (including review of physical and psychosocial issues) and review of pertinent imaging, consideration of the role of radiotherapy and other palliative interventions, and communication with patients and families regarding radiotherapy and other care recommendations, such as symptom management, goals of care conversations, family meetings, and collaborative management with the patient's care team. Since the inception of SPRO, the palliative radiotherapy service has seen an increase in the number of weekly consults from 10 (pre-SPRO) to 16, of which ~60% are inpatient consultations. The dedicated service has been well received by referring and participating clinicians and has improved workflows and satisfaction among participating radiation oncologists.

Fundamentally, the key question with any palliative radiotherapy program is: what value is added by the service compared with traditional palliative radiotherapy referrals? The SPRO program from Dana-Farber Cancer Institute evaluated palliative care needs among patients referred for palliative radiotherapy and found that 82% of patients had at least 2 areas of palliative care domains that were relevant to their care, including physical symptoms, care coordination, psychosocial distress, and goals of care.[35] These issues are best addressed through a collaborative relationship with medical oncology and palliative care teams, ensuring that patients' symptoms, psychosocial concerns and values/goals are addressed in the context of their care. Innovative models allow improved integration with palliative care and palliative radiotherapy, allowing direct communication, sometimes even facilitating palliative care consultation during the palliative radiotherapy process.[36] Other programs have looked specifically to create mechanisms that incentivize use of the shortest possible and appropriate course of palliative radiation.[37,38] Such programs show sustained high rates of use of single-fraction radiotherapy for patients with uncomplicated bone metastases, improving the overall quality of care for patients receiving palliative radiotherapy.

Overall, the growth of dedicated rapid access palliative radiotherapy clinics worldwide[39,40] has shown positive outcomes related to patient, work flow, and health care outcomes including[41]:

- Rapid reduction in pain and other cancer-related symptoms
- Improved patient-reported outcomes
- Enhanced patient access to supportive services
- Decreased radiotherapy waiting times
- Reduced emergency visits and hospital admissions
- Improved radiation oncologist workload
- Increased referrals to palliative care
- Improved opportunities for education and research
- Evidence-based radiotherapy practice
- Decreased health care cost

For these reasons, a dedicated palliative radiotherapy service was started at the University of Pennsylvania in 2012, initially with a nurse practitioner seeing inpatient consults and subsequently with dedicated attending physician and resident coverage. The program saw a 50% increase in the number of inpatient and outpatient consults, leading to the development of a standardized outpatient rapid-access clinic for adults with metastatic disease who would benefit from an urgent assessment of the potential benefit of palliative radiotherapy. The goal of this clinic is to facilitate access to palliative radiation for a variety of cancer-related symptoms (mainly pain); to accelerate the process of consultation, treatment planning, and radiation delivery; to minimize the number of visits; and to avoid treatment delays and emergency admissions. Referrals from multidisciplinary team members are triaged by a palliative radiation oncology nurse. The patients are assessed initially by either a registered nurse or a senior radiation oncology resident rotating on the palliative service, followed by a palliative radiation oncologist. If palliative radiotherapy is indicated, the patient is simulated following the clinic visit in a dedicated time slot, with a plan to start the radiation treatment within 24 hours. When necessary, the clinic also expedites patient access to other supportive services and clinicians in the multidisciplinary team, such as medical oncology, orthopedic surgery, neurosurgery, dietitian, palliative team for symptom management, and psychosocial services.[42]

In addition to the development of dedicated palliative radiotherapy clinics, several efforts are underway to assess generalist palliative care skills among radiation oncologists and to help radiation oncologists to provide primary palliative care for patients referred for palliative radiotherapy.[43-45] These efforts are seeking to establish formalized guidelines for palliative care education for radiation oncologists, thereby narrowing any potential gaps between care provided in palliative radiotherapy clinics and that provided by general radiation oncologists.

PROGNOSTICATION AND COMMUNICATION WITH PATIENTS AND FAMILIES

Although it has been described that prognosis can affect patient and family medical decision making,[46] the impact of prognosis on clinical decision making in palliative radiotherapy has been less well studied. Part of the challenge is that prognosis for patients with advanced cancer referred for radiotherapy has changed dramatically. For example, a study comparing patients referred to the Rapid Response Palliative Radiotherapy Clinic in Toronto for bone metastases in 1999 and again from 2014 to 2017 showed significant improvement in median overall survival from 4.5 months for the 1999 cohort to 15.3 months for the cohort from the mid-2010s.[39] Moreover, studies of patients with brain metastases have shown that prognosis has improved dramatically over the past 20 years, with median survival in the best recursive partition analysis classification being slightly more than 6 months, whereas further refinement of the diagnosis-specific graded prognostic assessment[47] shows that patients with the best outcomes have a median survival of more than 2 years. Studies have shown that radiation oncologists, like other clinicians, are unable to always predict survival and, as a result, have trouble tailoring palliative radiotherapy courses specifically based on patient survival.[48] How, then, should prognosis and communication about prognosis be incorporated into the care of patients referred for palliative radiotherapy?

Many patients with advanced metastatic disease have limited anticipated survival. Studies beyond palliative radiotherapy have shown that discussions about advanced illness can affect anxiety, depression, and quality of life.[49-51] Studies from various palliative radiotherapy programs have been able to develop models for prognostication for patients with advanced cancer, including the Number of Risk Factors model,[52,53] the TEACHH (Type of cancer, Eastern Cooperative Oncology Group performance status, Age, prior palliative Chemotherapy, prior Hospitalizations, and Hepatic metastases) model[54,55] and the NEAT (number of active tumors [N], Eastern Cooperative Oncology Group performance status [E], albumin [A] and primary tumor site [T]) model.[56] Other prognostic models explore survival for patients with brain metastases and spinal cord compression. See **Table 2** for a comparison of the prognostic models.

INTEGRATION OF PALLIATIVE RADIOTHERAPY WITH SYSTEMIC THERAPY

The growing repertoire of targeted and immune therapies has expanded the options for patients who develop metastatic disease. Although extensive evaluation of their safety profile in combination with radiotherapy in the metastatic setting is lacking, the few published studies and reviews overall seem to show general tolerability when these new systemic agents are used in close proximity with radiotherapy, although there are certain exceptions. Toxicities from the combination of radiation with agents targeting vascular endothelial growth factor (VEGF) are commonly cited. Bevacizumab in combination with GI radiotherapy shows increased risk of GI bleeding,[57,58] as well as fistula formation when combined with thoracic radiation.[59] Other agents that inhibit VEGF, such as the multitarget tyrosine kinase inhibitors sorafenib and sunitinib, also show increased in-field GI toxicity when combined with palliative radiotherapy doses.[60,61] In addition, serious and fatal in-field toxicities have been seen when using anti-VEGF agents following SBRT in the GI tract (for review, see

Ref.[62]). Anti-VEGF agents with cranial radiation does produce some increased toxicity, although not to the same extent as that of the GI tract, and have been combined even in high doses for glioblastoma with acceptable toxicity.[63,64] Drugs targeting epidermal growth factor receptor (eg, cetuximab, erlotinib, gefitinib) seem to have low toxicity when combined with palliative radiotherapy to the thorax,[65,66] central nervous system (CNS),[67] and the GI tract.[68] Anaplastic lymphoma kinase (ALK) inhibitors, when combined with radiotherapy (ablative doses or protracted courses), do not seem to add toxicity.[67,69,70] Anti-Human Epidermal Growth Factor Receptor 2 agents (eg, trastuzumab, pertuzumab), when combined with radiotherapy, do not seem to increase toxicity.[71–73] B-raf proto-oncogene (BRAF) inhibitors (eg, dabrafenib, vemurafenib) combined with radiotherapy have well-documented toxicities, in particular radiodermatitis.[74,75] This reaction can be severe, with a European Collaborative Oncology Group (ECOG) consensus recommendation to hold the medication for 3 days or longer before fractionated radiotherapy and 1 day or longer before/after SRS.[74] There are limited published data describing experience combining poly-(ADP-ribose) polymerase (PARP) inhibitors (eg, palbociclib) with radiotherapy; however, a recent study in patients with symptomatic metastases reports the combination seems to be limited to mild grade 2 toxicities.[76]

Immune therapy is now established for patients with metastatic disease in most tumors, and the combination with radiation is an evolving paradigm.[77] Studies are emerging on its safety and tolerability when combined with radiotherapy in the neoadjuvant, concurrent, and adjuvant setting. There is even a potential survival benefit with combining immune therapies with brain radiotherapy in melanoma.[78] In general, the use of immune therapy with palliative radiation doses (to the CNS, thorax, abdomen/pelvis, skin) seems to adds only mild toxicity depending on the site irradiated; however, this generally resolves following completion of radiotherapy.[79–82] The experience in combining radiotherapy with adoptive cell therapies, such as chimeric antigen receptor T-cell therapy (CART) or dendritic cell therapies, is limited. Overall, radiotherapy may reduce the toxicity associated with certain immune therapies (ie, CART) by decreasing disease burden, whereas it could augment response to other therapies (ie, anti–programmed cell death protein 1/programmed death-ligand 1 agents) through increased antigen exposure. These questions remain to be answered.

RADIOTHERAPY NEAR THE END OF LIFE

Several systematic reviews and recent studies have evaluated the use of radiotherapy in the last 30 days of life.[83–85] Park and colleagues[83] describe that although only 10% to 15% of patients received radiotherapy in the last 30 days of life, 50% of those patients died during treatment, 69% completed their last treatment 10 days before death, and half of patients identified spent greater than 60% of their remaining life receiving radiotherapy. Poor performance status has consistently been identified as one of the strongest predictors for death.[85–89] A recent study from University of California, San Francisco also found that older age, lower body mass index, and inpatient status at the time of consultation were independent risk factors for death within 30 days.[85] The application of tools to estimate survival is essential to help clinicians decide the best treatment course (discussed earlier). Furthermore, patients enrolled in hospice care are less likely to receive protracted treatment courses within the last 30 days of life,[85,90] and early referrals to or discussions about hospice should be made for this patient population if a relationship has not already been established. Because of prognostic uncertainty, it will never be possible to eliminate radiotherapy use near the end of life, but it will continue to be important to provide short courses of radiotherapy for patients with short life expectancy to maximize the chance of benefit and minimize the likelihood of unnecessary burden.

SUMMARY

Palliative radiotherapy is a safe, effective treatment option for many symptoms of advanced cancer, often delivered with few side effects. The growth of dedicated palliative radiotherapy services has helped to provide optimal clinical care for patients with advanced cancer and has helped to spur research into the optimal use of palliative radiotherapy as well as opportunities for continued work in education and research. As the landscape of advanced cancer care changes with improvements in systemic therapy, so too are there changes in the world of palliative radiotherapy. Many questions remain regarding palliative care and radiation oncology:

- What is the optimal timing for palliative radiotherapy, particularly for patients with longer anticipated survival?
- When is radiotherapy near the end of life indicated?
- What is the role of advanced techniques for patients receiving palliative radiotherapy?
- What are the optimal models for integration of palliative care and radiation oncology, ensuring that the radiotherapy consultation assesses patients in a holistic manner?
- How do clinicians optimally communicate with patients and families about prognosis, values, priorities, and goals of care?
- How do clinicians ensure that all radiation oncologists have the basic palliative care skills to care for patients with advanced cancer, both with long anticipated survival and near the end of life?

The development of dedicated palliative radiotherapy programs in the inpatient and outpatient settings has begun to answer some of these questions. More program development, quality improvement initiatives, and clinical studies will be important to continue to advance the science and the art of palliative radiotherapy.

DISCLOSURE STATEMENT

The authors have nothing to disclose.

REFERENCES

1. Jones J. A brief history of palliative radiation oncology. In: Lutz S, Chow E, Hoskin P, editors. Radiation oncology in palliative cancer care. First. West Sussex: Wiley-Blackwell; 2013. p. 3–14.
2. Lutz ST, Jones J, Chow E. Role of radiation therapy in palliative care of the patient with cancer. J Clin Oncol 2014;32(26):2913–9.
3. Lutz S, Balboni T, Jones J, et al. Palliative radiation therapy for bone metastases: update of an ASTRO evidence-based guideline. Pract Radiat Oncol 2017; 7(1):4–12.
4. Tsao MN, Khuntia D, Mehta MP. Brain metastases: what's new with an old problem? Curr Opin Support Palliat Care 2012;6(1):85–90.
5. Moeller B, Balagamwala EH, Chen A, et al. Palliative thoracic radiation therapy for non-small cell lung cancer: 2018 update of an American Society for Radiation

Oncology (ASTRO) evidence-based guideline. Pract Radiat Oncol 2018;8(4): 245–50.

6. Johnstone C, Rich SE. Bleeding in cancer patients and its treatment: a review. Ann Palliat Med 2018;7(2):265–73.

7. Danjoux C, Chow E, Drossos A, et al. An innovative rapid response radiotherapy program to reduce waiting time for palliative radiotherapy. Support Care Cancer 2006;14(1):38–43.

8. Chen E, Nguyen J, Cramarossa G, et al. Symptom clusters in patients with advanced cancer: sub-analysis of patients reporting exclusively non-zero ESAS scores. Palliat Med 2012;26(6):826–33.

9. Johnstone C. Palliative radiation oncology programs: design, build, succeed! Ann Palliat Med 2019;8(3):264–73.

10. Gorman D, Balboni T, Taylor A, et al. The supportive and palliative radiation oncology service: a dedicated model for palliative radiation oncology care. J Adv Pract Oncol 2015;6(2):135–40. Available at: http://www.ncbi.nlm.nih.gov/pubmed/26649246. Accessed August 28, 2019.

11. Blackhall LJ, Read P, Stukenborg G, et al. CARE track for advanced cancer: impact and timing of an outpatient palliative care clinic. J Palliat Med 2016; 19(1):57–63.

12. Wilson DD, Alonso CE, Sim AJ, et al. STAT RT: a prospective pilot clinical trial of Scan-Plan-QA-Treat stereotactic body radiation therapy for painful osseous metastases. Ann Palliat Med 2019;8:1207.

13. Butala AA, Lo SS, Jones JA. Advanced radiotherapy for metastatic disease—a major stride or a futile effort? Ann Palliat Med 2019;8(3):337–51.

14. van Oorschot B, Rades D, Schulze W, et al. Palliative radiotherapy–new approaches. Semin Oncol 2011;38(3):443–9.

15. Jones JA, Simone CB II. Palliative radiotherapy for advanced malignancies in a changing oncologic landscape: guiding principles and practice implementation. Ann Palliat Med 2014;3(3):192–202. Available at: http://www.amepc.org/apm/article/view/4147/5062. Accessed September 22, 2014.

16. Spencer K, Parrish R, Barton R, et al. Palliative radiotherapy. BMJ 2018;360:k821.

17. Sharma S, Hertan L, Jones J. Palliative radiotherapy: current status and future directions. Semin Oncol 2014. https://doi.org/10.1053/j.seminoncol.2014.09.021.

18. Danielson B, Fairchild A. Beyond palliative radiotherapy: a pilot multidisciplinary brain metastases clinic. Support Care Cancer 2012;20(4):773–81.

19. Jung H, Sinnarajah A, Enns B, et al. Managing brain metastases patients with and without radiotherapy: initial lessons from a team-based consult service through a multidisciplinary integrated palliative oncology clinic. Support Care Cancer 2013; 21(12):3379–86.

20. Tsao MN, Rades D, Wirth A, et al. Radiotherapeutic and surgical management for newly diagnosed brain metastasis(es): an American Society for Radiation Oncology evidence-based guideline. Pract Radiat Oncol 2012;2(3):210–25.

21. Barzilai O, Versteeg AL, Sahgal A, et al. Survival, local control, and health-related quality of life in patients with oligometastatic and polymetastatic spinal tumors: a multicenter, international study. Cancer 2019;125(5):770–8.

22. Laufer I, Rubin DG, Lis E, et al. The NOMS framework: approach to the treatment of spinal metastatic tumors. Oncologist 2013;18(6):744–51.

23. Aloia TA, Vauthey J-N, Loyer EM, et al. Solitary colorectal liver metastasis: resection determines outcome. Arch Surg 2006;141(5):460–7.

24. Lee BC, Lee HG, Park IJ, et al. The role of radiofrequency ablation for treatment of metachronous isolated hepatic metastasis from colorectal cancer. Medicine (Baltimore) 2016;95(39):e4999.
25. Gomez DR, Blumenschein GRJ, Lee JJ, et al. Local consolidative therapy versus maintenance therapy or observation for patients with oligometastatic non-small-cell lung cancer without progression after first-line systemic therapy: a multicentre, randomised, controlled, phase 2 study. Lancet Oncol 2016;17(12): 1672–82.
26. Palma DA, Olson R, Harrow S, et al. Stereotactic ablative radiotherapy versus standard of care palliative treatment in patients with oligometastatic cancers (SABR-COMET): a randomised, phase 2, open-label trial. Lancet 2019; 393(10185):2051–8.
27. Gomez DR, Tang C, Zhang J, et al. Local consolidative therapy vs. maintenance therapy or observation for patients with oligometastatic non-small-cell lung cancer: long-term results of a multi-institutional, phase II, randomized study. J Clin Oncol 2019;37(18):1558–65.
28. Lam TC, Tseng Y. Defining the radiation oncologist's role in palliative care and radiotherapy. Ann Palliat Med 2019;8(3):246–63.
29. Nguyen Q-N, Chun SG, Chow E, et al. Single-fraction stereotactic vs conventional multifraction radiotherapy for pain relief in patients with predominantly nonspine bone metastases. JAMA Oncol 2019;5(6):872.
30. Chang S, May P, Goldstein NE, et al. A palliative radiation oncology consult service's impact on care of advanced cancer patients. J Palliat Med 2018;21(4): 438–44.
31. Stavas MJ, Pagan JD, Varma S, et al. Building a palliative radiation oncology program: from bedside to B.E.D. Pract Radiat Oncol 2017;7(3):203–8.
32. Mitin T, Thomas CR, Jaboin JJ. PRADO: a palliative care model for every radiation oncology practice. Int J Radiat Oncol Biol Phys 2017;99(3):518–9.
33. McKee MJ, Keith K, Deal AM, et al. A multidisciplinary breast cancer brain metastases clinic: the University of North Carolina experience. Oncologist 2016; 21(1):16–20.
34. Tseng YD, Krishnan MS, Jones JA, et al. Supportive and palliative radiation oncology service: impact of a dedicated service on palliative cancer care. Pract Radiat Oncol 2014;4(4):247–53.
35. Parker GM, LeBaron VT, Krishnan M, et al. Burden of palliative care issues encountered by radiation oncologists caring for patients with advanced cancer. Pract Radiat Oncol 2017;7(6):e517–24.
36. Wilson D, Sheng K, Yang W, et al. STAT-RAD: a potential real-time radiation therapy workflow. In: Natanasabapathi G, editor. Modern practices in radiation therapy. London: InTech; 2012. p. 1–19. https://doi.org/10.5772/2019.
37. Olson RA, Tiwana MS, Barnes M, et al. Use of single- versus multiple-fraction palliative radiation therapy for bone metastases: population-based analysis of 16,898 courses in a Canadian Province. Int J Radiat Oncol Biol Phys 2014; 89(5):1092–9.
38. Olson RA, Tiwana M, Barnes M, et al. Impact of using audit data to improve the evidence-based use of single-fraction radiation therapy for bone metastases in British Columbia. Int J Radiat Oncol Biol Phys 2016;94(1):40–7.
39. Razvi Y, Chan S, Zhang L, et al. A review of the rapid response radiotherapy program in patients with advanced cancer referred for palliative radiotherapy over two decades. Support Care Cancer 2019;27(6):2131–4.

40. Dennis K, Linden K, Balboni T, et al. Rapid access palliative radiation therapy programs: an efficient model of care. Future Oncol 2015;11(17):2417–26.
41. Lefresne S, Olson R, Cashman R, et al. Prospective analysis of patient reported symptoms and quality of life in patients with incurable lung cancer treated in a rapid access clinic. Lung Cancer 2017;112:35–40.
42. Davis E, Jones J, Proud C. Development of the rapid access radiotherapy clinic at the University of Pennsylvania. Chicago: Society of Radiation Oncology Administrators; 2019.
43. Wei RL, Mattes MD, Yu J, et al. Attitudes of radiation oncologists toward palliative and supportive care in the United States: report on national membership survey by the American Society for Radiation Oncology (ASTRO). Pract Radiat Oncol 2017;7(2):113–9.
44. Krishnan M, Racsa M, Jones J, et al. Radiation oncology resident palliative education. Pract Radiat Oncol 2017;7(6):e439–48.
45. Wei RL, Colbert LE, Jones J, et al. Palliative care and palliative radiation therapy education in radiation oncology: a survey of US radiation oncology program directors. Pract Radiat Oncol 2017;7(4):234–40.
46. Gilligan T, Coyle N, Frankel RM, et al. Patient-clinician communication: American Society of Clinical Oncology Consensus guideline. J Clin Oncol 2017;35(31):3618–32.
47. Nieder C, Marienhagen K, Dalhaug A, et al. Prognostic models predicting survival of patients with brain metastases: integration of lactate dehydrogenase, albumin and extracranial organ involvement. Clin Oncol (R Coll Radiol) 2014;26(8):447–52.
48. Gripp S, Mjartan S, Boelke E, et al. Palliative radiotherapy tailored to life expectancy in end-stage cancer patients: reality or myth? Cancer 2010;116(13):3251–6.
49. Bernacki R, Paladino J, Neville BA, et al. Effect of the serious illness care program in outpatient oncology. JAMA Intern Med 2019;179(6):751.
50. Hoerger M, Epstein RM, Winters PC, et al. Values and options in cancer care (VOICE): study design and rationale for a patient-centered communication and decision-making intervention for physicians, patients with advanced cancer, and their caregivers. BMC Cancer 2013;13:188.
51. Jackson VA, Jacobsen J, Greer JA, et al. The cultivation of prognostic awareness through the provision of early palliative care in the ambulatory setting: a communication guide. J Palliat Med 2013;16(8):894–900.
52. Chow E, Abdolell M, Panzarella T, et al. Predictive model for survival in patients with advanced cancer. J Clin Oncol 2008;26(36):5863–9.
53. Glare P, Shariff I, Thaler HT. External validation of the number of risk factors score in a palliative care outpatient clinic at a comprehensive cancer center. J Palliat Med 2014;17(7):797–802.
54. Dosani M, Tyldesley S, Bakos B, et al. The TEACHH model to predict life expectancy in patients presenting for palliative spine radiotherapy: external validation and comparison with alternate models. Support Care Cancer 2018;26(7):2217–27.
55. Krishnan MS, Epstein-Peterson Z, Chen Y-H, et al. Predicting life expectancy in patients with metastatic cancer receiving palliative radiotherapy: the TEACHH model. Cancer 2014;120(1):134–41.
56. Zucker A, Tsai CJ, Loscalzo J, et al. The NEAT predictive model for survival in patients with advanced cancer. Cancer Res Treat 2018;50(4):1433–43.

57. Lordick F, Geinitz H, Theisen J, et al. Increased risk of ischemic bowel complications during treatment with bevacizumab after pelvic irradiation: report of three cases. Int J Radiat Oncol Biol Phys 2006;64(5):1295–8.

58. Crane CH, Ellis LM, Abbruzzese JL, et al. Phase I trial evaluating the safety of bevacizumab with concurrent radiotherapy and capecitabine in locally advanced pancreatic cancer. J Clin Oncol 2006;24(7):1145–51.

59. Spigel DR, Hainsworth JD, Yardley DA, et al. Tracheoesophageal fistula formation in patients with lung cancer treated with chemoradiation and bevacizumab. J Clin Oncol 2010;28(1):43–8.

60. Murray L, Longo J, Wan J, et al. Phase I dose escalation study of concurrent palliative radiation therapy with sorafenib in three anatomical cohorts (Thorax, Abdomen, Pelvis): the TAP study. Radiother Oncol 2017;124(1):74–9.

61. Peters NAJB, Richel DJ, Verhoeff JJC, et al. Bowel perforation after radiotherapy in a patient receiving sorafenib. J Clin Oncol 2008;26(14):2405–6.

62. Pollom EL, Deng L, Pai RK, et al. Gastrointestinal toxicities with combined antiangiogenic and stereotactic body radiation therapy. Int J Radiat Oncol Biol Phys 2015;92(3):568–76.

63. Chinot OL, Wick W, Mason W, et al. Bevacizumab plus radiotherapy-temozolomide for newly diagnosed glioblastoma. N Engl J Med 2014;370(8): 709–22.

64. Chinot OL, de La Motte Rouge T, Moore N, et al. AVAglio: phase 3 trial of bevacizumab plus temozolomide and radiotherapy in newly diagnosed glioblastoma multiforme. Adv Ther 2011;28(4):334–40.

65. Iyengar P, Kavanagh BD, Wardak Z, et al. Phase II trial of stereotactic body radiation therapy combined with erlotinib for patients with limited but progressive metastatic non-small-cell lung cancer. J Clin Oncol 2014;32(34):3824–30.

66. Swaminath A, Wright JR, Tsakiridis TK, et al. A phase II trial of erlotinib and concurrent palliative thoracic radiation for patients with non-small-cell lung cancer. Clin Lung Cancer 2016;17(2):142–9.

67. Hendriks LEL, Schoenmaekers J, Zindler JD, et al. Safety of cranial radiotherapy concurrent with tyrosine kinase inhibitors in non-small cell lung cancer patients: a systematic review. Cancer Treat Rev 2015;41(7):634–45.

68. Valentini V, De Paoli A, Gambacorta MA, et al. Infusional 5-fluorouracil and ZD1839 (Gefitinib-Iressa) in combination with preoperative radiotherapy in patients with locally advanced rectal cancer: a phase I and II Trial (1839IL/0092). Int J Radiat Oncol Biol Phys 2008;72(3):644–9.

69. Gan GN, Weickhardt AJ, Scheier B, et al. Stereotactic radiation therapy can safely and durably control sites of extra-central nervous system oligoprogressive disease in anaplastic lymphoma kinase-positive lung cancer patients receiving crizotinib. Int J Radiat Oncol Biol Phys 2014;88(4):892–8.

70. Ni J, Li G, Yang X, et al. Optimal timing and clinical value of radiotherapy in advanced ALK-rearranged non-small cell lung cancer with or without baseline brain metastases: implications from pattern of failure analyses. Radiat Oncol 2019;14(1):44.

71. Halyard MY, Pisansky TM, Dueck AC, et al. Radiotherapy and adjuvant trastuzumab in operable breast cancer: tolerability and adverse event data from the NCCTG phase III trial N9831. J Clin Oncol 2009;27(16):2638–44.

72. Belkacemi Y, Gligorov J, Ozsahin M, et al. Concurrent trastuzumab with adjuvant radiotherapy in HER2-positive breast cancer patients: acute toxicity analyses from the French multicentric study. Ann Oncol 2008;19(6):1110–6.

73. Ajgal Z, de Percin S, Dieras V, et al. Combination of radiotherapy and double blockade HER2 with pertuzumab and trastuzumab for HER2-positive metastatic or locally recurrent unresectable and/or metastatic breast cancer: assessment of early toxicity. Cancer Radiother 2017;21(2):114–8.

74. Anker CJ, Grossmann KF, Atkins MB, et al. Avoiding severe toxicity from combined BRAF inhibitor and radiation treatment: consensus guidelines from the Eastern Cooperative Oncology Group (ECOG). Int J Radiat Oncol Biol Phys 2016;95(2):632–46.

75. Schulze B, Meissner M, Wolter M, et al. Unusual acute and delayed skin reactions during and after whole-brain radiotherapy in combination with the BRAF inhibitor vemurafenib. Two case reports. Strahlenther Onkol 2014;190(2):229–32.

76. Chowdhary M, Sen N, Chowdhary A, et al. Safety and efficacy of palbociclib and radiation therapy in patients with metastatic breast cancer: initial results of a novel combination. Adv Radiat Oncol 2019;4(3):453–7.

77. Gong J, Le TQ, Massarelli E, et al. Radiation therapy and PD-1/PD-L1 blockade: the clinical development of an evolving anticancer combination. J Immunother Cancer 2018;6(1):46.

78. Tetu P, Allayous C, Oriano B, et al. Impact of radiotherapy administered simultaneously with systemic treatment in patients with melanoma brain metastases within MelBase, a French multicentric prospective cohort. Eur J Cancer 2019;112:38–46.

79. Pike LRG, Bang A, Ott P, et al. Radiation and PD-1 inhibition: favorable outcomes after brain-directed radiation. Radiother Oncol 2017;124(1):98–103.

80. Bang A, Wilhite TJ, Pike LRG, et al. Multicenter evaluation of the tolerability of combined treatment with PD-1 and CTLA-4 immune checkpoint inhibitors and palliative radiation therapy. Int J Radiat Oncol Biol Phys 2017;98(2):344–51.

81. Fareed M, Krishnan M, Balboni T, et al. Indications, barriers and paths to advancement in palliative radiation oncology. Applied Radiation Oncology 2018;7(2):18–25. Available at: https://appliedradiationoncology.com/articles/indications-barriers-and-paths-to-advancement-in-palliative-radiation-oncology. Accessed August 1, 2018.

82. Schoenfeld JD, Nishino M, Severgnini M, et al. Pneumonitis resulting from radiation and immune checkpoint blockade illustrates characteristic clinical, radiologic and circulating biomarker features. J Immunother Cancer 2019;7(1):112.

83. Park KR, Lee CG, Tseng YD, et al. Palliative radiation therapy in the last 30 days of life: a systematic review. Radiother Oncol 2017;125(2):193–9.

84. Jones JA, Lutz ST, Chow E, et al. Palliative radiotherapy at the end of life: a critical review. CA Cancer J Clin 2014;64(5):295–310.

85. Wu SY, Singer L, Boreta L, et al. Palliative radiotherapy near the end of life. BMC Palliat Care 2019;18(1):29.

86. Zhang Z, Gu X-L, Chen M-L, et al. Use of palliative chemo- and radiotherapy at the end of life in patients with cancer: a retrospective cohort study. Am J Hosp Palliat Care 2017;34(9):801–5.

87. Angelo K, Norum J, Dalhaug A, et al. Development and validation of a model predicting short survival (death within 30 days) after palliative radiotherapy. Anticancer Res 2014;34(2):877–85. Available at: http://www.ncbi.nlm.nih.gov/pubmed/24511026. Accessed September 21, 2014.

88. Ellsworth SG, Alcorn SR, Hales RK, et al. Patterns of care among patients receiving radiation therapy for bone metastases at a large academic institution. Int J Radiat Oncol Biol Phys 2014;89(5):1100–5.

89. Anshushaug M, Gynnild MA, Kaasa S, et al. Characterization of patients receiving palliative chemo- and radiotherapy during end of life at a regional cancer center in Norway. Acta Oncol 2014;1–8. https://doi.org/10.3109/0284186X.2014.948061.
90. Guadagnolo BA, Liao K-P, Elting L, et al. Use of radiation therapy in the last 30 days of life among a large population-based cohort of elderly patients in the United States. J Clin Oncol 2013;31(1):80–7.

Radiation Oncology Emergencies

Mannat Narang, Pranshu Mohindra, MD, Mark Mishra, MD, William Regine, MD, Young Kwok, MD*

KEYWORDS

- Radiation oncology emergency • Palliative thoracic radiation
- Spinal cord compression • Superior vena cava syndrome • Hemoptysis
- Airway obstruction • Atelectasis

KEY POINTS

- Corticosteroids and surgical consultation must be started promptly initiated in patients suspected of or diagnosed with spinal cord compression.
- A randomized trial has unequivocally demonstrated that direct decompression and stabilization of spinal cord compression leads to improved ambulatory rate.
- Chemotherapy should be promptly initiated in pediatric spinal cord compression patients unless there is a rapid progression of neurologic status that requires surgery.
- Palliative thoracic radiation is highly effective in hemoptysis and superior vena cava syndrome. The roles of metal stents for superior vena cava syndrome and continuous positive airway pressure for atelectasis before radiation remain undefined.
- Neurologic emergencies like pending brain herniation or hydrocephalus from brain metastasis or leptomeningeal carcinomatosis require urgent neurosurgical intervention before radiation.

INTRODUCTION

Radiation oncology emergencies arise most commonly in patients with metastatic disease. As cancer therapies and survivals of such patients improve over time, it is likely that the incidence of these emergencies will increase. As with other emergencies, radiation oncology emergencies require quick and accurate diagnosis. Treatment necessitates prompt multidisciplinary teamwork, including efficient mobilization of radiation oncology staff as well as coordination of other medical specialties. This article focuses on the most common emergencies encountered by the radiation oncologist, including malignant spinal cord compression, superior vena cava (SVC) syndrome, hemoptysis, and airway compromise.

Disclosure Statement: The authors have nothing to disclose.
Department of Radiation Oncology, University of Maryland School of Medicine, 22 South Greene Street, Baltimore, MD 21201, USA
* Corresponding author.
E-mail address: ykwok@umm.edu

Hematol Oncol Clin N Am 34 (2020) 279–292
https://doi.org/10.1016/j.hoc.2019.09.004
0889-8588/20/Published by Elsevier Inc.

SPINAL CORD COMPRESSION

Malignant spinal cord compression affects 5% to 10% of all patients with cancer. More than 20,000 cases of metastatic spinal cord compression (MSCC) are diagnosed annually in the United States.[1,2] It is considered a true medical emergency. Up to one-third will survive beyond 1 year. Therefore, aggressive therapy should always be considered to preserve or improve quality of life.[3]

Pathophysiology

MSCC develops primarily through:

a. Continued growth and expansion of vertebral metastasis into the epidural space (**Fig. 1**);
b. Neural foramina invasion by a paraspinal mass (**Fig. 2**);
c. Destruction and collapse of vertebral cortical bone followed by retropulsion of bony fragments into the epidural space (**Fig. 3**); or
d. Rarely primary hematogenous seeding to the epidural space.

Epidural tumor extension causes epidural venous plexus compression, which leads to intramedullary edema (**Fig. 4**). This increase in vascular permeability and edema cause increased pressure on small arterioles. Capillary blood flow diminishes as the disease progresses, leading to white matter ischemia, ultimately leading to white matter infarction and permanent cord damage.[4]

Clinical Presentation, Diagnosis, and Prognosis

The vast majority of patients with MSCC have a cancer history. The most common tumor types are breast cancer, lung cancer, and prostate cancer.[5] New-onset back pain or radicular symptoms in patients with cancer need to be taken seriously and worked up promptly. Even without a prior cancer diagnosis, MSCC should be suspected in any high-risk patient (eg, long-time smokers) who presents with progressively

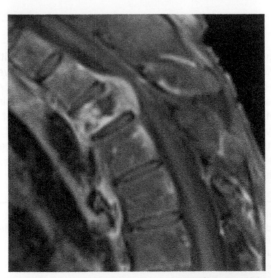

Fig. 1. Vertebral body metastasis with direct tumor growth into epidural space. The post-contrast sagittal T1-weighted MRI demonstrates an enhancing tumor in the epidural space that causes cord compression.

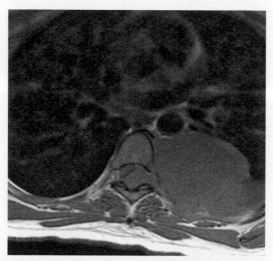

Fig. 2. Neuroforaminal invasion by a paraspinal mass. The axial T1-weighted MRI demonstrates a large paraspinal mass with invasion through the neuroforamen into the epidural space causing cord compression.

worsening back pain, incontinence, or paraplegia. The most common level of the MSCC involvement is in the thoracic spine (60%–80%), followed by lumbar (15%–30%) and cervical spine (<10%); multiple levels can be involved in up to one-half of patients.[5] Back pain is the most common presenting symptom (70%–94%), followed

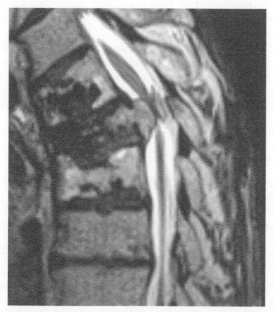

Fig. 3. Retropulsion of bony elements after vertebral collapse. The sagittal T2-weighted MRI demonstrates a collapsed vertebral leading to retropulsion of a large bony element that causes cord compression.

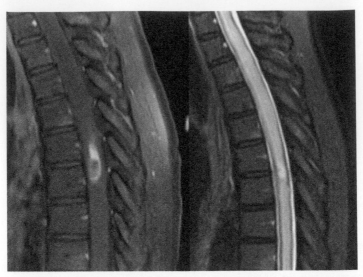

Fig. 4. Intramedullary metastasis. The sagittal T1-weighted MRI (*left*) demonstrates an intramedullary metastasis. This causes a significant amount of edema as seen in the sagittal short T1 inversion recovery-weighted MRI (*right*).

by weakness (61%–91%), sensory deficits (46%–90%), and autonomic dysfunction (40%–57%).[5]

MRI is the standard modality for spine imaging.[6,7] Because patients can have synchronous, multifocal MSCC, an MRI of the entire spine with and without contrast should be promptly performed. A high-resolution computed tomography scan or computed tomography myelogram of the spine should be performed for those with contraindications to MRI.

One of the most important prognostic factors predicting ambulatory outcome is the rapidity of symptom onset but others include radiosensitive histology (eg, multiple myeloma, germ cell tumors, small cell carcinoma) and pretherapy ambulatory function.[8] In a prospective study, Rades and colleagues separated patients into 3 groups according to the time to motor deficits before radiation therapy (RT):

- 1 to 7 days (group A),
- 8 to 14 days (group B), and
- More than 14 days (group C).

The ambulatory rates after therapy for groups A, B, and C were 35%, 55%, and 86% (*P* < .001), respectively. The symptom improvement rates for groups A, B, and C were 10%, 29%, and 86% (*P* = .026), respectively.[8] Rapid deterioration is predictive of irreversible cord infarction. Therefore, prompt diagnosis and treatment are essential.

Corticosteroids

Corticosteroids must be started as soon as possible in anyone suspected of having MSCC because it effectively decreases cord edema and can serve as an effective bridge to definitive treatment. Sorensen and colleagues[9] randomized patients with MSCC to a 96 mg intravenous (IV) bolus of dexamethasone followed by 96 mg orally per day for 3 days and a 10-day taper versus no corticosteroid therapy. This study demonstrated 3-month and 6-month ambulatory rates of 81% versus 63% and 59% versus 33% ($P < .05$), respectively, in favor of high-dose dexamethasone. Vecht and colleagues[10] randomized patients with MSCC to 10 mg versus 100 mg IV loading doses, followed in both arms by the same oral regimen of 16 mg/d. There was no difference between the 2 arms with respect to pain reduction, ambulation, or bladder function.

Very high doses of corticosteroids are associated with significant side effects. Heimdal and colleagues[11] reported a 14.3% incidence of serious gastrointestinal side effects in 28 consecutive patients treated with 96 mg of IV dexamethasone per day. Subsequently, the dexamethasone dose was decreased to 16 mg/d for the next 38 consecutive patients. There were no incidences of serious side effects ($P < .05$) and the ambulatory rates were not different.

Based on these data, a loading dose of 10 mg of IV dexamethasone followed by a maintenance dose of 4 to 6 mg every 6 to 8 hours should be sufficient before being tapered. Patients can be safely switched to an oral regimen after 24 to 48 hours because there is very good oral bioavailability of corticosteroids. Furthermore, patients should be started on a proton pump inhibitor for gastrointestinal prophylaxis.[12] In the rare case when non-Hodgkin lymphoma is suspected in MSCC, dexamethasone should either be delayed or lowered to minimum effective dose until a biopsy can be promptly performed.

Surgery

Radiation for nonradiosensitive tumors typically takes several days to have an effect and does not stabilize the spine. In contrast, surgery allows for immediate cord decompression and provides an opportunity to stabilize the spine. An early trial by Young and colleagues[13] randomized 29 patients with MSCC to decompressive laminectomy followed by RT versus RT alone. Although this randomized trial did not show a benefit to surgery before RT, it is difficult to draw any conclusion because of the small sample size. Earlier studies used posterior laminectomy in conjunction with RT; however, most lesions involve the anterior portion of the vertebral body. Therefore, a laminectomy as done in the randomized trial by Young and colleagues[13] may actually worsen the stability of the spine.

Authors have advocated the use of direct surgical decompression, tumor debulking, and spinal stabilization before RT. Patchell and colleagues[14] reported the first phase III randomized trial testing the efficacy of direct decompressive surgery in patients with MSCC (**Table 1**). The study compared RT alone (standard 30 Gy in 10 fraction) versus circumferential decompressive and stabilization surgery within 24 hours of diagnosis followed by the same RT (within 2 weeks of surgery). The trial was terminated early when early stopping rules were met regarding the primary end point of ambulation after treatment (84% vs 57%). This trial definitively demonstrated an advantage to surgery for every end point at statistically significant levels. For nonambulatory patients, the combined treatment led to a significantly higher chance of regaining the ability to walk after therapy (62% vs 19%), and the combined treatment led to a significantly higher chance of maintaining ambulation (94% vs 74%) in ambulatory patients.

If operable, patients should undergo surgical decompression and stabilization followed by RT. Even for radiosensitive tumors, surgery can often stabilize the spine. Therefore, all patients with MSCC require an evaluation by a surgeon.

Radiotherapy

Although a total of 30 Gy in 10 fractions is the most frequently used fractionation schedule, multiple fractionation schemes have been reported. In one of the largest

Table 1
Key findings of a phase III study of patients with metastatic spinal cord compression by Patchell and colleagues

	Surgery + Radiation (n = 50)	Radiation Alone (n = 51)	P Value
Primary end point			
Ability to walk after treatment			
Rate	84% (42/50)	57% (29/51)	.001
Time[c]	122 d	13 d	.003
Secondary end points[c]			
Maintenance of continence	156 d	17 d	.016
Maintenance of ASIA score[a]	566 d	72 d	.001
Maintenance of Frankel score[a]	566 d	72 d	.0006
Overall survival	126 d	100 d	.033
Other end points			
Mean daily morphine[b]	0.4 mg	4.8 mg	.002
Mean daily dexamethasone[b]	1.6 mg	4.2 mg	.0093
In patients ambulatory at study entry			
Ability to walk (maintaining)			
Rate	94% (32/34)	74% (26/34)	.024
Time[c]	153 d	54 d	.024
In patients nonambulatory at study entry			
Ability to walk (regaining)			
Rate	62% (10/16)	19% (3/16)	.012
Time[c]	59 d	0 d	.04

Abbreviation: ASIA, American Spinal Injury Association.
 [a] Measures of spinal function after injury.
 [b] Converted into equivalent doses.
 [c] Reported time (days) are median values.
 (*Data from* Patchell RA, Tibbs PA, Regine WF, et al. Direct decompressive surgical resection in the treatment of spinal cord compression caused by metastatic cancer: a randomised trial. Lancet 2005;366(9486):646.)

and most cited studies to date, Rades and colleagues[15] published a retrospective series of 1304 patients with MSCC treated with radiation. The patients were separated into 5 schedules: 8 Gy × 1 in 1 day (n = 261, group 1), 4 Gy × 5 in 1 week (n = 279, group 2), 3 Gy × 10 in 2 weeks (n = 274, group 3), 2.5 Gy × 15 in 3 weeks (n = 233, group 4), and 2 Gy × 20 in 4 weeks (n = 257, group 5). All of the groups had similar posttreatment ambulatory rates (63% to 74%) and motor function improvements (26% to 31%). However, in-field recurrence rates were much lower for the protracted schedules. The 2-year in-field recurrence rates for groups 1, 2, 3, 4, and 5 were 24%, 26%, 14%, 9%, and 7% (P<.001), respectively. They recommend that a single fraction of 8 Gy should be used in patients with MSCC with limited survival expectations, and that fractionated regimens should be used for all other patients.

Maranzano and colleagues[16] have reported on 2 randomized trials evaluating short, RT schedules. It is very difficult to interpret these results because none of these trials included a fractionation that would be considered a standard (ie, 30 Gy in 10 fractions). A more relevant randomized trial was reported by Rades and colleagues[17] comparing a short course regimen of 20 Gy in 5 fractions with 30 Gy in 10 fractions in patients with MSCC and a poor to intermediate survival prognosis. The primary end point was motor function response rate showing improvement or no progression of motor deficits at 1 month. The 1-month response rates were similar for both RT regimens (87.2%–89.6%; P = .73), and the 3- and 6-month response rates after treatment were also similar. Local progression-free survival and overall survival (median, 3.2 months) were similar for both arms. Based on this trial's results, 20 Gy in 5 fractions was deemed noninferior to 30 Gy in 10 fractions, and should be strongly considered for patients with a poor prognosis in whom limiting treatment time and discomfort should be a high priority.

For patients receiving palliative RT for MSCC from solid tumors, 30 Gy in 10 fractions is considered the standard of care. Shorter fractionation schedules, such as 8 Gy × 1 or 4 Gy × 5, should only be reserved for those with clear evidence of progressive disease refractory to systemic therapy in whom survival expectations are poor. If the patient is found to have a good performance status, oligometastatic disease, and controlled primary disease, then consideration should be made to escalate the total dose beyond 30 Gy because in an effort to achieve greater long-term gross tumor control. Special techniques such as intensity-modulated RT or fractionated stereotactic body RT (SBRT) should be considered to safely escalate the total dose. Investigators at Memorial Sloan Kettering have described the NOMS (neurologic, oncologic, mechanical instability, systemic disease) decision framework for the treatment of spinal metastasis. A significant component of NOMS is the use of SBRT. How advanced techniques such as SBRT and the NOMS algorithm fit into the treatment of MSCC can only be ascertained through prospective validation with randomized trials like STEREOCORD (SBRT vs surgery followed by RT).[18–20]

Pediatric Spinal Cord Compression

Histologic subtypes commonly encountered in children (eg, neuroblastoma, Wilms' tumor, and Ewing sarcoma) rarely occur in adults. In adults, most cases of MSCC are caused by direct invasion into the epidural space by metastatic vertebral body tumors, although in children most are caused by direct neural foraminal invasion, causing the characteristic dumbbell tumor. Chemotherapy plays a central role in the treatment of pediatric MSCC.[21]

Neuroblastoma is the most common histology of pediatric MSCC. The French Society of Pediatric Oncology protocol NBL-90 included 42 nonmetastatic neuroblastoma patients with intraspinal extension and consequent MSCC.[22] All patients were treated with initial chemotherapy, and this resulted in intraspinal tumor shrinkage, avoidance of surgery, and neurologic deficit improvement in 58%, 60%, and 92% of the patients, respectively. Severe neurologic sequelae occurred in only 6 patients (15%).

Emergent surgery should be offered to any pediatric patient with rapid neurologic progression at initial presentation or while on chemotherapy. In most circumstances, this treatment should be followed by definitive chemotherapy. In stable or mildly symptomatic patients, chemotherapy can obviate the need for emergent surgery, which is often associated with long-term skeletal deformities. RT should be reserved only for those who require palliation for progressive disease after multiple systemic regimens, or those who progress neurologically despite the initial treatment with chemotherapy or surgery.

Intramedullary Spinal Cord Metastasis

Intramedullary spinal cord metastasis (ISCM) is rare, representing only 1% of all intra-medullary tumors. It is most commonly secondary to a lung primary (54%), followed by breast cancer (11%).[23] Although back pain is common in more than 90% of patients with MSCC, back or neck pain was seen in only 38% with ISCM. However, high sensory deficits (79%), sphincter dysfunction (60%), and weakness (91%) are more common in ISCM. The most striking difference between ISCM and MSCC is the high incidence of synchronous brain metastasis (41%) in patients presenting with ISCM. An MRI of the brain should be obtained.

The treatment of ISCM should be approached very similarly to MSCC, except for the role of surgery. Most surgeons are reluctant to operate in ISCM because surgery carries a high morbidity rate. Corticosteroids as well as RT should be initiated promptly. Unfortunately, a diagnosis of ISCM portends a poor prognosis with median survival of only 1.0 to 5.5 months.[24]

THORACIC EMERGENCIES

Primary lung cancer afflicts more than 225,000 Americans each year and even more patients have metastatic disease to the lung.[25] Many of these patients develop symptoms associated with their intrathoracic disease that are directly life threatening or can impact their quality of life. The most immediate life-threatening conditions are hemoptysis, SVC syndrome, and airway obstruction. The role of RT in alleviating these symptoms is described here.

Hemoptysis

Hemoptysis is a life-threatening symptom of progressive intrathoracic disease. It can start as small amounts of bleeding from friable endobronchial tumor or a tumor eroding into a small intrapleural vessel, or a dramatic, copious, and often fatal amount of blood from a tumor eroding into one of the major vessels of the thorax.[26,27] The first step in the management of hemoptysis in patients with cancer is to ascertain its cause and exact location. In non–life-threatening hemoptysis, bronchoscopy establishes the diagnosis and location of the bleeding source, which facilitates targeting with RT. In massive hemoptysis, the role of bronchoscopy is both diagnostic and allows the opportunity to control the bleeding and stabilize the patient. In patients who have an established diagnosis of malignancy, such as lung cancer, the source and even location of the bleeding can be ascertained from a high-resolution computed tomography scan. Once the location is established and/or the acute bleed is stabilized, RT should be initiated as soon as possible.[28]

In a report from the University of Maryland, 568 patients were irradiated for intrathoracic disease, 113 of them for hemoptysis.[29] Symptomatic improvement of hemoptysis was achieved in 84% of all patients. A multi-institutional study performed by the RTOG reached a similar conclusion.[30] RTOG 73-02 randomized 409 patients with inoperable advanced non-small cell lung carcinoma (NSCLC) to a 40 Gy split course, 30 Gy continuous and 40 Gy continuous, 93 patients reported hemoptysis upon entering the study and 76% reported relief upon completion of RT. In the meta-analysis by Fairchild and colleagues,[31] the complete and overall response rates with palliative RT were 73.7% and 81.2%, respectively.

Superior Vena Cava Syndrome

The management of SVC syndrome is highly dependent on the clinical presentation. The majority of patients with SVC syndrome present without respiratory or hemodynamic instability. They usually present with engorged chest wall veins that can be appreciated both clinically and radiographically. This engorgement is reflective of collateral vessel formation and of a slowly progressing, chronic disease process. It is essential to obtain a tissue diagnosis and perform the appropriate staging workup in these clinically stable patients. The most likely malignant etiologies are small cell lung cancer, NSCLC, and lymphoma. Selection of appropriate treatment for SVC syndrome is driven by histology, stage, and the degree of emergent need. In some cases, a patient presents with a rapidly developing syndrome marked by respiratory or hemodynamic instability. For these, RT is an appropriate emergent treatment option. Ninety-seven percent of all cases of SVC obstruction are related to malignant disease.[29]

Recently, there has been more experience of inserting endovascular stenting before palliative RT, especially in those with instability and rapidly progressing SVC syndrome. Stents can immediately relieve obstruction, whereas responses from RT may take several days to weeks. Lanciego and colleagues[32] have demonstrated complete and overall response rates of 59.1% and 69.7%, respectively, with self-expandable metal stents. In a review by Rowell and Gleeson,[33] the effectiveness steroids and the optimal timing of stent insertion remain uncertain. Given this controversy, Wilson and colleagues[34] at the Princess Margaret Hospital initiated a randomized trial comparing palliative RT versus immediate stenting followed by palliative RT. This trial however closed early secondary to poor accrual.

The effectiveness of RT in palliating SVC syndrome has been well established. In a report by Slawson and colleagues,[35] 64 patients with SVC syndrome secondary to lung cancer were irradiated using 3 different RT schedules that included 20 to 25 Gy in 1 week, 20 to 30 Gy in 1 to 2 weeks, and 8 to 10 Gy per fraction for 1 to 3 fractions separated by 1 week. The complete and overall response rates were 86% and 92%, respectively. In a retrospective report from Belgium, 76% of patients with NSCLC responded to therapy with the majority responding within 3 days.[36] Patients with chemotherapy-refractory or recurrent small cell lung cancer responded 94% of the time. Armstrong and colleagues[37] have reported similar results in a retrospective analysis of 125 patients. High initial dose RT (3–4 Gy daily for 3 fractions) yielded good symptomatic relief in less than 2 weeks in 70% of patients.

Airway Obstruction

Despite recent advances in the management of lung cancer, control of disease within the thorax remains challenging. Experiences with RT in palliating atelectasis and/or dyspnea have shown only modest results.[30,38–42] Therefore, patients who require emergent management of airway compromise should not be managed initially with RT. A patient who is medically unstable because of airway compromise will receive much faster and more effective palliation from bronchoscopic stenting and/or laser ablation of endobronchial tumors. In a report from the University of Maryland, patients with atelectasis of a lobe or an entire lung treated with RT only rarely achieved re-aeration of the affected area.[38] Only 23% of patients had palliation of their atelectasis with RT. If, however, the patient was experiencing dyspnea without atelectasis, the chance of successful symptomatic palliation was 60%. Similarly, an Italian group demonstrated a 64% response rate; however, only 13% had their dyspnea completely resolve with RT.[40]

In RTOG 73-02, palliation of dyspnea occurred in 40% of patients.[30] In the prospective trial reported by Cross and associates,[40] patients received 2 fractions of 8.5 Gy 1 week apart. Dyspnea improved in only 30% of patients.[40] In addition to the relatively poor overall response of atelectasis and dyspnea to RT, the time to palliation of symptoms is less than ideal. For example, Cross and coworkers reported that no patient experienced relief until 1 week after the completion of RT. Thus, RT is an inadequate modality for the initial management of emergent airway compromise. However, given that up to 60% of patients may eventually experience palliation of dyspnea with RT, it should always be considered as way to improve the quality of life.

Recently, Appel and colleagues[43] reported the first case of using continuous positive airway pressure to re-expand a collapsed right upper lobe before RT. By re-expanding and increasing the lung volume, the gross tumor volume, clinical target volume, and planning target volume decreased by 46%, 45%, and 38%, respectively. Before this case report, Al Mutairi and colleagues[44] demonstrated in a randomized trial the beneficial effects of early use of continuous positive airway pressure in patients with acute atelectasis after cardiac surgery. Multiple and larger experiences are required before continuous positive airway pressure can be recommended in the routine treatment of airway obstruction from cancer.

Dose and Fractionation

Multiple retrospective and prospective randomized studies have compared different dose and fractionation regimens with respect to efficacy, durability, and survival. Toy and colleagues[45] examined 12 prospective randomized trials comparing dose regimens, which ranged from 10 Gy in 1 fraction to 60 Gy in 39 fractions. All but 2 of the studies reviewed concluded that there was no difference in symptom control among the various dose regimens studied. With respect to survival, 2 studies showed a significant survival benefit for patients treated with higher dose regimens.[46] In addition, the Medical Research Council study showed a more rapid palliation of symptoms with 17 Gy in 2 fractions (1 week apart) when compared with 39 Gy in 13 fractions. The authors of the review concluded that the majority of patients should receive short courses (1 or 2 fractions) of hypofractionated RT, and that selected patients with good performance status should be considered for higher dose regimens. In patients for whom RT is being used emergently, a high-dose short hypofractionated regimen using 4 to 8 Gy fractions offers the same likelihood and potentially more rapid palliation than the more standard fractionated courses such as 30 Gy in 10 fractions. Furthermore, a short course may improve patient safety by minimizing the time an unstable patient spends in the radiation oncology department.

In patients with good performance status whose palliation is not an emergent issue, more standard fractionation schemes are appropriate. Kramer and colleagues[47] randomized 297 patients with advanced lung cancer requiring palliation to the standard 30 Gy in 10 fractions versus 16 Gy in 2 fractions. The standard 30 Gy offered a more prolonged symptom relief and a longer 1-year overall survival (19.6% vs 10.9%; $P = .03$).[48] In a review of 13 randomized trials involving 3473 patients, Fairchild and colleagues[31] observed that an RT dose of 35 Gy(10)BED [eg, 30 Gy in 10 fractions = 35 Gy(10)BED vs 20 Gy in 5 fractions = 29.6 Gy(10)BED] is associated with greater symptoms improvement (65.4% vs 77.1%; $P = .003$), higher 1-year survival (26.5% vs 21.7%; $P = .002$), and lower retreatment rate, although it is associated with a higher dysphagia rate (20.5% vs 14.9%; $P = .01$).

Use of Concurrent Chemotherapy

The use of concurrent chemotherapy with palliative thoracic RT is controversial. Concurrent chemotherapy should not be given to those with limited life-expectancy. Recently, the American Society for Radiation Oncology (ASTRO) updated their consensus recommendations regarding the radiation management for NSCLC.[49] In the rare stage III NSCLC patient receiving palliative hypofractionated RT, ASTRO recommends a platinum doublet chemotherapy to be given concurrently. The recommendation was based on 3 randomized trials. However, ASTRO does not recommend concurrent chemoradiation for stage IV NSCLC based on the lack of level I evidence.

Other emergencies
There are other situations that may require emergent attention from the radiation oncologist. Patients presenting with massive gastrointestinal or gynecologic hemorrhage must immediately be hemodynamically stabilized before palliative RT can be urgently initiated. A standard fractionation such as 30 Gy in 10 fractions is highly effective in controlling the hemorrhage.[50,51] Shorter regimens like the QUAD SHOTS (14 Gy in 4 fractions, twice daily for 2 consecutive days), originally described for palliation of incurable head and neck cancer, have also been described to be very effective in pelvic tumors.[52,53] Conditions such as pending brain herniation or hydrocephalus from brain metastasis require urgent neurosurgical intervention before radiation because, save for radiosensitive tumors, a response to palliative RT can be prolonged. Leptomeningeal carcinomatosis on the other hand is typically treated with radiation alone since the prognosis is very poor.

SUMMARY

RT is an important and effective treatment modality when used in the management of oncologic emergencies. Optimal management hinges on efficient multidisciplinary evaluation and communication to arrive at a treatment plan, which is tailored to the individual patient. Therapeutic interventions include corticosteroids, surgery, chemotherapy, RT, and/or bronchoscopic intervention. Radiation dose and fractionation schedule should be tailored to the disease setting and life expectancy of the patient.

REFERENCES

1. Byrne TN. Spinal cord compression from epidural metastases. N Engl J Med 1992;327(9):614–9.

2. Quinn JA, DeAngelis LM. Neurologic emergencies in the cancer patient. Semin Oncol 2000;27(3):311–21.

3. Maranzano E, Bellavita R, Rossi R, et al. Short-course versus split-course radiotherapy in metastatic spinal cord compression: results of a phase III, randomized, multicenter trial. J Clin Oncol 2005;23(15):3358–65.

4. Kato A, Ushio Y, Hayakawa T, et al. Circulatory disturbance of the spinal cord with epidural neoplasm in rats. J Neurosurg 1985;63(2):260–5.

5. Prasad D, Schiff D. Malignant spinal-cord compression. Lancet Oncol 2005;6(1): 15–24.

6. Loughrey GJ, Collins CD, Todd SM, et al. Magnetic resonance imaging in the management of suspected spinal canal disease in patients with known malignancy. Clin Radiol 2000;55(11):849–55.

7. Loblaw DA, Laperriere NJ. Emergency treatment of malignant extradural spinal cord compression: an evidence-based guideline. J Clin Oncol 1998;16(4): 1613–24.

8. Rades D, Heidenreich F, Karstens JH. Final results of a prospective study of the prognostic value of the time to develop motor deficits before irradiation in metastatic spinal cord compression. Int J Radiat Oncol Biol Phys 2002;53(4):975–9.

9. Sorensen S, Helweg-Larsen S, Mouridsen H, et al. Effect of high-dose dexamethasone in carcinomatous metastatic spinal cord compression treated with radiotherapy: a randomised trial. Eur J Cancer 1994;30A(1):22–7.

10. Vecht CJ, Haaxma-Reiche H, van Putten WL, et al. Initial bolus of conventional versus high-dose dexamethasone in metastatic spinal cord compression. Neurology 1989;39(9):1255–7.

11. Heimdal K, Hirschberg H, Slettebo H, et al. High incidence of serious side effects of high dose dexamethasone treatment in patients with epidural spinal cord compression. J Neurooncol 1992;12(2):141–4.

12. Lanza FL, Chan FK, Quigley EM, Practice Parameters Committee of the American College of Gastroenterology. Guidelines for prevention of NSAID-related ulcer complications. Am J Gastroenterol 2009;104(3):728–38.

13. Young RF, Post EM, King GA. Treatment of spinal epidural metastases. Randomized prospective comparison of laminectomy and radiotherapy. J Neurosurg 1980;53(6):741–8.

14. Patchell RA, Tibbs PA, Regine WF, et al. Direct decompressive surgical resection in the treatment of spinal cord compression caused by metastatic cancer: a randomised trial. Lancet 2005;366(9486):643–8.

15. Rades D, Stalpers LJ, Veninga T, et al. Evaluation of five radiation schedules and prognostic factors for metastatic spinal cord compression. J Clin Oncol 2005; 23(15):3366–75.

16. Maranzano E, Trippa F, Casale M, et al. 8Gy single-dose radiotherapy is effective in metastatic spinal cord compression: results of a phase III randomized multicentre Italian trial. Radiother Oncol 2009;93(2):174–9.

17. Rades D, Segedin B, Conde-Moreno AJ, et al. Radiotherapy with 4 Gy x 5 Versus 3 Gy x 10 for metastatic epidural spinal cord compression: final results of the SCORE-2 Trial (ARO 2009/01). J Clin Oncol 2016;34(6):597–602.

18. Suppli MH, Rosenschold PM, Pappot H, et al. Stereotactic radiosurgery versus decompressive surgery followed by postoperative radiotherapy for metastatic spinal cord compression (STEREOCORD): study protocol of a randomized non-inferiority trial. J Radiosurg SBRT 2016;4(1):S1–9.

19. Laufer I, Rubin DG, Cox BW, et al. The NOMS framework: approach to the treatment of spinal metastatic tumors. Oncologist 2013;18(6):744–51.

20. Barzilai O, Laufer I, Yamada Y, et al. Integrating evidence-based medicine for treatment of spinal metastases into a decision framework: neurologic, oncologic, mechanicals stability, and systemic disease. J Clin Oncol 2017;35(1):2419–27.

21. Klein SL, Sanford RA, Muhlbauer MS. Pediatric spinal epidural metastases. J Neurosurg 1991;74(1):70, 75.

22. Plantaz D, Rubie H, Michon J, et al. The treatment of neuroblastoma with intraspinal extension with chemotherapy followed by surgical removal of residual disease. A prospective study of 42 patients–results of the NBL 90 Study of the French Society of Pediatric Oncology. Cancer 1996;78(2):311–9.

23. Kalayci M, Cagavi F, Gul S, et al. Intramedullary spinal cord metastases: diagnosis and treatment - an illustrated review. Acta Neurochir (Wien) 2004; 146(12):1347–54 [discussion: 1354].

24. Lee SS, Kim MK, Sym SJ, et al. Intramedullary spinal cord metastases: a single-institution experience. J Neurooncol 2007;84(1):85–9.

25. Siegal RL, Miller KD, Jemal A. Cancer statistics, 2019. CA Cancer J Clin 2019. https://doi.org/10.3322/caac.21555.

26. Larici AR, Franchi P, Occhipinti M, et al. Diagnosis and management of hemoptysis. Diagn Interv Radiol 2014;20(4):299–309.

27. Earwood JS. Hemoptysis: evaluation and management. Am Fam Physician 2015; 9(4):243–9.
28. Razazi K, Parrot A, Khalil A, et al. Severe Hemoptysis in patients with nonsmall cell lung carcinoma. Eur Respir J 2015;45:756–64.
29. Lokich JJ, Goodman R. Superior vena caval syndrome. Clinical management. JAMA 1975;231:58–61.
30. Simpson JR, Francis ME, Perez-Tamayo R, et al. Palliative radiotherapy for inoperable carcinoma of the lung: final report of a RTOG multi-institutional trial. Int J Radiat Oncol Biol Phys 1985;11(4):751–8.
31. Fairchild A, Harris K, Barnes E, et al. Palliative thoracic radiotherapy for lung cancer: a systematic review. J Clin Oncol 2008;26(24):4001–11.
32. Lanciego C, Pangua C, Chacón JI, et al. Endovascular stenting as the first step in the overall management of malignant superior vena cava syndrome. AJR Am J Roentgenol 2009;193(2):549–58.
33. Rowell NP, Gleeson FV. Steroids, radiotherapy, chemotherapy and stents for superior vena caval obstruction in carcinoma of the bronchus: a systematic review. Clin Oncol (R Coll Radiol) 2002;14(5):338–51.
34. Wilson P, Bezjak A, Asch M, et al. The difficulties of a randomized study in superior vena caval obstruction. J Thorac Oncol 2007;2(6):514–9.
35. Slawson RG, Prempree T, Viravathana T, et al. Radiation therapy for superior vena caval syndrome due to lung cancer. Md State Med J 1981;30(11):68–70.
36. Egelmeers A, Goor C, van Meerbeeck J, et al. Palliative effectiveness of radiation therapy in the treatment of superior vena cava syndrome. Bull Cancer Radiother 1996;83(3):153–7.
37. Armstrong BA, Perez CA, Simpson JR, et al. Role of irradiation in the management of superior vena cava syndrome. Int J Radiat Oncol Biol Phys 1987;13(4): 531–9.
38. Slawson RG, Scott RM. Radiation therapy in bronchogenic carcinoma. Radiology 1979;132(1):175–6.
39. Lupattelli M, Maranzano E, Bellavita R, et al. Short-course palliative radiotherapy in non-small-cell lung cancer: results of a prospective study. Am J Clin Oncol 2000;23(1):89–93.
40. Cross CK, Berman S, Buswell S, et al. Prospective study of palliative hypofractionated radiotherapy (8.5 Gy x 2) for patients with symptomatic non-small-cell lung cancer. Int J Radiat Oncol Biol Phys 2004;58(4):1098–105.
41. Lutz ST, Huang DT, Ferguson CL, et al. A retrospective quality of life analysis using the lung cancer symptom scale in patients treated with palliative radiotherapy for advanced nonsmall cell lung cancer. Int J Radiat Oncol Biol Phys 1997;37(1): 117–22.
42. Langendijk JA, ten Velde GPM, Aaronson NK, et al. Quality of life after palliative radiotherapy in non-small cell lung cancer: a prospective study. Int J Radiat Oncol Biol Phys 2000;47(1):149–55.
43. Appel S, Weizman N, Davidson T, et al. Reexpansion of atelectasis caused by use of continuous positive airway pressure (CPAP) before radiation therapy (RT). Adv Radiat Oncol 2016;1(2):136–40.
44. Al Mutairi F, Fallows S, Mason-Whitehead E, et al. The effect of early use of continuous positive airway pressure (CPAP) therapy to treat acute atelectasis after cardiac surgery: randomized study. Eur Respir J 2011;38:3250.
45. Toy E, Macbeth F, Coles B, et al. Palliative thoracic radiotherapy for non-small-cell lung cancer: a systematic review. Am J Clin Oncol 2003;26(2):112–20, 70.

46. Reinfuss M, Glinski B, Kowalska T, et al. Radiotherapy for stage III, inoperable, asymptomatic non-small cell lung cancer. Final results of a prospective randomized study (240 patients). Cancer Radiother 1999;3:475–9.
47. Kramer GW, Wanders SL, Noordijk EM, et al. Results of the Dutch National study of the palliative effect of irradiation using two different treatment schemes for non-small-cell lung cancer. J Clin Oncol 2005;23(13):2962–70.
48. Lee KA, Dunne M, Small C, et al. (ICORG 05-03): prospective randomized non-inferiority phase III trial comparing two radiation schedules in malignant spinal compression (not proceeding with surgical decompression);the quality of life analysis. Acta Oncol 2018;57(7):965–72.
49. Moeller B, Balagamwala E, Chen A, et al. Palliative thoracic radiation therapy for non-small cell lung cancer: 2018 Update of an American Society for Radiation Oncology (ASTRO) evidence-based guideline. Pract Radiat Oncol 2018;8(4): 245–50.
50. Sapienza LG, Ning MS, Jhingra A, et al. Short-course palliative radiation therapy leads to excellent bleeding control: a single centre retrospective study. Clin Transl Radiat Oncol 2018;14:40–6.
51. Kondoh C, Shitara K, Nomura M, et al. Efficacy of palliative radiotherapy for gastric bleeding in patients with unresectable advanced gastric cancer: a retrospective cohort study. BMC Palliat Care 2015;14:37.
52. Corry J, Peters L, D'Costa I, et al. The 'QUAD SHOT'-a phase II study of palliative radiotherapy for incurable head and neck cancer. Radiother Oncol 2005;77(2): 137–42.
53. Lin M, Kondalsamy-Chennakesavan S, Bernshaw D, et al. Carcinoma of the cervix in elderly patients treated with radiotherapy; patterns of care and treatment outcomes. J Gynecol Oncol 2016;27(6):e59.

Imaging for Response Assessment in Radiation Oncology: Current and Emerging Techniques

Sonja Stieb, MD, Kendall Kiser, MS, Lisanne van Dijk, PhD,
Nadia Roxanne Livingstone, BA, Hesham Elhalawani, MD, MSc,
Baher Elgohari, MD, MSc, Brigid McDonald, BS, Juan Ventura, BS,
Abdallah Sherif Radwan Mohamed, MD, MSc,
Clifton David Fuller, MD, PhD*

KEYWORDS

- CT • MRI • PET • Functional imaging • Response assessment • Tumor
- Organs at risk • Radiation oncology

KEY POINTS

- Computed tomography, MRI, and PET are the current state-of-the-art imaging methods in radiation oncology for treatment response assessment, depending on cancer site.
- New and promising imaging techniques like functional MRI and radiomics are currently investigated for prediction of treatment response in tumors and organs at risk.
- Still, more research needs to be conducted to implement these new imaging techniques into clinical routine.

INTRODUCTION

Computed tomography (CT), magnetic resonance imaging (MRI), and positron emission tomography (PET) play a major role in the assessment of tumor response. Moreover, these imaging modalities are increasingly used to evaluate treatment-related changes in normal tissue and correlate these findings with treatment-related toxicity. Especially in radiation oncology, the prediction of tumor response and radiation-induced normal tissue damage arouses more and more interest. The aim is to adapt therapy in cases of more aggressive tumors or severe changes in organs at risk (OARs). For example, a patient found to have less oxygenated, radioresistant tumor regions at a mid-treatment hypoxia PET scan might be a candidate for an additional

Disclosure Statement: See last page of article.
Department of Radiation Oncology, The University of Texas MD Anderson Cancer Center, 1515 Holcombe Boulevard, Houston, TX 77030, USA
* Corresponding author.
E-mail address: CDFuller@mdanderson.org

Hematol Oncol Clin N Am 34 (2020) 293–306
https://doi.org/10.1016/j.hoc.2019.09.010
0889-8588/20/© 2019 Elsevier Inc. All rights reserved.

boost dose to the tumor.[1] On the other hand, a patient with a rapidly responding tumor might benefit from treatment adaptation to spare normal tissues.[2]

Because CT is increasingly used to dictate patient positioning during radiotherapy, many CT images are produced daily, which has prompted many investigators to search for predictors of tumor control and normal tissue toxicity in CT, for example, with radiomics analysis.[3] In contrast, MRI has not been afforded the same attention as CT because MRI cannot be directly used for modeling dose deposition. However, with advantages of no radiation dose and superior soft tissue contrast compared with CT, and with the rising availability of combined MR linear accelerators (MR Linacs) that facilitate online imaging during irradiation, MRI is also a promising alternative for response assessment already during the course of radiotherapy.

In this article, the authors delve into current and emerging imaging techniques using CT, MRI, and PET for assessment of tumor response and OAR toxicity. Other emerging methods for assessing tumor treatment response such as circulating tumor DNA or nanotechnologies are not nearly so ubiquitous in today's clinic as is imaging. Imaging – already a staple of clinical decision-making – is the most sensible opportunity for timely adoption of practice-changing tumor response clinical assessment tools.

IMAGING APPLICATIONS FOR TUMOR RESPONSE ASSESSMENT
CT Approaches

Tumor response in CT is principally assessed by the Response Evaluation Criteria in Solid Tumors (RECIST) criteria.[4] Simplified, a complete response is therein defined as disappearance of all so-called target lesions. Stable disease is the proper term if the sum of the longest diameter of target lesions is less than 30% decreased (otherwise partial response) and less than 20% increased (otherwise progressive disease). It is an inherent and important limitation, however, that RECIST's response evaluation is only 2-dimensional.

Another use for CT imaging is quantitative characterization of tumor function using dynamic contrast-enhanced CT (DCE-CT). DCE-CT scans are repeatedly acquired for approximately 40 seconds after injecting iodine-based contrast agents.[5] DCE-CT has gained popularity among radiation oncologists as a valuable tool to spatially map tumor vascular attributes like perfusion, permeability, and blood flow.[6] DCE-CT has shown promise in early and longitudinal assessment of tumor response to radiation therapy,[7] multiparametric functional imaging characterization of radioresistant tumor subvolumes, and adaptive radiotherapy.[5,8,9] Studies assessing chronologic changes in quantitative DCE-CT metrics like transfer coefficient (K-trans) and relative tumor blood volume (rTBV) have reported a dose and treatment modality–dependent correlation in various cancer sites, such as head and neck cancers (HNCs) and non–small-cell lung cancer (NSCLC).[10,11] Nonetheless, as with all quantitative imaging biomarkers, the development of clinically applicable DCE-CT biomarker profiles in radiation oncology hinges on standardization and reproducibility assurance efforts that address technical validation and robustness issues.[12]

Dual-energy CT (DE-CT) uses 2 x-ray sources of nonidentical energies to acquire signal, rather than a single x-ray source used in traditional, single-energy CT (SE-CT) (Fig.1).[13] Because tissue x-ray attenuation varies with photon energy, dual-photon energies capture greater information about tissue density than does SE-CT.[14] The most common use for DE-CT is to extract iodine contrast maps and correlate them with a variable of interest.[15] For example, Bahig and colleagues[16] described the first attempt to correlate DE-CT–derived iodine tissue concentration with oncologic outcomes in HNC. Primary gross tumor volume (GTV) maximum voxel-wise iodine concentration, primary GTV kurtosis, nodal GTV volume, and nodal GTV iodine concentration standard deviation each predicted worse locoregional recurrence risk in a cohort of 25 patients with laryngeal and hypopharyngeal cancer. DE-CT–derived iodine content also has the ability to differentiate metastatic, inflamed, and healthy lymph nodes.[17] Iodine maps derived by DE-CT may complement RECIST's 2-dimensional limitation by identifying cases in which tumor viability has indeed decreased despite no change in tumor size.[15] Furthermore, they may also prove useful for risk-stratifying radiotherapy patients before radiation[18].

An evolving approach is the use of radiomics features, which encompass a wide range of mineable multidimensional values that quantitatively describe tumor shape, intensity, and texture.[19] Predictive radiomics biomarkers have been demonstrably informative in HNC, gastric cancer, and lung cancer, among others.[20] In a study by Ramella and colleagues,[21] a combined signature of semantic and radiomics features derived from baseline CT could be correlated to rate of volumetric changes at subsequent time points in NSCLC. A similar study found a gray-level co-occurrence matrix texture feature improved the capacity of a clinicopathological model to predict tumor shrinkage at mid-treatment course.[22] Other studies tracked the kinetics of radiomics features from sequential in-treatment CT images and demonstrated an association with subsequent response to radiation in HNC and NSCLC.[23,24]

MRI Approaches

MRI is superior to CT for tumor response assessment in soft tissues when motion artifacts and tissue/air interfaces leading to susceptibility artifacts are negligible. As is the case for CT, the RECIST criteria[4] are commonly used for response assessment of solid tumors on MRI.

Other MRI response criteria have been implemented, including criteria that are specific to certain anatomic subsites and/or tumors (such as glioma). Similar to the RECIST criteria, they are based on lesion sizes as well. For example, the criteria of Macdonald and colleagues[25] assess the size of contrast-enhancing tumor in T1 sequences, whereas an updated version of the Response Assessment for Neuro-Oncology (RANO) criteria were introduced in 2010[26] to allow for incorporation of T2/Flair changes as well.

Newer imaging techniques, like MR perfusion and spectroscopy, are still not adopted by these criteria, although they are more accurate at differentiating

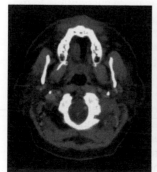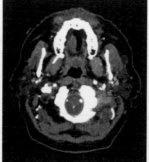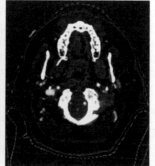

Fig. 1. Example of a patient with a lung adenocarcinoma metastasis at the left skull base (*red arrow*). Left: 140 keV DE-CT (window level: −100–250 HU); middle: 60 keV DE-CT (window level: −100–250 HU); right: Iodine map of DE-CT (window level: −10–100 HU).

between true progression and treatment-induced changes.[27] This is especially a problem with the increasing use of immunotherapy.[28] High-grade glioma usually presents with increased vasculature, and the relative blood volume is greater in tumor progression or recurrence than in necrosis or pseudoprogression. This can be measured by dynamic susceptibility contrast (DSC) perfusion MRI.[29] Machine learning approaches have achieved some success at differentiating disease progression from pseudoprogression using diffusion-weighted imaging (DWI)[30] and DSC perfusion MRI.[31] Arterial spin labeling measures perfusion using magnetically labeled blood as an endogenous tracer. Using magnetic resonance spectroscopy, active tumor tissue is defined as having an elevated choline level[32]; lipid-lactate peaks, a decrease in N-acetyl-aspartate, and a lack of choline elevation, however, is suspect for radiation necrosis.[33,34]

Functional MRI has further potential to predict for tumor response. For example, high apparent diffusion coefficient (ADC) values pretreatment derived from DWI associate with poor outcomes in HNC.[35,36] Treatment responders showed a higher increase in ADC during the first weeks of radiotherapy than nonresponders or partial responders.[35] DCE imaging is comparably more invasive because it uses an intravenous contrast agent and is inconsistent in its response prediction for most of the parameters. K-trans seems most reliable, with higher values correlating with better tumor response.[37–39] In recent years, nanoparticles have been investigated as MRI contrast agents. Negatively charged superparamagnetic iron oxide nanoparticles, for example, can produce good image contrast, but concern exists that long-term retention of the particles could harm organ function.[40] Other approaches include Blood Oxygen Level Dependent (BOLD) imaging, which leverages the paramagnetic nature of deoxyhemoglobin to visualize a decrease in $T2^*$.[41] As tumor hypoxia is known to adversely affect the outcome after radiotherapy and/or chemotherapy, BOLD imaging may also be a predictive imaging biomarker.

MRI radiomics features may become a convenient tool for phenotyping tumors and normal tissues and integrating spatially driven parameters to guide therapy and outcome.[42] In breast cancer, radiomics models have predicted tumor response to neoadjuvant and adjuvant therapy.[43,44] Similarly, in HNC radiomics, models have predicted local control and survival.[45,46] MRI has more acquisition parameters than CT (such as pulse sequence, echo time, relaxation time), which means that the task of standardizing reproducible features is even more challenging for MRI than CT.[47] Different vendor sequences or perhaps different Tesla magnets could complicate the reproducibility of extracted features.[48] Because MRI is more susceptible to motion artifact than CT, feature reproducibility may also depend on immobilization during acquisition. Effort is clearly needed to standardize different inconsistencies in MRI radiomics starting from imaging acquisition, imaging processing, model building, and model validation. This is a necessary step to integrate functional quantitative imaging data into clinical decision making tools toward personalized medicine.

PET Approaches

Utilization of PET for tumor response assessment has become a key component for monitoring disease progression and for restaging (**Fig. 2**).[49,50] PET visualizes metabolic activity within the body in ways that CT and MRI may be limited.[51] The addition of this functional imaging modality presents a need for new standardized guidelines and criteria in tumor response assessment to provide patients with consistent quality care.

The first set of standardized tumor response guidelines for PET was defined by the European Organization for Research and Treatment of Cancer (EORTC) in 1999.[52] These recommendations consider both clinical and subclinical measurements in treatment response interpretation. In 2009, the PET Response Criteria in Solid Tumors (PERCIST) criteria were introduced, which modifies the RECIST criteria to include metabolic activity with PET with fludeoxyglucose F 18 (^{18}F FDG-PET) as an additional criterion to anatomic findings.[53] PET standardized uptake values (SUV) are a quantitative metric for categorizing tumor response, progression, or stabilization of disease.

A review of the EORTC and PERCIST response criteria showed strong agreement between the two despite their different approaches.[54] The review was limited by small patient cohorts, heterogeneous patient populations, heterogenous equipment, and other factors, so it is still necessary to investigate differences between the two on a larger, homogeneous patient population to validate possible interchangeability and use for practice.

PET/CT has become standard for response assessment in most lymphomas.[55] According to the Lugano Classification, a complete response is defined as complete metabolic response of initially FDG-avid lymphoma independent of residual masses, whereas progressive disease is considered in case of increased FDG uptake compared with baseline values or the appearance of new FDG-avid lesions consistent with lymphoma.[55]

To limit the incidence of false-positive PET readings due to normal tissue damage and immune response caused by radiation therapy, response assessment must be delayed for some period after treatment.[56] Local inflammation and radiotherapy changes will be FDG-avid and limit the positive predictive value for local residual tumor. However, PET remains a strong diagnostic tool for identifying distant metastatic disease and progression. A 16-week FDG-PET reassessment in locally advanced HNC showed good diagnostic accuracy and can be used to guide management with the high negative probability of complete response.[57] Although FDG is the most commonly used and studied radiotracer to monitor tumor response, others have shown some utility. 18F-fluorothymidine (18F-FLT), is promising as a more reliable tracer in measuring tumor proliferation than 18F-FDG, but is limited by its relatively low uptake in cells and is even more hindered by radiotherapy and cytotoxic chemotherapy.[58]

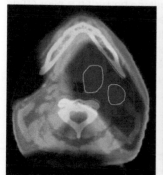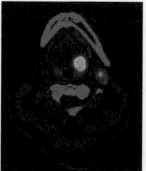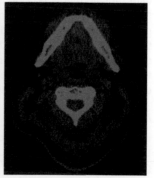

Fig. 2. Example of a patient with T2 base of tongue (BOT) tumor and ipsilateral neck lymph node. Left: Treatment plan with BOT tumor delineated in green, lymph node in yellow, and clinical target volume in red; middle: PET/CT before treatment (window level for PET: 0.5–22 SUV); right: corresponding PET/CT slice 3 months after radiochemotherapy (window level for PET: 0.5–22 SUV).

Cancer cells have been noted to adapt metabolically to hypoxic environments despite functioning mitochondria and the presence of oxygen. This phenomenon, known as the Warburg Effect,[59] contributes to therapy resistance and tumor progression.[60] Measurement of hypoxia has historically been performed by assessing the oxygen partial pressure (P_{O_2}) through a polarographic needle electrode that is invasive and limited to a small portion of the tumor.[61] However, cellular hypoxia measurements can now be performed with PET/CT using radiotracers like 18F-fluoroazomycin arabinoside (FAZA) and 18F-fluoromisonidazole (FMISO). Both tracers fall under the nitroimidazole family, which work by the reduction of its NO2-group in the hypoxic environment, leading to covalent binding with macromolecules in the cell.[62] As a second-generation hypoxia PET radiotracer, FAZA has improved contrast when compared with the more widely used FMISO. The potential of both tracers to predict treatment outcome has been shown in several studies,[63] but must be further examined before implementing into clinical use.

IMAGING APPLICATIONS FOR ORGANS AT RISK ASSESSMENT
CT Approaches

Advanced treatment options such as proton therapy[64,65] and MR-guided radiation[66] create new opportunities to spare normal tissues. As life expectancy for cancer survivors increases, so does demand for predicting the development of treatment-induced side effects. OAR morphologic changes may be informative for this goal,[67,68] but so may other image parameters, such as intensity on CT.[69,70]

Just as radiomics has been investigated for monitoring tumor response, it also may be serviceable for monitoring OARs.[19,71] Aerts and colleagues[72] were the first to perform a large extraction of radiomics features from tumors, including intensity, morphologic, and texture features, to predict survival. Since then, a wealth of radiomics studies have investigated tumor features, yet radiomics is comparatively less used to investigate normal tissue response or toxicity. van Dijk and colleagues[73] showed that radiomics texture features were associated with radiation-induced side effects in addition to dosimetric parameters and could improve current normal tissue complication probability models. Radiomics features from images taken during treatment have been exploited to predict radiation-induced xerostomia,[67,69,74] and Cunliffe and colleagues[70] showed that the change in lung texture during treatment correlated with radiation-induced pneumonitis. Colen and colleagues[75] showed in a pilot study that radiomics analysis may also predict immunotherapy-induced toxicities. As mentioned in the previous discussion of radiomics for tumor response assessment, the development of radiomics for predicting of normal tissue toxicity is still in its early stages. Larger, more robust image validation sets and feature parameter standardization are needed. Nevertheless, current and past studies have highlighted the potential of radiomics to improve conventional toxicity modeling.

MRI Approaches

Like CT, MRI can be used to identify radiation-induced changes in size of the structures. For example, several studies have reported on a volume loss of the salivary glands during radiotherapy.[76] Muscles on the other hand have been described to increase in thickness in a dose-dependent manner.[77] Volumetric changes can be easily measured in standard anatomic T1 or T2 sequences. Functional MRI like DWI or intravoxel incoherent motion imaging can quantify extracellular water as a biomarker for edema. DWI is one of the most reported functional MR sequences used for estimation of damage in OAR. Exemplarily, the ADC of the salivary glands increased during the course of radiotherapy and could be correlated with the degree of xerostomia.[78] Another functional MR sequence commonly used is DCE imaging, which gives details about vasculature that can be affected in the case of radiation-induced inflammation, but more research is necessary to consistently report on the changes and correlate them with outcomes. A dedicated sequence to describe the fatty degeneration of tissue is DIXON, but this sequence has only rarely been used for OAR assessment so far (**Fig. 3**).[79] To better compare study results between different institutions, reporting percentage changes could be helpful. This could compensate for some interinstitutional variability caused by different MRI machines, radiofrequency coils, and image acquisition parameters. Nevertheless, segmentation of OARs can also influence normal tissue complication probability outputs,[80] as can post-processing methods.[81]

MRI radiomics has been explored for predicting normal tissue toxicities as well. One study correlated fat content in parotid glands and xerostomia at 12 months post-therapy.[82] Another study investigated femoral bone damage after radiotherapy by exploring radiomics features extracted from different MRI sequences.[83] As extensively discussed in the MRI for tumor response assessment section, standardization of radiomics acquisition and post-processing is crucial.

PET/SPECT Approaches

PET/CT and single-photon emission CT (SPECT)/CT are imaging modalities that are not currently used clinically for OAR toxicity assessment. However, there is potential for both modalities to quantify toxicity using the anatomic information from the CT and the functional information from the PET or SPECT to help clinicians ascertain the damage to normal tissue by providing metabolic[84] or perfusion[85] information.

For example, 18F-FDG-PET has been used to investigate radiation-induced normal tissue toxicity to the parotid gland; a decrease in 18F-FDG-uptake post-radiotherapy correlated with the development of late xerostomia.[86]

68Ga–prostate-specific membrane antigen (PSMA) is another radionuclide that can be used to quantify metabolic activity in prostate cancer and in salivary and lacrimal glands.[87] PSMA-PET/CT further allows for visualization of seromucous glands in the soft palate, pharyngeal wall, nasal mucosa, and supraglottic larynx, which is not possible with other imaging modalities.[87] This is a significant step along the path to quantifying radiation-induced metabolic activity changes in these minor glands.

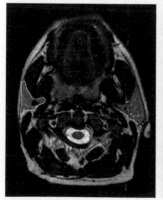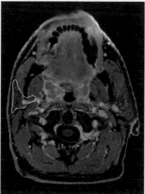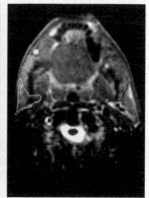

Fig. 3. A 54-year old patient with bilateral tonsil cancer stage IVA. Parotid gland structures are highlighted in yellow and pink and were rigidly propagated from T2 image (*left*) to DIXON (*middle*) and ADC map (*right*).

Another possible application for PET/CT in OAR assessment was described for the prediction of radiation-induced lung toxicity (RILT).[88] Petit and colleagues[88] found that patients were more likely to develop RILT if the lung voxels with the highest 18F-FDG uptake in the pretreatment scan received 2 Gy or more. In another study, SPECT/CT was used to evaluate the association between perfusion and radiation dose in patients who developed radiation pneumonitis after treatment.[85]

Furthermore, PET/CT, using 15O-H_2O as tracer, can be used to detect perfusion changes in the heart after breast radiotherapy and thus also help to identify radiation-induced heart damage.[89] Similarly, patients showed a significantly higher 18F-FDG uptake in myocardial regions within the radiation field as opposed to nonirradiated regions.[90]

SUMMARY

CT, MRI, PET or a combination of these modalities, is commonly used for response assessment after radiotherapy, depending on treatment site. With the recent technical advances, newer imaging methods and quantitative approaches have become increasingly available, such as DE-CT, functional MRI, and radiomics. Despite promising results regarding the prediction of tumor response and toxicity with newer techniques, larger studies are yet lacking to clinically validate them and thereafter scale them to the standard of care.

DISCLOSURE

S. Stieb is funded by the Swiss Cancer League (BIL KLS-4300-08-2017). L. van Dijk received funding from the NOW Rubicon Award and N.R. Livingstone a National Institutes of Health (NIH)/National Institute of Dental and Craniofacial Research (NIDCR) diversity supplement (3R01DE025248-03). C.D. Fuller received funding from NIDCR Award (1R01DE025248-01/R56DE025248) and Academic-Industrial Partnership Award (R01 DE028290), the National Science Foundation (NSF), Division of Mathematical Sciences, Joint NIH/NSF Initiative on Quantitative Approaches to Biomedical Big Data Grant (NSF 1557679), the NIH Big Data to Knowledge (BD2K) Program of the National Cancer Institute (NCI) Early Stage Development of Technologies in Biomedical Computing, Informatics, and Big Data Science Award (1R01CA214825), the NCI Early Phase Clinical Trials in Imaging and Image-Guided Interventions Program (1R01CA218148), the NIH/NCI Cancer Center Support Grant (CCSG) Pilot Research Program Award from the University of Texas MD Anderson CCSG Radiation Oncology and Cancer Imaging Program (P30CA016672), the NIH/NCI Head and Neck Specialized Programs of Research Excellence Developmental Research Program Award (P50 CA097007) and the National Institute of Biomedical Imaging and Bioengineering Research Education Program (R25EB025787). C.D. Fuller has received direct industry grant support, speaking honoraria and travel funding from Elekta AB.

REFERENCES

1. Vera P, Thureau S, Chaumet-Riffaud P, et al. Phase II study of a radiotherapy total dose increase in hypoxic lesions identified by (18)F-Misonidazole PET/CT in patients with non-small cell lung carcinoma (RTEP5 study). J Nucl Med 2017;58(7):1045–53.
2. Mohamed ASR, Bahig H, Aristophanous M, et al. Prospective in silico study of the feasibility and dosimetric advantages of MRI-guided dose adaptation for human papillomavirus positive oropharyngeal cancer patients compared with standard IMRT. Clin Transl Radiat Oncol 2018;11:11–8.

3. Fave X, Mackin D, Yang J, et al. Can radiomics features be reproducibly measured from CBCT images for patients with non-small cell lung cancer? Med Phys 2015;42(12):6784–97.

4. Eisenhauer EA, Therasse P, Bogaerts J, et al. New response evaluation criteria in solid tumours: revised RECIST guideline (version 1.1). Eur J Cancer 2009;45(2): 228–47.

5. Thorwarth D. Functional imaging for radiotherapy treatment planning: current status and future directions—a review. Br J Radiol 2015;88(1051):20150056.

6. O'Connor JP, Tofts PS, Miles KA, et al. Dynamic contrast-enhanced imaging techniques: CT and MRI. Br J Radiol 2011;84(Spec No 2):S112–20.

7. Coolens C, Driscoll B, Chung C, et al. Automated voxel-based analysis of volumetric dynamic contrast-enhanced CT data improves measurement of serial changes in tumor vascular biomarkers. Int J Radiat Oncol Biol Phys 2015; 91(1):48–57.

8. Cao Y, Pan C, Balter JM, et al. Liver function after irradiation based on computed tomographic portal vein perfusion imaging. Int J Radiat Oncol Biol Phys 2008; 70(1):154–60.

9. Even AJG, Reymen B, La Fontaine MD, et al. Clustering of multi-parametric functional imaging to identify high-risk subvolumes in non-small cell lung cancer. Radiother Oncol 2017;125(3):379–84.

10. Abramyuk A, Hietschold V, Appold S, et al. Radiochemotherapy-induced changes of tumour vascularity and blood supply estimated by dynamic contrast-enhanced CT and fractal analysis in malignant head and neck tumours. Br J Radiol 2015;88(1045):20140412.

11. Hwang SH, Yoo MR, Park CH, et al. Dynamic contrast-enhanced CT to assess metabolic response in patients with advanced non-small cell lung cancer and stable disease after chemotherapy or chemoradiotherapy. Eur Radiol 2013; 23(6):1573–81.

12. Shukla-Dave A, Obuchowski NA, Chenevert TL, et al. Quantitative imaging biomarkers alliance (QIBA) recommendations for improved precision of DWI and DCE-MRI derived biomarkers in multicenter oncology trials. J Magn Reson Imaging 2019;49(7):e101–21.

13. van Elmpt W, Landry G, Das M, et al. Dual energy CT in radiotherapy: current applications and future outlook. Radiother Oncol 2016;119(1):137–44.

14. Grajo JR, Patino M, Prochowski A, et al. Dual energy CT in practice: basic principles and applications. Appl Radiol 2016;45(7):6–12.

15. Agrawal MD, Pinho DF, Kulkarni NM, et al. Oncologic applications of dual-energy CT in the abdomen. Radiographics 2014;34(3):589–612.

16. Bahig H, Lapointe A, Bedwani S, et al. Dual-energy computed tomography for prediction of loco-regional recurrence after radiotherapy in larynx and hypopharynx squamous cell carcinoma. Eur J Radiol 2019;110:1–6.

17. Tawfik AM, Razek AA, Kerl JM, et al. Comparison of dual-energy CT-derived iodine content and iodine overlay of normal, inflammatory and metastatic squamous cell carcinoma cervical lymph nodes. Eur Radiol 2014;24(3):574–80.

18. Lapointe A, Bahig H, Blais D, et al. Assessing lung function using contrast-enhanced dual-energy computed tomography for potential applications in radiation therapy. Med Phys 2017;44(10):5260–9.

19. Lambin P, Rios-Velazquez E, Leijenaar R, et al. Radiomics: extracting more information from medical images using advanced feature analysis. Eur J Cancer 2012;48(4):441–6.

20. Liu Z, Wang S, Dong D, et al. The applications of radiomics in precision diagnosis and treatment of oncology: opportunities and challenges. Theranostics 2019; 9(5):1303–22.

21. Ramella S, Fiore M, Greco C, et al. A radiomic approach for adaptive radiotherapy in non-small cell lung cancer patients. PLoS One 2018;13(11):e0207455.

22. Sicilia R, Cordelli E, Ramella S, et al. Exploratory radiomics for predicting adaptive radiotherapy in non-small cell lung cancer. Paper presented at: 2018 IEEE 31st International Symposium on Computer-Based Medical Systems (CBMS). Karlstad University, June 18–21, 2018.

23. Paul J, Yang C, Wu H, et al. Early assessment of treatment responses during radiation therapy for lung cancer using quantitative analysis of daily computed tomography. Int J Radiat Oncol Biol Phys 2017;98(2):463–72.

24. Elhalawani HE, Mohamed ASR, Volpe S, et al. PO-0991: serial tumor radiomic features predict response of head and neck cancer treated with radiotherapy. Radiother Oncol 2018;127:S551.

25. Macdonald DR, Cascino TL, Schold SC Jr, et al. Response criteria for phase II studies of supratentorial malignant glioma. J Clin Oncol 1990;8(7):1277–80.

26. Wen PY, Macdonald DR, Reardon DA, et al. Updated response assessment criteria for high-grade gliomas: response assessment in neuro-oncology working group. J Clin Oncol 2010;28(11):1963–72.

27. van Dijken BRJ, van Laar PJ, Holtman GA, et al. Diagnostic accuracy of magnetic resonance imaging techniques for treatment response evaluation in patients with high-grade glioma, a systematic review and meta-analysis. Eur Radiol 2017; 27(10):4129–44.

28. Okada H, Weller M, Huang R, et al. Immunotherapy response assessment in neuro-oncology: a report of the RANO working group. Lancet Oncol 2015; 16(15):e534–42.

29. Hu LS, Baxter LC, Smith KA, et al. Relative cerebral blood volume values to differentiate high-grade glioma recurrence from posttreatment radiation effect: direct correlation between image-guided tissue histopathology and localized dynamic susceptibility-weighted contrast-enhanced perfusion MR imaging measurements. AJNR Am J Neuroradiol 2009;30(3):552–8.

30. Hu X, Wong KK, Young GS, et al. Support vector machine multiparametric MRI identification of pseudoprogression from tumor recurrence in patients with resected glioblastoma. J Magn Reson Imaging 2011;33(2):296–305.

31. Cha J, Kim ST, Kim HJ, et al. Differentiation of tumor progression from pseudoprogression in patients with posttreatment glioblastoma using multiparametric histogram analysis. AJNR Am J Neuroradiol 2014;35(7):1309–17.

32. Kamada K, Houkin K, Abe H, et al. Differentiation of cerebral radiation necrosis from tumor recurrence by proton magnetic resonance spectroscopy. Neurol Med Chir (Tokyo) 1997;37(3):250–6.

33. Kazda T, Bulik M, Pospisil P, et al. Advanced MRI increases the diagnostic accuracy of recurrent glioblastoma: single institution thresholds and validation of MR spectroscopy and diffusion weighted MR imaging. Neuroimage Clin 2016;11: 316–21.

34. Kimura T, Sako K, Tohyama Y, et al. Diagnosis and treatment of progressive space-occupying radiation necrosis following stereotactic radiosurgery for brain metastasis: value of proton magnetic resonance spectroscopy. Acta Neurochir (Wien) 2003;145(7):557–64 [discussion: 564].

35. Kim S, Loevner L, Quon H, et al. Diffusion-weighted magnetic resonance imaging for predicting and detecting early response to chemoradiation therapy of squamous cell carcinomas of the head and neck. Clin Cancer Res 2009;15(3):986–94.
36. Lombardi M, Cascone T, Guenzi E, et al. Predictive value of pre-treatment apparent diffusion coefficient (ADC) in radio-chemotherapy treated head and neck squamous cell carcinoma. Radiol Med 2017;122(5):345–52.
37. Ng SH, Lin CY, Chan SC, et al. Clinical utility of multimodality imaging with dynamic contrast-enhanced MRI, diffusion-weighted MRI, and 18F-FDG PET/CT for the prediction of neck control in oropharyngeal or hypopharyngeal squamous cell carcinoma treated with chemoradiation. PLoS One 2014;9(12):e115933.
38. Ng SH, Lin CY, Chan SC, et al. Dynamic contrast-enhanced MR imaging predicts local control in oropharyngeal or hypopharyngeal squamous cell carcinoma treated with chemoradiotherapy. PLoS One 2013;8(8):e72230.
39. Kim S, Loevner LA, Quon H, et al. Prediction of response to chemoradiation therapy in squamous cell carcinomas of the head and neck using dynamic contrast-enhanced MR imaging. AJNR Am J Neuroradiol 2010;31(2):262–8.
40. Wallyn J, Anton N, Akram S, et al. Biomedical imaging: principles, technologies, clinical aspects, contrast agents, limitations and future trends in nanomedicines. Pharm Res 2019;36(6):78.
41. Buxton RB. The physics of functional magnetic resonance imaging (fMRI). Rep Prog Phys 2013;76(9):096601.
42. Avanzo M, Stancanello J, El Naqa I. Beyond imaging: the promise of radiomics. Phys Med 2017;38:122–39.
43. Liu Z, Li Z, Qu J, et al. Radiomics of multiparametric MRI for pretreatment prediction of pathologic complete response to neoadjuvant chemotherapy in breast cancer: a multicenter study. Clin Cancer Res 2019;25(12):3538–47.
44. Xiong Q, Zhou X, Liu Z, et al. Multiparametric MRI-based radiomics analysis for prediction of breast cancers insensitive to neoadjuvant chemotherapy. Clin Transl Oncol 2019. [Epub ahead of print].
45. Zhang LL, Huang MY, Li Y, et al. Pretreatment MRI radiomics analysis allows for reliable prediction of local recurrence in non-metastatic T4 nasopharyngeal carcinoma. EBioMedicine 2019;42:270–80.
46. Zhuo EH, Zhang WJ, Li HJ, et al. Radiomics on multi-modalities MR sequences can subtype patients with non-metastatic nasopharyngeal carcinoma (NPC) into distinct survival subgroups. Eur Radiol 2019;29(10):5590–9.
47. Duron L, Balvay D, Vande Perre S, et al. Gray-level discretization impacts reproducible MRI radiomics texture features. PLoS One 2019;14(3):e0213459.
48. Zhao B, Tan Y, Tsai WY, et al. Reproducibility of radiomics for deciphering tumor phenotype with imaging. Sci Rep 2016;6:23428.
49. Ben-Haim S, Ell P. 18F-FDG PET and PET/CT in the evaluation of cancer treatment response. J Nucl Med 2009;50(1):88–99.
50. Yao M, Graham MM, Smith RB, et al. Value of FDG PET in assessment of treatment response and surveillance in head-and-neck cancer patients after intensity modulated radiation treatment: a preliminary report. Int J Radiat Oncol Biol Phys 2004;60(5):1410–8.
51. Bussink J, van Herpen CM, Kaanders JH, et al. PET-CT for response assessment and treatment adaptation in head and neck cancer. Lancet Oncol 2010;11(7):661–9.
52. Young H, Baum R, Cremerius U, et al. Measurement of clinical and subclinical tumour response using [18F]-fluorodeoxyglucose and positron emission tomography: review and 1999 EORTC recommendations. European Organization for

Research and Treatment of Cancer (EORTC) PET Study Group. Eur J Cancer 1999;35(13):1773–82.

53. Wahl RL, Jacene H, Kasamon Y, et al. From RECIST to PERCIST: evolving considerations for PET response criteria in solid tumors. J Nucl Med 2009;50(Suppl 1): 122S–50S.

54. Kim JH. Comparison of the EORTC criteria and PERCIST in solid tumors: a pooled analysis and review. Oncotarget 2016;7(36):58105–10.

55. Cheson BD, Fisher RI, Barrington SF, et al. Recommendations for initial evaluation, staging, and response assessment of Hodgkin and non-Hodgkin lymphoma: the Lugano classification. J Clin Oncol 2014;32(27):3059–68.

56. Laing RE, Nair-Gill E, Witte ON, et al. Visualizing cancer and immune cell function with metabolic positron emission tomography. Curr Opin Genet Dev 2010;20(1): 100–5.

57. Prestwich RJ, Subesinghe M, Gilbert A, et al. Delayed response assessment with FDG-PET-CT following (chemo) radiotherapy for locally advanced head and neck squamous cell carcinoma. Clin Radiol 2012;67(10):966–75.

58. Weber WA. Monitoring tumor response to therapy with 18F-FLT PET. J Nucl Med 2010;51(6):841–4.

59. Liberti MV, Locasale JW. The Warburg effect: how does it benefit cancer cells? Trends Biochem Sci 2016;41(3):211–8.

60. Wilson WR, Hay MP. Targeting hypoxia in cancer therapy. Nat Rev Cancer 2011; 11(6):393–410.

61. Sun X, Niu G, Chan N, et al. Tumor hypoxia imaging. Mol Imaging Biol 2011;13(3): 399–410.

62. Lopci E, Grassi I, Chiti A, et al. PET radiopharmaceuticals for imaging of tumor hypoxia: a review of the evidence. Am J Nucl Med Mol Imaging 2014;4(4): 365–84.

63. Stieb S, Eleftheriou A, Warnock G, et al. Longitudinal PET imaging of tumor hypoxia during the course of radiotherapy. Eur J Nucl Med Mol Imaging 2018;45(12): 2201–17.

64. Langendijk JA, Lambin P, De Ruysscher D, et al. Selection of patients for radiotherapy with protons aiming at reduction of side effects: the model-based approach. Radiother Oncol 2013;107(3):267–73.

65. Lomax A. Intensity modulation methods for proton radiotherapy. Phys Med Biol 1999;44(1):185–205.

66. Pollard JM, Wen Z, Sadagopan R, et al. The future of image-guided radiotherapy will be MR guided. Br J Radiol 2017;90(1073):20160667.

67. van Dijk LV, Brouwer CL, van der Laan HP, et al. Geometric image biomarker changes of the parotid gland are associated with late xerostomia. Int J Radiat Oncol Biol Phys 2017;99(5):1101–10.

68. Broggi S, Fiorino C, Dell'Oca I, et al. A two-variable linear model of parotid shrinkage during IMRT for head and neck cancer. Radiother Oncol 2010;94(2): 206–12.

69. Wu H, Chen X, Yang X, et al. Early prediction of acute xerostomia during radiation therapy for head and neck cancer based on texture analysis of daily CT. Int J Radiat Oncol Biol Phys 2018;102(4):1308–18.

70. Cunliffe A, Armato SG 3rd, Castillo R, et al. Lung texture in serial thoracic computed tomography scans: correlation of radiomics-based features with radiation therapy dose and radiation pneumonitis development. Int J Radiat Oncol Biol Phys 2015;91(5):1048–56.

71. Gillies RJ, Kinahan PE, Hricak H. Radiomics: images are more than pictures, they are data. Radiology 2016;278(2):563–77.
72. Aerts HJ, Velazquez ER, Leijenaar RT, et al. Decoding tumour phenotype by noninvasive imaging using a quantitative radiomics approach. Nat Commun 2014;5:4006.
73. van Dijk LV, Brouwer CL, van der Schaaf A, et al. CT image biomarkers to improve patient-specific prediction of radiation-induced xerostomia and sticky saliva. Radiother Oncol 2017;122(2):185–91.
74. Rosen BS, Hawkins PG, Polan DF, et al. Early changes in serial CBCT-measured parotid gland biomarkers predict chronic xerostomia after head and neck radiation therapy. Int J Radiat Oncol Biol Phys 2018;102(4):1319–29.
75. Colen RR, Fujii T, Bilen MA, et al. Radiomics to predict immunotherapy-induced pneumonitis: proof of concept. Invest New Drugs 2018;36(4):601–7.
76. Stieb S, Elgohari B, Fuller CD. Repetitive MRI of organs at risk in head and neck cancer patients undergoing radiotherapy. Clin Transl Radiat Oncol 2019;18:131–9.
77. Popovtzer A, Cao Y, Feng FY, et al. Anatomical changes in the pharyngeal constrictors after chemo-irradiation of head and neck cancer and their dose-effect relationships: MRI-based study. Radiother Oncol 2009;93(3):510–5.
78. Zhang Y, Ou D, Gu Y, et al. Evaluation of salivary gland function using diffusion-weighted magnetic resonance imaging for follow-up of radiation-induced xerostomia. Korean J Radiol 2018;19(4):758–66.
79. Zhou N, Chu C, Dou X, et al. Early evaluation of radiation-induced parotid damage in patients with nasopharyngeal carcinoma by T2 mapping and mDIXON Quant imaging: initial findings. Radiat Oncol 2018;13(1):22.
80. Brouwer CL, Steenbakkers RJ, Gort E, et al. Differences in delineation guidelines for head and neck cancer result in inconsistent reported dose and corresponding NTCP. Radiother Oncol 2014;111(1):148–52.
81. Zeilinger MG, Lell M, Baltzer PA, et al. Impact of post-processing methods on apparent diffusion coefficient values. Eur Radiol 2017;27(3):946–55.
82. van Dijk LV, Thor M, Steenbakkers R, et al. Parotid gland fat related Magnetic Resonance image biomarkers improve prediction of late radiation-induced xerostomia. Radiother Oncol 2018;128(3):459–66.
83. Abdollahi H, Mahdavi SR, Shiri I, et al. Magnetic resonance imaging radiomic feature analysis of radiation-induced femoral head changes in prostate cancer radiotherapy. J Cancer Res Ther 2019;15(Supplement):S11–9.
84. Mawlawi O, WR, Wong WH. Principles of PET/CT. In: Kim EE, Lee MC, Inoue R, et al, editors. Clinical PET. Springer; 2004. ISBN 9781441923554. p. 41-61.
85. Farr KP, Khalil AA, Moller DS, et al. Time and dose-related changes in lung perfusion after definitive radiotherapy for NSCLC. Radiother Oncol 2018;126(2):307–11.
86. Cannon B, Schwartz DL, Dong L. Metabolic imaging biomarkers of postradiotherapy xerostomia. Int J Radiat Oncol Biol Phys 2012;83(5):1609–16.
87. Klein Nulent TJW, Valstar MH, de Keizer B, et al. Physiologic distribution of PSMA-ligand in salivary glands and seromucous glands of the head and neck on PET/CT. Oral Surg Oral Med Oral Pathol Oral Radiol 2018;125(5):478–86.
88. Petit SF, van Elmpt WJ, Oberije CJ, et al. [(1)(8)F]fluorodeoxyglucose uptake patterns in lung before radiotherapy identify areas more susceptible to radiation-induced lung toxicity in non-small-cell lung cancer patients. Int J Radiat Oncol Biol Phys 2011;81(3):698–705.

89. Zyromska A, Malkowski B, Wisniewski T, et al. (15)O-H2O PET/CT as a tool for the quantitative assessment of early post-radiotherapy changes of heart perfusion in breast carcinoma patients. Br J Radiol 2018;91(1088):20170653.

90. Unal K, Unlu M, Akdemir O, et al. 18F-FDG PET/CT findings of radiotherapy-related myocardial changes in patients with thoracic malignancies. Nucl Med Commun 2013;34(9):855–9.

The Evolution (and Future) of Stereotactic Body Radiotherapy in the Treatment of Oligometastatic Disease

Benjamin E. Onderdonk, MD[1], Stanley I. Gutiontov, MD[1],
Steven J. Chmura, MD, PhD*

KEYWORDS

- Oligometastases • Radiation • Stereotactic body radiotherapy • SBRT • SABR
- Immunotherapy

KEY POINTS

- Oligometastases represent a unique metastatic phenotype, which may represent a disease state curable with local therapies.
- Stereotactic body radiotherapy is being investigated in numerous prospective trials seeking to confirm the oligometastatic state in disease-specific sites.
- There is interest in combining stereotactic body radiotherapy with other novel immunomodularity and targeted agents to improve the therapeutic ratio.

BACKGROUND

The de novo oligometastatic disease state was first formally proposed as an intermediate phenotype between localized and widespread cancer in 1995.[1] Previously, patients with metastatic disease were grouped together and usually considered incurable. However, in contrast with widespread metastatic disease, studies of patients with a limited burden of metastatic disease have demonstrated a potential for cure with aggressive local treatments to metastatic sites. Historical case reports and surgical series of patients with a limited burden of metastatic disease who have undergone metastatectomy have shown improved survival outcomes.[2-11] Most notable were improvements in 5-year survival after resection of liver metastases from colorectal cancer.[2] Moreover, pulmonary metastectomy for various tumor histologies has resulted in improved survival outcomes.[10]

Disclosure Statement: The authors have nothing to disclose.
Department of Radiation and Cellular Oncology, University of Chicago, 5758 S Maryland Avenue, Chicago, IL 60637, USA
[1] Authors contributed equally to work.
* Corresponding author.
E-mail address: schmura@radonc.uchicago.edu

Hematol Oncol Clin N Am 34 (2020) 307–320
https://doi.org/10.1016/j.hoc.2019.09.003
0889-8588/20/© 2019 Elsevier Inc. All rights reserved.

hemonc.theclinics.com

More recent data have demonstrated benefits in cancer-specific outcomes with ablative radiotherapy to sites of oligometastases. Beside the de novo oligometastatic state, the terms oligorecurrence and oligoprogression have also been coined. Oligorecurrence has been described as the metachronous development of a limited burden of metastatic disease after treatment has been delivered to the primary tumor.[12] Oligoprogression has been identified as a state of widespread metastatic disease with minimal progression in a limited number of metastatic sites.[13] With this history in mind, evidence regarding the biology of oligometastases in different tumor histologies is emerging, and prospective clinical trials are investigating treatment of metastatic sites to determine which patients, if any, may obtain a benefit from metastasis-directed therapies. Our review focuses on the biology of extracranial de novo oligometastases and oligorecurrence, the current state of prospective clinical data, our current management paradigm, and suggested future directions for the field.

BIOLOGY OF OLIGOMETASTASIS

The mechanism for the development of metastatic disease was first postulated in 1889.[14] This seed-and-soil model depended on a favorable interaction between the tumor cells and the host organ. Tumor cells that leave the primary site must pass through physical boundaries (ie, basement membranes), survive in circulation, and colonize distant organs. This colonization occurs in a relatively plastic tumor microenvironment where hypoxia, macrophages, and innate and adaptive immune signals play key roles in the selection of tumor clones that may survive and continue to grow.[15,16] Recently, different genes have been identified and categorized as initiator, promotor, and virulence genes and incorporated into this metastatic framework for various histologic subtypes.[17-19]

The biology of a de novo oligometastatic phenotype is now supported by preclinical data. For instance, the time from initiation of carcinogenesis to the development of a primary tumor has been shown to be a relatively slow process[20] and metastases develop late in the course of oncogenesis.[21] Tumor models also demonstrate varying degrees of metastatic potential of clonogens within a heterogeneous tumor.[22,23] Moreover, the initial notion of the primary tumor giving rise to metastatic tumors has changed as newer data have emerged regarding the ability of metastatic tumors to give rise to further metastases. For example, in androgen-deprived metastatic prostate cancer, 1 study demonstrated a Darwinian evolutionary process.[24] Multiple subclones within a single primary tumor formed the initial metastatic presentation. By sequencing multiple subclones in 10 patients, they demonstrated the existence of polyclonal seeding. Further analysis demonstrated that 1 metastatic clone commonly gave rise to further metastases. Studies such as these demonstrate the rationale for early intervention in the metastatic cascade to prevent further dissemination of disease.

However, despite strong clinical and emerging molecular data supporting the existence of an oligometastatic state, the ability to accurately predict which patients are truly oligometastatic and therefore would benefit the most from ablative therapies is still developing. Our group published a multi-institutional pooled analysis of oligometastatic patients demonstrating a relationship between survival and primary tumor histology, number of organs involved, lymph node involvement, liver involvement, and adrenal involvement.[25] Several other studies have identified the number of metastases,[26] the synchronicity of metastases,[27] the disease-free interval to metastases,[10] and the absence of lymph node metastases as useful variables in the classification of oligometastatic disease.

More recently, there has been significant progress in defining molecular features suggestive of oligometastases. Lussier,[28,29] Uppal,[30] and Oshima and colleagues[31] have demonstrated that the microRNA expression profile (and in particular the 14q32 microRNA levels) of metastases from a variety of tumor types correlated strongly with long-term recurrence-free survival and that reactivation of epigenetically silenced 14q32 microRNA could suppress metastatic potential in mice. The TRACERx Renal Consortium classified primary and matched metastatic renal cell carcinomas according to intratumoral heterogeneity and somatic copy number alterations and found that these factors were predictive of outcome.[32] Other studies have demonstrated distinct immune profiles within metastases, with immune-activated lesions being associated with improved outcomes as compared with immune-depleted lesions.[33,34]

As these and other molecular profiles indicating an oligometastatic phenotype are discovered and validated, we expect an increased ability to select patients for prospective trials of ablative therapies. Furthermore, Pitroda and Weichselbaum[35] have recently proposed that integrated staging systems combining clinical, molecular, and host parameters will enhance our ability to assess metastatic disease in the near future. Both of these developments will in turn grow the evidence base supporting the application of ablative therapies for oligometastatic disease.

CURRENT STATE OF PROSPECTIVE CLINICAL DATA

As imaging modalities continue to improve, the ability to detect subsequent de novo oligometastatic disease will increase and the population eligible for aggressive local therapies will grow. Surgical resection, although invasive, may serve this purpose and is being incorporated into prospective trials. In contrast, ablative techniques such as stereotactic body radiotherapy (SBRT) have emerged as a prominent and safe modality for metastasis-directed therapy across tumor histologies, metastatic locations, and seems to result in long-term disease control. Thus, SBRT may be a more feasible and applicable form of local metastasis-directed therapy than surgery. Here, we review the prospective data supporting the use of ablative radiation therapy for metastatic sites (metastasis-directed therapy, **Table 1**) and also local therapy to the primary tumor in the oligometastatic state.

The first phase I cooperative group trial NRG BR001 reporting early results demonstrated safety of high-dose multisite SBRT for oligometastases.[36] In this trial, 36 patients with breast, non-small cell lung cancer (NSCLC), or prostate cancer were enrolled. A median of 3 metastatic sites per patient were treated with high-dose SBRT (45 Gy in 3 fractions or 50 Gy in 5 fractions). With quality assurance of the delivered plans reaching 100%, there were no dose-limiting toxicities. Based on the results of this trial, the doses of SBRT were deemed safe and have been incorporated into other prospective phase II/III trials.

In addition to these phase I data, several phase II trials with recent results suggest that disease control translates into a progression-free survival (PFS) as well as an overall survival (OS) benefit, further increasing the excitement for essential and currently enrolling phase III trials. In the setting of oligometastatic NSCLC, 2 phase II trials have been published. The first enrolled 74 patients with stage IV NSCLC with 3 or fewer metastatic lesions after first-line chemotherapy and randomized them to local consolidative therapy (radiotherapy or surgery) with or without subsequent maintenance therapy versus maintenance therapy (which could include observation) alone.[37] Radiotherapy treatment was allowed to be concurrent chemoradiation, hypofractionated radiation, or SBRT, with 48% of patients receiving hypofractionation or SBRT. The study was terminated early owing to improved outcomes in the consolidative therapy arm, with a median PFS of 11.9 months versus 3.9 months (hazard ratio [HR], 0.35; $P = .0054$) at the cost of 20% grade 3 toxicity. With an updated median follow-up of 38.8 months, the PFS benefit was durable (14.2 months vs 4.4 months, $P = .022$) and a marked OS benefit was also seen (41.2 months vs 17.0 months; $P = .017$).[38] The second study in this setting

Table 1
Prospective phase II studies of metastasis-directed therapy in oligometastatic cancer

Study	Inclusion Criteria	No. of Patients and Follow-up	Intervention	Outcome	Toxicity
Gomez et al,[37] 2018	NSCLC with 1–3 metastases following first-line chemotherapy	N = 74; 38.8 mo	Maintenance therapy (including observation) with or without local consolidative therapy (radiotherapy or surgery)	PFS 14.2 mo vs 4.4 mo (P = .022) OS 41.2 mo vs 17.0 mo (P = .017)	20% grade 3
Iyengar et al,[39] 2018	NSCLC with 1–5 metastases	N = 29; 9.6 mo (closed early owing to PFS benefit on unplanned interim analysis)	Maintenance chemotherapy ± SBRT to all sites	PFS 9.7 mo vs 3.5 mo (P = .01)	No difference in toxicity between arms (29% grade 3 on SBRT arm)
Ost et al,[26] 2018	Oligorecurrent prostate with 1–3 metastases	N = 62; 3 y	Metastasis-directed therapy (surgery or SBRT) vs surveillance	ADT-free survival 21 mo vs 13 mo (P = .11)	No grade 2+
SABR-COMET (Palma et al,[40] 2019)	All histologies, controlled primary and 1–5 metastases	N = 99; 26 mo	SBRT to all metastatic sites vs palliative standard of care treatments (2:1 randomization)	OS 41 vs 28 mo (HR, 0.57, P = .090, meeting prespecified 2-sided alpha of 0.20) PFS 12 vs 6 mo (HR, 0.47, P = .0012)	29% grade 2 + in SBRT arm vs 9% in control arm 4.5% (3 cases) of grade 5 toxicity in SBRT arm

Abbreviation: ADT, androgen deprivation therapy.

enrolled 29 patients with stage IV NSCLC with 5 or fewer metastases, randomizing them to SBRT plus maintenance chemotherapy versus maintenance chemotherapy alone, with a wide range of acceptable SBRT fractionation.[39] This study was closed early owing to unplanned interim analysis demonstrating an improvement in median PFS in the SBRT arm of 9.7 months versus 3.5 months in the chemotherapy alone arm (P = .01), without a difference in toxicity.

In the setting of prostate cancer, a prospective phase II study enrolled 62 patients with oligorecurrent disease, defined as 3 or fewer lesions on choline PET/computed tomography (CT) and randomized them to either surveillance or metastasis-directed therapy (surgery or SBRT with 30 Gy in 3 fractions) with a primary end point of androgen deprivation therapy-free survival.[26] At a median follow-up time of 3 years, the median androgen deprivation therapy-free survival time was 21 months in the intervention arm versus 13 months in the control arm (P = .11) with no grade 2+ toxicity, suggesting that this approach should be explored further in phase III trials.

The most recent phase II results come from the non-site-specific, multicenter SABR-COMET trial.[40] This trial enrolled 99 patients with a controlled primary tumor and 5 or fewer metastases, randomizing patients in a 1:2 fashion to palliative standard of care treatments alone versus standard of care plus SBRT to all metastatic sites, with OS as the primary end point. After a median follow-up of 26 months in the SBRT group, the median OS was 41 months in the SBRT group versus 28 months in the control group (HR, 0.57; P = .090), meeting the prespecified 2-sided alpha of 0.20 and demonstrating a full 13-month OS benefit. There was a doubling of median PFS from 6.0 months to 12 months (HR, 0.47; P = .0012). However, unlike in the preceding studies, there was limited radiotherapy quality assurance, which likely resulted in the 4.5% rate of grade 5 toxicity in the SBRT arm owing to 1 case each of radiation pneumonitis, pulmonary abscess, and subdural hemorrhage in the setting of surgical repair of an SBRT-related gastric ulcer (vs 0% in the control arm).

Beyond metastasis-directed therapy, targeting the primary tumor in early metastatic disease states is being increasingly studied. The STAMPEDE phase III trial examined patients with newly diagnosed metastatic prostate cancer who were randomized to standard of care with or without the addition of local hypofractionated radiation to the prostate.[41] The local radiation group demonstrated an improvement in failure-free survival (HR, 0.76; P<.0001) in all comers. Patients were classified as high metastatic burden if they had 4 or more bone metastases with 1 or more outside of the vertebrae or pelvis, or visceral metastases on whole-body scintigraphy and CT or MRI; all other patients were considered low metastatic burden. On prespecified subgroup analysis of low metastatic burden patients, an improvement in failure-free survival (HR, 0.59; P < .0001) and OS (HR, 0.90; P = .007) was demonstrated in low metastatic burden patients. Another similar prospective randomized trial (HORRAD) examined standard of care hormonal therapy with or without local radiation therapy to the prostate in metastatic patients.[42] In this trial, there was an improvement in median time to prostate-specific antigen (PSA) progression of 15 months (radiation arm) versus 12 months (standard arm) (HR, 0.78; P = .02), but no difference in OS (HR, 0.90; P = .4). In patients with a low metastatic burden (<5 metastatic sites on bone scintigraphy), there was a trend for improved OS in the local radiation arm (HR, 0.68; 95% confidence interval, 0.42–1.10). These results have spurred other prospective trials examining local radiation. For example, SWOG 1802 is examining the addition of aggressive local therapy in addition to standard systemic therapy versus standard systemic therapy alone. Furthermore, several ongoing phase III trials using ablative radiation are investigating whether aggressive local therapies may lead to improved survival in patients with limited metastatic disease (Table 2).

As phase III trials evaluating SBRT alone for oligometastases accrue, there is early clinical interest in examining the role of SBRT combined with immunotherapy and other novel molecular targets in an attempt to improve the systemic response of immunotherapy. This paradigm of using local radiation to enhance a distant response in an unirradiated lesion is commonly referred to as the abscopal response. One of these randomized phase II trials presented at ASCO 2018 demonstrated a doubling in objective response rate in patients with advanced NSCLC in patients receiving SBRT to a single metastatic site (8 Gy ×3) followed by sequential pembrolizumab.[43] Meanwhile, another randomized phase II trial in patients with advanced head and neck cancer used SBRT to a single metastatic site (9 Gy ×3) between doses of nivolumab and failed to demonstrate an improvement in PFS.[44] The difference between the 2 outcomes may lay in the timing of SBRT followed by immunotherapy, where the SBRT acts as a primer to the immune system. Moreover, SBRT is being investigated in combination with modulation of novel molecular targets such as CSF-1R (NCT03431948) and 4-1BB (NCT00461110; NCT03431948) to modulate the tumor microenvironment. As these early prospective data emerge, multisite cytoreductive SBRT combined with immunotherapy and/or molecular targets may prove beneficial in some patients.

Currently, SBRT to oligometastases remains well-tolerated, but concern for increased toxicity is raised with multisite SBRT. One approach to decrease toxicity has been to decrease the dose to adjacent organs at risk. In patients receiving immunotherapy, local control of irradiated metastases may be achieved through high-dose irradiation of the tumor center with a concomitant lower dose to the periphery.[45] Another method to decrease toxicity may be through adaptive radiation planning, although this method remains logistically challenging.

In conclusion, several phase II studies have demonstrated significant promise in the treatment of oligometastatic disease with SBRT, setting the stage for more site-specific phase III trials. These trials may help to demonstrate the existence of the oligometastatic state across histologies, define the most meaningful end points in this treatment setting (eg, PFS, OS, deferral of systemic treatment, etc), and establish a new paradigm in cancer treatment. Furthermore, there are several early clinical prospective trials examining SBRT with immunotherapy with conflicting responses spurring interest in further study as well as tumor microenvironment modulation through novel molecular targets. Finally, numerous avenues exist to decrease the toxicity of multisite SBRT and thereby improve our therapeutic ratio in this growing patient population.

THE EVOLVING STANDARD OF CARE

With the recent publication of several previously outlined phase II trials demonstrating marked improvements in PFS and, in some cases OS, of locally ablative therapy in a variety of oligometastatic settings, there is a strong rationale and impetus for further investigation of this approach. However, the conclusions of the emerging phase II trials should be approached with a certain caution mixed in with the well-founded optimism. Although a possible paradigm shift in the standard of care is on the horizon with a move toward regional, potentially curative treatment for patients with oligometastatic disease, there remain many unanswered questions that currently accruing phase III trials are expected to answer.

It is important to note that the gold standard in cancer clinical trial design is the phase III randomized controlled trial, and in those disease sites in which such trials have been possible they have determined the standard of care. Furthermore, phase II results are often overturned by their phase III counterparts, as was seen recently in the publication of RTOG 1016 which failed to demonstrate non-inferiority of cetuximab radiotherapy as

Table 2
Ongoing SBRT phase III oligometastatic cancer trials

Study	ClinicalTrials.Gov Identifier	Oligometastatic Definition	Estimated Enrollment	Status	Intervention
NRG BR002	NCT02364557	≤4 metastases (breast)	402	Recruiting	SBRT/surgical resection and systemic therapy (at physician discretion) vs standard of care treatment
STEREO-STEIN	NCT02089100	1–5 metastases (breast)	280	Recruiting	SBRT + standard of care vs standard of care (no specific local therapy other than palliation)
NRG LU002	NCT03137771	1–3 metastases (NSCLC)	300	Recruiting	SBRT + maintenance chemotherapy vs maintenance chemotherapy
OMEGA	NCT03827577	1–3 metastases (NSCLC)	195	Not yet recruiting	SBRT/surgical resection and standard medical treatment vs standard of care treatment
SARON	NCT02417662	1–3 metastases (NSCLC)	340	Recruiting	Radiotherapy (SBRT or conventional) to primary + SBRT to metastases + standard chemotherapy vs standard chemotherapy alone
PCS IX	NCT02685397	1–5 metastases (prostate)	130	Recruiting	SBRT/LHRH agonist/enzalutamide vs LHRH agonist/enzalutamide
CORE	NCT02759783	1–3 metastases (prostate, breast, NSCLC)	245	Active, not recruiting	SBRT + standard of care vs standard of care
SABR-COMET-3	NCT03862911	1–3 metastases (all histologies)	201	Not yet recruiting	SBRT and chemotherapy (at physician discretion) vs standard of care treatment
SABR-COMET-10	NCT03721341	4–10 metastases (all histologies)	159	Recruiting	SBRT and systemic therapy: chemotherapy, immunotherapy, hormonal therapy, or observation (at physician discretion) vs standard of care treatment

Abbreviation: LHRH, luteinizing hormone-releasing hormone.

compared with standard platinum-based chemoradiation in human papillomavirus-positive oropharyngeal carcinoma.[46] Conversely, recent phase III trials investigating various molecular therapies have led to US Food and Drug Administration approval of agents improving OS by 2 months,[47] whereas the remarkable doubling of PFS and 13-month improvement in OS across histologies in the SABR-COMET trial led to the authors' conclusion that "further research should aim to provide support for the overall survival benefits for tumor-specific groups in formal phase 3 trials."

Indeed, one of the major concerns with this goal has been an inability to accrue sufficient numbers of oligometastatic patients to tumor-specific studies. However, recent advances in imaging and systemic therapy are increasing the number of patients with oligometastatic and oligoprogressive disease, respectively. Specifically, the addition of PET/CT to standard systemic workup for patients with stage I to III lung cancer has demonstrated an ability to detect metastatic disease in an additional 19% of patients, which could be targeted with aggressive local treatments,[48] and the use of tyrosine kinase inhibitors in epidermal growth factor receptor mutant NSCLC seems to be increasing the proportion of patients with oligoprogression.[49] Many similar changes occurring across disease sites can be expected to markedly increase the pool of eligible patients, both for accrual on phase III protocols and for careful treatment off protocol (see Our Approach to the Oligometastatic Patient).

One of the open questions in the field concerns the radiation dose and fractionation, which has major repercussions on the safety and synergy of SBRT with modern systemic therapies. Although the radiation dose to achieve excellent local tumor control using SBRT is becoming better defined through phase II protocols,[50] the rates of grade 5 toxicity have varied in recent publications (0% on BR001 vs 5% on SABR-COMET). Although SBRT is generally safe when delivered with excellent quality assurance, the risks need to be better defined.

SBRT will likely play a greater role in the modern oncologic armamentarium, and there is therefore a growing need to establish the optimal dose that synergizes with immunotherapy and other novel systemic agents. This is of the utmost importance and is unlikely to be defined by phase II protocols. Just as there have been several influential phase III dose escalation studies in the definitive, conventionally fractionated setting,[51,52] the second generation of phase III, ablative oligometastatic trials will need to discover the ideal dose and fractionation schemes to optimize site-specific outcomes.

Finally, tumor biology heavily influences outcome and treatment response, and although SABR-COMET may be the strongest randomized clinical evidence to date of an oligometastatic state, it is difficult to draw site-specific conclusions because all primary tumor sites were eligible for enrollment. There have been several site-specific phase II studies reported in the literature, and the results of their phase III counterparts including but not limited to NRG BR002 and NRG LU002 are eagerly awaited.

OUR APPROACH TO THE OLIGOMETASTATIC PATIENT AND CONCLUDING THOUGHTS

As we await the phase III data, an important question arises: what is the optimal management of the patient with oligometastatic cancer given the currently available literature? Although a full discussion of our evolving approach is beyond the scope of this review, consideration of a few points may be instructive (see the Flow Diagram).

It is essential to first note that the current standard of care for the majority of cases of asymptomatic, extracranial oligometastatic disease is systemic therapy alone without the addition of local ablative therapy.

With that in mind, our first preference is to enroll eligible patients into clinical trials, and we would strongly recommend enrollment on the aforementioned phase III studies outlined in **Table 2** if possible. If this is not an option and there are no site-specific phase I/II protocols incorporating multisite SBRT with or without systemic therapy at our institution, we then evaluate whether the patient meets the inclusion criteria of the major phase II studies discussed in this review. If this is the case (see cases 1–3, presented elsewhere in this article, for examples), we then discuss treatment with multisite SBRT in sequence with standard of care systemic therapy. Of note, careful multidisciplinary discussion is essential at each of these decision points and will optimize outcomes.

In conclusion, given the remarkable signal of clinical efficacy on recently reported phase II trials, an excellent safety profile, and the potential mechanistic synergy with current cutting-edge systemic therapies, ablative therapy for oligometastatic disease with SBRT holds great promise. Although a growing number of patients can likely be treated safely with this approach off study assuming excellent quality assurance, the enrollment of patients with oligometastatic cancer on current and opening phase III protocols is of the utmost importance. The conclusive demonstration of benefits in cancer-specific outcomes, the ability to begin to address pressing dosimetric and biologic questions, and the widespread acceptance of a new paradigm for cancer therapy await.

FLOW DIAGRAM: OUR APPROACH TO THE OLIGOMETASTATIC PATIENT

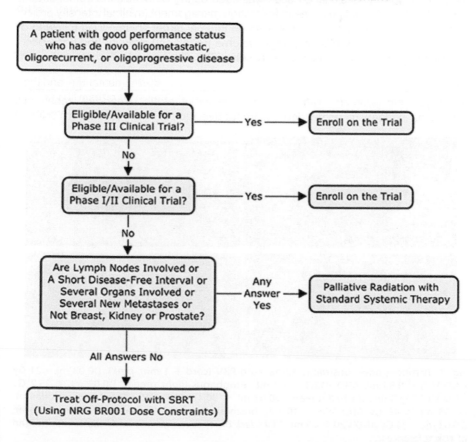

CASES

Case 1

A 70-year-old man in excellent health with a history of prostatic adenocarcinoma (pT2N0, Gleason 3 + 4, preoperative PSA of 11 ng/dL, postoperative PSA of <0.05 ng/dL) who underwent radical prostatectomy 5 years prior developed subsequent biochemical recurrence (PSA of 0.7 ng/dL and PSA doubling time of 12 months). An 18F-flucyclovine PET/CT scan demonstrated oligorecurrent disease with a single bony lesion to T1 for which he received SBRT using a volumetric modulated arc therapy plan to 30 Gy in 3 fractions. Given epidural extension, CT myelogram was performed on the day of simulation to aid in delineation of the target as well as the spinal cord (+1 mm to planning organ at risk volume [PRV]) and thecal sac, and Exac-Trac, cone beam CT, kV confirmation, and triggered kVs every 45° were used during treatment to verify set-up (**Fig. 1**).

Case 2

A 55-year-old woman with metastatic ER+/PR+/HER2- invasive ductal carcinoma of the breast on AI + CDK4/6 inhibitor therapy with stable disease for 2 years presents with a single oligoprogressive liver lesion. She refused chemotherapy owing to previous intolerance and received SBRT using a volumetric modulated arc therapy plan to 45 Gy in 3 fractions. Fiducials were placed by interventional radiology to aid in treatment delivery, 4-dimensional CT scan was used during CT simulation demonstrating minimal motion abrogating the need for motion management (minimal intensity projection scan used for target delineation with an internal target volume [ITV] followed by 5 mm expansion to the planning target volume [PTV]), and daily kV and cone beam CT were used during treatment to verify setup (**Fig. 2**).

Case 3

A 45-year-old woman with de novo oligometastatic clear-cell renal cell carcinoma underwent right-sided cytoreductive radical nephrectomy (pT3N0M1)

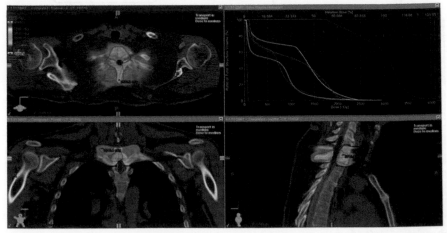

Fig. 1. Pertinent dose constraints: spinal cord PRV (cord + 1 mm, *pink*): D0.03 mL ≤21 Gy AND V18 ≤ 0.35 mL AND V12.3 ≤ 1.2 mL; esophagus (*light green*): D0.03 mL ≤ 25.2 Gy AND V17.7 ≤ 5 mL; trachea (*green*): D0.03 mL ≤ 30 Gy AND V15 ≤ 4 mL; Aorta (*salmon*): D0.03 mL ≤ 45 Gy AND V39 ≤ 10 mL; brachial plexus PRV (plexus + 2 mm; *orange*): D0.03 mL ≤ 24 Gy AND V20.4 ≤ 3 mL. PTV (*dark blue*) coverage was sacrificed to meet organ at risk tolerances.

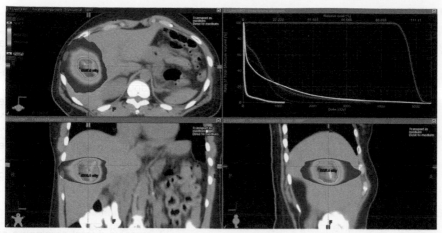

Fig. 2. Pertinent dose constraints: liver – ITV (*yellow*): mean volume spared (MVS) 17.1 Gy ≥ 700 mL; bile duct (*orange*): V36 ≤ 0.03 mL; ipsilateral kidney (*blue*): V12.3 ≤ 130 mL; duodenum (*lime*): V23 ≤ 0.03 mL AND V15 ≤ 10 mL. All were met with excellent PTV (*red*) coverage.

and received SBRT to a left central lung lesion, 50 Gy in 5 fractions. A 4-dimensional CT scan was used during CT simulation demonstrating minimal motion abrogating the need for motion management (maximum intensity projection scan used for target delineation with an ITV followed by 3 mm expansion to PTV)), and daily kV and cone beam CT were used during treatment to verify setup (**Fig. 3**).

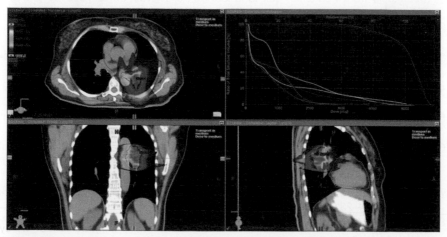

Fig. 3. Pertinent dose constraints: proximal bronchial tree (*Aqua*): D0.03 mL ≤ 52.5 Gy; heart (*salmon*): D0.03 mL ≤ 38 Gy AND V32 ≤ 15 mL; ipsilateral lung (*Blue*) mean volume spared (MVS): 12.5 Gy ≥ 1500 mL AND MVS 13.5 Gy ≥ 1000 mL; great vessel (*Green*): D0.03 mL ≤ 53 Gy AND V47 less than 10 mL; esophagus (*Brown*): D0.03 mL ≤ 52.5 Gy; PTV (*Red*) coverage was sacrificed to meet organ at risk tolerances.

REFERENCES

1. Hellman S, Weichselbaum RR. Oligometastases. J Clin Oncol 1995;13(1):8–10.
2. Rees M, Tekkis PP, Welsh FK, et al. Evaluation of long-term survival after hepatic resection for metastatic colorectal cancer: a multifactorial model of 929 patients. Ann Surg 2008;247(1):125–35.
3. Fong Y, Fortner J, Sun RL, et al. Clinical score for predicting recurrence after hepatic resection for metastatic colorectal cancer: analysis of 1001 consecutive cases. Ann Surg 1999;230(3):309–18 [discussion: 318–21].
4. Carpizo DR, D'Angelica M. Liver resection for metastatic colorectal cancer in the presence of extrahepatic disease. Ann Surg Oncol 2009;16(9):2411–21.
5. Elias D, Cavacanti de Albuquerque A, Eggenspieler P, et al. Resection of liver metastases from a noncolorectal primary: indications and results based on 147 monocentric patients. J Am Coll Surg 1998;187(5):487–93.
6. de Jong MC, Pulitano C, Ribero D, et al. Rates and patterns of recurrence following curative intent surgery for colorectal liver metastasis: an international multi-institutional analysis of 1669 patients. Ann Surg 2009;250(3):440–8.
7. Choong PF, Pritchard DJ, Rock MG, et al. Survival after pulmonary metastasectomy in soft tissue sarcoma. Prognostic factors in 214 patients. Acta Orthop Scand 1995;66(6):561–8.
8. Casiraghi M, De Pas T, Maisonneuve P, et al. A 10-year single-center experience on 708 lung metastasectomies: the evidence of the "international registry of lung metastases. J Thorac Oncol 2011;6(8):1373–8.
9. Petersen RP, Hanish SI, Haney JC, et al. Improved survival with pulmonary metastasectomy: an analysis of 1720 patients with pulmonary metastatic melanoma. J Thorac Cardiovasc Surg 2007;133(1):104–10.
10. Pastorino U, Buyse M, Friedel G, et al. Long-term results of lung metastasectomy: prognostic analyses based on 5206 cases. J Thorac Cardiovasc Surg 1997; 113(1):37–49.
11. Mercier O, Fadel E, de Perrot M, et al. Surgical treatment of solitary adrenal metastasis from non-small cell lung cancer. J Thorac Cardiovasc Surg 2005; 130(1):136–40.
12. Niibe Y, Hayakawa K. Oligometastases and oligo-recurrence: the new era of cancer therapy. Jpn J Clin Oncol 2010;40(2):107–11.
13. Cheung P. Stereotactic body radiotherapy for oligoprogressive cancer. Br J Radiol 2016;89(1066):20160251.
14. Paget S. The distribution of secondary growths in cancer of the breast. 1889. Cancer Metastasis Rev 1989;8(2):98–101.
15. Fidler IJ. The organ microenvironment and cancer metastasis. Differentiation 2002;70(9–10):498–505.
16. Axelson H, Fredlund E, Ovenberger M, et al. Hypoxia-induced dedifferentiation of tumor cells–a mechanism behind heterogeneity and aggressiveness of solid tumors. Semin Cell Dev Biol 2005;16(4–5):554–63.
17. Chiang AC, Massague J. Molecular basis of metastasis. N Engl J Med 2008; 359(26):2814–23.
18. Gupta GP, Massague J. Cancer metastasis: building a framework. Cell 2006; 127(4):679–95.
19. Nguyen DX, Massague J. Genetic determinants of cancer metastasis. Nat Rev Genet 2007;8(5):341–52.
20. Brown PO, Palmer C. The preclinical natural history of serous ovarian cancer: defining the target for early detection. PLoS Med 2009;6(7):e1000114.

21. Yachida S, Jones S, Bozic I, et al. Distant metastasis occurs late during the genetic evolution of pancreatic cancer. Nature 2010;467(7319):1114–7.
22. Li Y, Tang ZY, Ye SL, et al. Establishment of cell clones with different metastatic potential from the metastatic hepatocellular carcinoma cell line MHCC97. World J Gastroenterol 2001;7(5):630–6.
23. Shindo-Okada N, Takeuchi K, Nagamachi Y. Establishment of cell lines with high- and low-metastatic potential from PC-14 human lung adenocarcinoma. Jpn J Cancer Res 2001;92(2):174–83.
24. Gundem G, Van Loo P, Kremeyer B, et al. The evolutionary history of lethal metastatic prostate cancer. Nature 2015;520(7547):353–7.
25. Hong JC, Ayala-Peacock DN, Lee J, et al. Classification for long-term survival in oligometastatic patients treated with ablative radiotherapy: a multi-institutional pooled analysis. PLoS One 2018;13(4):e0195149.
26. Ost P, Reynders D, Decaestecker K, et al. Surveillance or metastasis-directed therapy for oligometastatic prostate cancer recurrence: a prospective, randomized, multicenter phase II trial. J Clin Oncol 2018;36(5):446–53.
27. Ashworth AB, Senan S, Palma DA, et al. An individual patient data metaanalysis of outcomes and prognostic factors after treatment of oligometastatic non-small-cell lung cancer. Clin Lung Cancer 2014;15(5):346–55.
28. Lussier YA, Khodarev NN, Regan K, et al. Oligo- and polymetastatic progression in lung metastasis(es) patients is associated with specific microRNAs. PLoS One 2012;7(12):e50141.
29. Lussier YA, Xing HR, Salama JK, et al. MicroRNA expression characterizes oligometastasis(es). PLoS One 2011;6(12):e28650.
30. Uppal A, Wightman SC, Mallon S, et al. 14q32-encoded microRNAs mediate an oligometastatic phenotype. Oncotarget 2015;6(6):3540–52.
31. Oshima G, Poli EC, Bolt MJ, et al. DNA methylation controls metastasis-suppressive 14q32-encoded miRNAs. Cancer Res 2019;79(3):650–62.
32. Turajlic S, Xu H, Litchfield K, et al. Tracking cancer evolution reveals constrained routes to metastases: TRACERx renal. Cell 2018;173(3):581–94.e12.
33. Pitroda SP, Khodarev NN, Huang L, et al. Integrated molecular subtyping defines a curable oligometastatic state in colorectal liver metastasis. Nat Commun 2018; 9(1):1793.
34. Huang L, David O, Cabay RJ, et al. Molecular classification of lymph node metastases subtypes predict for survival in head and neck cancer. Clin Cancer Res 2019;25(6):1795–808.
35. Pitroda SP, Weichselbaum RR. Integrated molecular and clinical staging defines the spectrum of metastatic cancer. Nat Rev Clin Oncol 2019;16(9):581–8.
36. Al-Hallaq HA, Chmura SJ, Salama JK, et al. Benchmark Credentialing results for NRG-BR001: the first National cancer Institute-Sponsored trial of stereotactic body radiation therapy for multiple metastases. Int J Radiat Oncol Biol Phys 2017;97(1):155–63.
37. Gomez DR, Blumenschein GR Jr, Lee JJ, et al. Local consolidative therapy versus maintenance therapy or observation for patients with oligometastatic non-small-cell lung cancer without progression after first-line systemic therapy: a multicentre, randomised, controlled, phase 2 study. Lancet Oncol 2016; 17(12):1672–82.
38. Gomez DR, Tang C, Zhang J, et al. Local consolidative therapy Vs. Maintenance therapy or observation for patients with oligometastatic non-small-cell lung cancer: long-term results of a multi-institutional, phase II, randomized study. J Clin Oncol 2019;37(18):1558–65.

39. Iyengar P, Wardak Z, Gerber DE, et al. Consolidative radiotherapy for limited metastatic non-small-cell lung cancer: a phase 2 randomized clinical trial. JAMA Oncol 2018;4(1):e173501.

40. Palma DA, Olson R, Harrow S, et al. Stereotactic ablative radiotherapy versus standard of care palliative treatment in patients with oligometastatic cancers (SABR-COMET): a randomised, phase 2, open-label trial. Lancet 2019; 393(10185):2051–8.

41. Parker CC, James ND, Brawley CD, et al. Radiotherapy to the primary tumour for newly diagnosed, metastatic prostate cancer (STAMPEDE): a randomised controlled phase 3 trial. Lancet 2018;392(10162):2353–66.

42. Boeve LMS, Hulshof MCCM, Vis AN, et al. Effect on survival of androgen deprivation therapy alone compared to androgen deprivation therapy combined with concurrent radiation therapy to the prostate in patients with primary bone metastatic prostate cancer in a prospective randomised clinical trial: data from the HORRAD trial. Eur Urol 2019;75(3):410–8.

43. Theelen W, Peulen H, Lalezari F, et al. Randomized phase II study of pembrolizumab after stereotactic body radiotherapy (SBRT) versus pembrolizumab alone in patients with advanced non-small cell lung cancer: the PEMBRO-RT study. J Clin Oncol 2018;36(15_suppl):9023.

44. McBride SM, Sherman EJ, Tsai CJ, et al. A phase II randomized trial of nivolumab with stereotactic body radiotherapy (SBRT) versus nivolumab alone in metastatic (M1) head and neck squamous cell carcinoma (HNSCC). J Clin Oncol 2018; 36(15_suppl):6009.

45. Luke JJ, Lemons JM, Karrison TG, et al. Safety and clinical activity of pembrolizumab and multisite stereotactic body radiotherapy in patients with advanced solid tumors. J Clin Oncol 2018;36(16):1611–8.

46. Gillison ML, Trotti AM, Harris J, et al. Radiotherapy plus cetuximab or cisplatin in human papillomavirus-positive oropharyngeal cancer (NRG Oncology RTOG 1016): a randomised, multicentre, non-inferiority trial. Lancet 2019;393(10166): 40–50.

47. Llovet JM, Ricci S, Mazzaferro V, et al. Sorafenib in advanced hepatocellular carcinoma. N Engl J Med 2008;359(4):378–90.

48. MacManus MP, Hicks RJ, Matthews JP, et al. High rate of detection of unsuspected distant metastases by pet in apparent stage III non-small-cell lung cancer: implications for radical radiation therapy. Int J Radiat Oncol Biol Phys 2001;50(2):287–93.

49. Ng TL, Morgan RL, Patil T, et al. Detection of oligoprogressive disease in oncogene-addicted non-small cell lung cancer using PET/CT versus CT in patients receiving a tyrosine kinase inhibitor. Lung Cancer 2018;126:112–8.

50. Bezjak A, Paulus R, Gaspar LE, et al. Safety and efficacy of a five-fraction stereotactic body radiotherapy schedule for centrally located non-small-cell lung cancer: NRG oncology/RTOG 0813 trial. J Clin Oncol 2019;37(15):1316–25.

51. Minsky BD, Pajak TF, Ginsberg RJ, et al. INT 0123 (Radiation Therapy Oncology Group 94-05) phase III trial of combined-modality therapy for esophageal cancer: high-dose versus standard-dose radiation therapy. J Clin Oncol 2002;20(5): 1167–74.

52. Bradley JD, Paulus R, Komaki R, et al. Standard-dose versus high-dose conformal radiotherapy with concurrent and consolidation carboplatin plus paclitaxel with or without cetuximab for patients with stage IIIA or IIIB non-small-cell lung cancer (RTOG 0617): a randomised, two-by-two factorial phase 3 study. Lancet Oncol 2015;16(2):187–99.

Printed and bound by CPI Group (UK) Ltd, Croydon, CR0 4YY

03/10/2024

01040401-0010